PROGRESS IN BRAIN RESEARCH

VOLUME 31

MECHANISMS OF SYNAPTIC TRANSMISSION

PROGRESS IN BRAIN RESEARCH

PROGRESS IN BRAIN RESEARCH
VOLUME 31

MECHANISMS OF
SYNAPTIC TRANSMISSION

EDITED BY

K. AKERT AND P. G. WASER

Institute for Brain Research, and Pharmacological Institute, University of Zürich (Switzerland)

ELSEVIER PUBLISHING COMPANY
AMSTERDAM / LONDON / NEW YORK
1969

ELSEVIER PUBLISHING COMPANY
335 JAN VAN GALENSTRAAT,
P.O. BOX 211, AMSTERDAM, THE NETHERLANDS

ELSEVIER PUBLISHING CO. LTD.
BARKING, ESSEX, ENGLAND

AMERICAN ELSEVIER PUBLISHING COMPANY, INC.
52 VANDERBILT AVENUE, NEW YORK, N.Y. 10017

This volume contains the Proceedings of an International Symposium on

MECHANISMS OF SYNAPTIC TRANSMISSION

Morphological, Biochemical, Pharmacological and Physiological Aspects

held at Einsiedeln (Switzerland) in September 1968

under the auspices of the Swiss Society of the Natural Sciences

(146th annual convention)

LIBRARY OF CONGRESS CARD NUMBER 78–85149

STANDARD BOOK NUMBER 444-40777-4

WITH 168 ILLUSTRATIONS AND 14 TABLES

PRINTED IN THE NETHERLANDS

List of Contributors

K. AKERT, Institute for Brain Research, University of Zürich, Zürich (Switzerland).

J. AXELROD, Department of Health, Education and Welfare, National Institutes of Health, Bethesda, Md. 20014 (U.S.A.).

F. BAUMANN, Physiological Institute, University of Geneva, Geneva (Switzerland).

B. BLONDEL, Physiological Institute, University of Geneva, Geneva (Switzerland).

A. CARLSSON, Department of Pharmacology, University of Göteborg (Sweden).

J. P. CHENEVAL, Physiological Institute, University of Geneva, Geneva (Switzerland).

O. CREUTZFELDT, German Research Institute for Psychiatry, (Max-Planck-Institute), Munich (Germany).

D. R. CURTIS, The John Curtin School of Medical Research, The Australian National University, Department of Physiology, Canberra, A.C.T. 2600 (Australia).

M. DA PRADA, Medical Research Division, Hoffmann-La Roche Inc., Basle (Switzerland).

J. DIAMOND, Department of Physiology, University College, London (Great Britain).

M. DOLIVO, Physiological Institute, University of Lausanne, Lausanne (Switzerland).

J. DUNANT, Physiological Institute, University of Lausanne, Lausanne (Switzerland).

B. FILLOUX, Physiological Institute, University of Geneva, Geneva (Switzerland).

W. G. FORSSMANN, Department of Physiology, University of Geneva, Geneva (Switzerland).

A. G. GAIDE-HUGUENIN, Physiological Institute, University of Lausanne, Lausanne (Switzerland).

L. GIRARDIER, Physiological Institute, University of Geneva, Geneva (Switzerland).

V. GISIGER, Physiological Institute, University of Lausanne, Lausanne (Switzerland).

E. G. GRAY, University College, Department of Anatomy, London (Great Britain).

W. E. HAEFELY, Department of Experimental Medicine, Hoffmann-La Roche Inc., Basle (Switzerland).

L. HÖSLI, Department of Neurophysiology, Neurological Clinic of the University of Basle, Basle (Switzerland).

A. HYDE, Physiological Institute, University of Geneva, Geneva (Switzerland).

I. J. KOPIN, Department of Health, Education and Welfare, National Institutes of Health, Bethesda, Md. 20014 (U.S.A.).

H. LANGEMANN, Pharmacological Institute of the University, Zürich (Switzerland).

M. G. LARRABEE, Department of Biophysics, The Johns Hopkins University, Baltimore, Md. 21218 (U.S.A.)

W. LEUZINGER, Columbia University, College of Physicians & Surgeons, Department of Neurology, New York, N.Y. (U.S.A.).

W. LICHTENSTEIGER, Pharmacological Institute of the University, Zürich (Switzerland).

K. MAEKAWA, German Research Institute for Psychiatry, (Max-Planck-Institute), Munich (Germany).

A. MATTER, Physiological Institute, University of Geneva, Geneva (Switzerland).

H. MOOR, Botanical Institute, Laboratory for Electronmicroscopy, ETH, Zürich (Switzerland).

ELVIRA NICKEL, Pharmacological Institute, University of Zürich, Zürich (Switzerland).

K. PFENNINGER, Institute for Brain Research, University of Zürich, Zürich (Switzerland).

L. PIERI, Medical Research Division, Hoffmann-La Roche Inc., Basle (Switzerland).

A. PLETSCHER, Medical Research Division, Hoffmann-La Roche Inc., Basle (Switzerland).

J. M. POSTERNAK, Physiological Institute, University of Geneva, Medical School, Geneva (Switzerland).

J. G. RICHARDS, Medical Research Division, Hoffmann-La Roche Inc., Basle (Switzerland).

ANNA ROSINA, Physiological Institute, University of Milano, Milano (Italy).

CH. ROUILLER, Histological and Embryological Institute, University, Medical School, Geneva (Switzerland).

CLARA SANDRI, Institute for Brain Research, University of Zürich, Zürich (Switzerland).

T. C. SMITH, Laboratory of Neurophysiology, Intramural Research, National Institutes of Health, Bethesda, Md. 20014 (U.S.A.).

R. L. SNIPES, Medical Research Division, Hoffmann-La Roche Inc., Basle (Switzerland).

F. A. STEINER, Medical Research Division, Hoffmann-La Roche Inc., Basle (Switzerland).

L. TAUC, Centre d'Études de Physiologie Nerveuse, Centre National de la Recherche Scientifique, Laboratoire de Neurophysiologie Cellulaire, Paris (France).

J. TAXI, Faculté des Sciences, Laboratoire de Biologie Animale, C.P.E.M., Paris (France).

H. THOENEN, Medical Research Division, Hoffmann-La Roche Inc., Basle (Switzerland).

J. P. TRANZER, Medical Research Division, Hoffmann-La Roche Inc., Basle (Switzerland).

U. TRENDELENBURG, Harvard Medical School, Department of Pharmacology, Boston, Mass. 02115 (U.S.A.).

P. G. WASER, Pharmacological Institute of the University of Zürich, Zürich (Switzerland).

S. WEIDMANN, Physiological Institute of the University of Berne, Berne (Switzerland).

V. P. WHITTAKER, Department of Biochemistry, University, Cambridge (Great Britain).

G. M. YASARGIL, Physiological Institute of the University of Zürich, Zürich (Switzerland).

Other volumes in this series:

Preface

The synapse is undoubtedly the single most important specific structure of brain tissue. Its morphology, physiology, pharmacology and biochemistry formed the topic of an International Symposium held in Einsiedeln on September 29 and 30, 1968, under the auspices of the Swiss Society of the Natural Sciences on the occasion of its 148th annual convention. The specific aim of the conference was a synthesis of recent developments in this field presented in the form of concise reviews by well-known scientists. An additional number of speakers gave laboratory reports on selected topics.

The organizers of and contributors to the Symposium wish to extend their special thanks to the sponsoring agencies: the Swiss Federal Government, Department of Interior; the Swiss National Foundation for Scientific Research; Ciba A.G., Basel; J. R. Geigy A.G., Basel; F. Hoffmann-La Roche and Co., Basel, and Sandoz A.G., Basel.

His Excellency, Msgr. Raimund Tschudy kindly made the beautiful Fürstensaal of the Benedictine Abbey available for the conference, and Father Kanisius Zünd helped the Organizing Committee in making local arrangements for the personal comfort of speakers and guests.

Special thanks are due to Miss U. Fischer and Mrs. E. Hemmer for untiring secretarial assistance.

Zürich K. AKERT
March 1969 P. G. WASER

Contents

Opening Remarks

J. M. POSTERNAK

Institute of Physiology, University of Geneva (Switzerland)

In an article that appeared in "*Science*" five months ago, entitled "That was the molecular biology that was", Stent (1968), deliberating upon the frontiers of biological research, wrote: "There now seems to remain only one major frontier of biological inquiry for which reasonable molecular mechanisms cannot even be imagined: the higher nervous system". Crick (1966), in one of the lectures published under the title "*Of Molecules and Men*", considers our present knowledge of the nervous system to be "in an exceedingly primitive state". He adds that molecular biologists had been focusing their attention mainly on the borderline between the living and the non-living, and that they "were looking for rather simple explanations of rather simple processes". It is essential for the understanding of the brain function, however, to consider both the behaviour of the organism as a whole and the complex interactions involved in the making of that behaviour. Along with Crick one must of course quote Watson, who said during a talk held in Geneva a few years ago, that intelligent molecular biologists felt that the time had come to study the brain, but that he didn't consider himself sufficiently intelligent to tackle so complex a system.

Such scepticism is comprehensible when one takes into account the long road that lies ahead before the functions of the brain, in general, and the storage of information, in particular, can be described in terms of shape and organization of molecules. The study of synaptic mechanisms may well be one of the roads leading towards this end. This is indeed a subject in which the co-ordination of ultrastructural, physiological, biochemical and pharmacological research is particularly impressive.

The united efforts of biochemists, morphologists and physiologists have furthered the development of histochemical and fluoroscopic techniques, the control of their specificity, as well as the progress in autoradiography. This collaboration has moreover made possible the identification of subcellular fractions in synaptic regions, fractions now being studied with such effectiveness by biochemists.

Although this is far from suggesting that all the functional implications of the structural diversity of synaptic contacts are thereby apprehended, it does mean that investigators of ultrastructural and functional aspects have solid grounds for asking each other pertinent questions, a necessary condition of progress. By arranging each session so that it contains reports on morphological and on functional problems, the programme committee hopes to stimulate such interactions.

Many successful results have been obtained from experiments performed on

References p. 3

synaptic systems either functionally isolated *in vivo* or surviving *in vitro*, in a controlled environment. Although these systems are generally chosen for their apparent simplicity, they are often found to be of a structural, biochemical and functional complexity, initially unsuspected, that may lead to many a new finding. This increasing demand for "simple" systems is illustrated by numerous studies on intercellular contacts between cells in culture, whether these be of similar or of different types. Such models seem to pave the way for the study of the most fundamental question of how cells recognize one another, a process which appears to depend partly on membrane interaction. Moreover our knowledge both of the formation of synaptic contacts as well as of the intercellular relationships known as trophic actions is enhanced by studies of this type. They will no doubt contribute to our understanding of some of the mechanisms operating in the genesis of cerebral organization.

Finally, the spatial and temporal scales at which synaptic phenomena are studied deserve a mention. In electrophysiology, the spatial resolution obtainable by microelectrodes seems to have reached its limits. The use of capillary micro-electrodes for the micro-iontophoretic administration of active substances at proximity to the receptor membrane has proved most efficacious for testing candidates to the office of chemical mediator. On a spatial scale, morphologists are continuing to increase spatial resolution, whereas on a temporal scale, neurophysiologists are, on the contrary, showing more and more interest in the detection of long-term synaptic effects. The duration of some of such effects observed in relatively simple cellular systems is of the order of magnitude of the hour. The past history of certain synapses is becoming increasingly important for the understanding of their present reactions. Thus, physiologists are advancing from synchronous and short-term synaptic effects with a time scale graduated in milliseconds to diachronic neuronal interactions. The way lies open for a more thorough study of the plasticity of synaptic mechanisms. This symposium will probably reflect a great deal of these tendencies.

Now that the contents of the play about to be performed have been outlined, I'd like to add a word about the actors. The principal reports presented by distinguished speakers who have kindly accepted the committee's invitation to travel from abroad, will be accompanied by shorter contributions of a more local flavour. The place and the scenery may well influence the actors' performance.

The baroque style of this building evokes the artists' struggle to throw off the yoke of classical academicism. Favourable influences may emanate from the town itself, since it saw the birth and upbringing, towards the end of the fifteenth century, of a man who contributed considerably to the transition of medicine from mediaeval scholastics to a modern-age science, Paracelsus. Alchemist and physician, he was a forerunner of our age of symposia. A travelling scholar like many of you, he covered great distances, from Poland to Ireland, from Asia Minor to Sweden, for the purpose of exchanging ideas with his colleagues. He attended many an illustrious patient, such as Erasmus, before being appointed to the University of Basle where a reactionary faculty soon followed with a disapproving eye his attempts to reform the medical teaching of his time. He caused a scandal by lecturing in the vernacular rather than in latin, and by divulging his programme in a poster containing the following statement, quite revolutionary then: "If I want to prove anything, I shall not try to do it by quoting authorities, but by experiment and by reasoning thereon".

REFERENCES

CRICK, F., (1966); *Of Molecules and Men*. University of Washington Press. Washington.
STENT, G. S., (1968); That Was the Molecular Biology That Was. *Science*, **160**, 390–395.

Morphological and Cytochemical Studies on the Synapses in the Autonomic Nervous System

J. TAXI

*Laboratory of Animal Biology, Faculty of Sciences, and Centre for
Applied Electronic Microscopy, C.N.R.S., Paris (France)*

INTRODUCTION: QUESTIONS OF TERMINOLOGY

The use of the term synapse for certain neuroeffector connexions in the autonomic nervous system raises some questions of definition with which we shall first deal.

The concept of synapse *sensu stricto* was introduced by Foster and Sherrington (1897) for the interneuronal connexions only; it applies to discrete contacts physiologically and morphologically differentiated in respect of the transmission of the excitation; also the motor endplates obviously answer to this definition (Couteaux, 1947). At the ultrastructural level, the interneuronal synapses exhibit morphological differentiations both in the nerve endings, such as the synaptic vesicles, and the effector, such as the "thickening" of the postsynaptic membrane in the so-called "synaptic complexes" (Palay, 1956, 1959) or "active zones" (Couteaux, 1961). Moreover, the motor endplate is characterized by a special differentiation of the muscular membrane, the subneural apparatus of Couteaux.

On the contrary, in the tissues innervated by the autonomic nervous system, for instance in the smooth muscle, it is generally not possible to distinguish, with techniques presently available, limited areas morphologically differentiated both on the nerve side and on the effector side, which might be clearly recognized as synaptic contacts. Thus, although the reality of a nervous control on the effector has been established physiologically for many organs, the existence of synapses *sensu stricto* must be questioned, and it seems more probable that a diffuse effect of the transmitter is involved, this physiological mechanism being possible owing to the receptor properties of the whole effector membrane.

On account of the lack of morphological evidence and of precise physiological data on a true synaptic transmission, it appears inadequate to call synapses the neuroeffector connexions of the autonomic nervous system; but, as it is certain that the peripheral part of the autonomic nerve fibres is able to release a transmitter, this part can be called the "efficient part" of the sympathetic or parasympathetic fibres, and the study of its properties will normally take place with that of the presynaptic fibres *sensu stricto*.

References p. 17–20

MORPHOLOGY

(1) The vesicles in the peripheral fibres of the autonomic nervous system

There is no need to give here an extensive account on the morphology of the synapse in the autonomic nervous system. Detailed studies of the interneuronal and neuro-effector connexions were recently made by Elfvin (1963), Richardson (1962, 1964), Grillo (1966), Taxi (1961, 1965, 1967a), and general reviews on the synapses were published by Gray and Guillery (1966), Gray (1966) and Palay (1967). But it may be useful, at the beginning of this meeting, to remind you of some still controversial points of the morphology of these connexions.

The synaptic vesicles were the first highly characteristic component recognized in the presynaptic areas (Palade and Palay, 1954; De Robertis and Bennett, 1954). Since that time, it has been observed that several kinds of vesicles may be met in the terminal part of the axons, and a large agreement now seems realized on the existence of three fundamental types of vesicles (Richardson, 1962, 1964; Grillo and Palay, 1962; Grillo, 1966; Taxi, 1965, 1967a; Palay, 1967).

(*a*) The *synaptic vesicles*, 300–600 Å in diameter, appear empty or filled with a slightly dense, homogeneous material. Analyses made on fractionated brain by Whittaker (1960, 1965) and De Robertis *et al.* (1962) have brought good evidence that these vesicles are the storage site of acetylcholine.

(*b*) The *small granulated vesicles* (SGV), or small dense-core vesicles, recognized first by De Robertis and Pellegrino de Iraldi (1961), have about the same size as the synaptic vesicles, or they may be a little larger according to Palay (1967). They contain a granule which appears extremely dense after fixation by osmium tetroxide or by glutaraldehyde followed by osmium. These granules may have different sizes and different positions inside the vesicles, which are never completely filled with the dense material.

Pellegrino de Iraldi and De Robertis (1961) observed, in spite of a confusion between the nerve fibres and pinealocyte processes, that the dense cores disappear under the effect of reserpine. Moreover, Wolfe *et al.* (1962) showed that the fibres containing the SGV can be labelled by [3H]noradrenaline. Thus the SGV appear characteristic

---

Fig. 1. Sympathetic ganglion of the frog. ($\times$ 34 200.) In the presynaptic area of this ganglionic synapse fixed by osmium tetroxide, there is a large number of synaptic vesicles near the zone of "membrane thickening" and a great development of the endoplasmic reticulum in the other part of the presynaptic area. There is a kind of transitional zone between these two regions of the pre-synaptic area, suggesting a possible origin of the vesicles from the endoplasmic reticulum. N, ganglionic neuron; G, glial cell.

Fig. 2. Sympathetic ganglion of the frog. ($\times$ 40 000.) In this preparation fixed by glutaraldehyde followed by osmium tetroxide, a neuronal spine (S) is cut transversally inside a presynaptic area which occupies almost all the surface of the figure. Many vesicles have a more or less elongated form (arrows). In the top region, there are several large sections of agranular endoplasmic reticulum. G, glial cell.

Fig. 3. Sympathetic ganglion of the frog. ($\times$ 53 500.) In this presynaptic area fixed by osmium tetroxide, many vesicles have an elongated or dumb-bell form (arrows).

of the noradrenergic fibres; they are usually mixed with empty vesicles, which represent another form of the SGV, as shown by Tranzer and Thoenen (1967).

(c) The "*large granulated vesicles*" (LGV), or large dense-core vesicles, have a

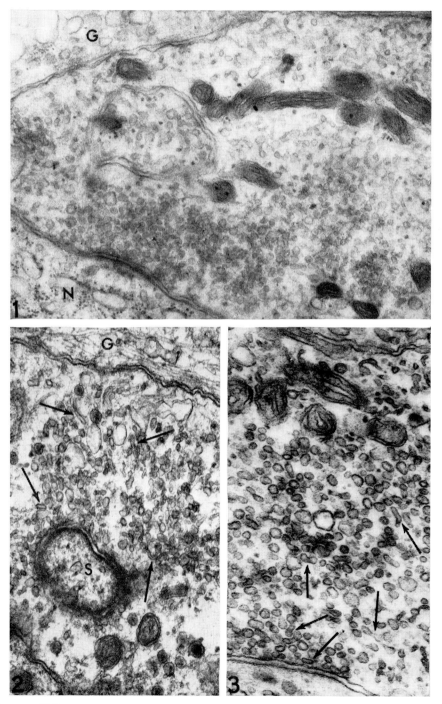

diameter which varies over a range from 600 to more than 1000 Å. Thus the smallest vesicles may be confused with the largest SGV, and the biggest reach the size of the neurosecretory granules. There are rather large variations in the density of the core, generally less dense than that of the SGV. These vesicles are present, and more or less numerous, in cholinergic fibres, such as preganglionic endings (Taxi, 1961), or in adrenergic ones, as peripheral sympathetic fibres (Richardson, 1962; Grillo and Palay, 1962). The dense core of these vesicles is not clearly modified under the action of reserpine (Bondareff and Gordon, 1965; Taxi, 1965; Clementi *et al.*, 1966).

There is perhaps a fourth type to be distinguished, according Uchizono (1965), the flattened or elongated vesicles, observed in certain synapses of the central nervous system, which would be related to an inhibitory function (see Gray's paper in this meeting, p. 141).

The first point with which we deal is related to this last question: it concerns a contribution of the aspects provided by the autonomic nervous system to the problem of the form of the synaptic vesicles and its possible meaning.

The sympathetic neurons of the frog or those of the ciliary ganglion of the chick have a large presynaptic apparatus originating from a single preganglionic fibre, which exhibits many synaptic contacts "en passant". It is not rare to observe in the synaptic areas of these synapses a mixture of typical, spherical synaptic vesicles and of elongated or tubular forms. Dumb-bell shapes are also seen (Figs. 2, 3). In many places there is a close relationship between the agranular endoplasmic reticulum and synaptic vesicles (Fig. 1), and forms which associate spherical and tubular parts (Fig. 4) are frequently found.

The various orientations of elongated vesicles allows us to exclude some sectioning artifact which, according Manolov (1967), could be responsible for the deformation of spherical vesicles in certain zones of the sections. According to Birks' observations (1965), osmium tetroxide fixation may cause a fragmentation of tubular structures in the presynaptic ending of the frog myoneural junctions, which results in vesicular, spherical forms. In our material, if the elongated vesicles appear more numerous and even predominant after aldehydic fixation (Fig. 2), they are not rare in osmium fixed preparations (Figs. 3, 4), as they are in the spinal cord of the same animal (Sotelo and Taxi, 1968). The aspects of elongated vesicles are much more frequent in this material than those of vesicles opening in or attached to the cell membrane, suggesting a mechanism of pinocytosis for the formation of synaptic vesicles. Such an origin cannot be excluded in the preganglionic nerve endings of the frog, but our observations suggest more a common nature and perhaps affiliation of the synaptic vesicles from the agranular endoplasmic reticulum, as Palay (1958) has expressed already.

The neoformation of tremendous amounts of vesicles after the ligature of a nerve, first observed on the splenic nerve of the cat by Kappeler and Mayor (1967), was recently reinvestigated by Pellegrino de Iraldi and De Robertis (1968) on the sciatic nerve of the rat. These last authors consider that the vesicles originate from the microtubules (= neurotubules) of the nerve fibres. This origin implies a fundamental modification of the membrane structure, as the microtubules have no unit membrane, but are only formed by protein, fibrillar subunits (Tilney and Porter, 1967). Such a transformation is not necessary to imagine if synaptic vesicles originate from the endoplasmic reticulum. On the other hand, the large variations in shape of the synaptic vesicles observed in one presynaptic area emphasize that, at least in this material, each form of vesicle is not related to a peculiar physiological function of the nerve ending.

(2) Permanence of postsynaptic differentiations after section of preganglionic fibres

The second point of pure morphology I would speak about is the permanence of the postsynaptic differentiations. In the ganglionic synapses of the frog, in addition to the "thickening" of the postsynaptic membrane, a subsynaptic layer may not infrequently be seen, always opposite a so-called "active zone" (Taxi, 1961). Such formations may be considered as an excellent criterion for recognizing "active zones" after section of preganglionic fibres and degeneration of presynaptic endings, which render more delicate the identification of the postsynaptic "membrane thickenings".

At the conclusion of several experiments on degeneration, we stated in 1962 that the subsynaptic formation may persist a short time, about five days, after the section of the rami communicantes, and then quickly disappears. As this point is of importance in the interpretation of the significance of the postsynaptic and subsynaptic formations, we asked Sotelo (1968) to make a new set of experiments on a larger scale. Sotelo was able to observe subsynaptic formations of normal aspect 7 days (Fig. 5) and up to 12 days after the section of the preganglionic nerves; at this time, the presynaptic arborization has completely disappeared (Fig. 6). Thus, if the postsynaptic membrane thickening and the subsynaptic layer appear as differentiations probably induced by a morphogenetic influence of the presynaptic fibre on the postganglionic neuron, their permanence during a long period after the section of preganglionic fibres suggests that they are not so closely related to the synaptic activity as we had thought previously. They are rather stable, if not definitive differentiations. The discrepancy between our first results and those obtained by Sotelo is probably due to individual variations in the degeneration processes. It seems probable that, in general, a part of the subsynaptic formations disappears and a part remains intact.

CYTOCHEMISTRY

(1) Radioautographic studies of the accumulation of some biogenic amines in the peripheral sympathetic fibres

We arrive now at the main activity of our laboratory during the last couple of years, which is concerned with cytochemistry. This investigation, dealing with the properties of uptake and storage of the peripheral, "efficient part" of the sympathetic nerve fibres, was made with the radioautographic method. This work started in collaboration with Droz, largely thanks to his technical experience in radioautography (Taxi and Droz, 1966a,b, 1967a,b).

This study was carried out in order to get, as far as possible, the cytochemical transposition at the electron-microscope level of the numerous biochemical, pharma-

cological and also histochemical data in light microscopy, these last established by
the fluorescence method of Falck and Hillarp for catecholamines.

All the compounds studied were injected into the vena jugularis externa at a dose
of 5 mC for a rat weighing 80–100 g. More technical details may be found in Taxi
and Droz (1968).

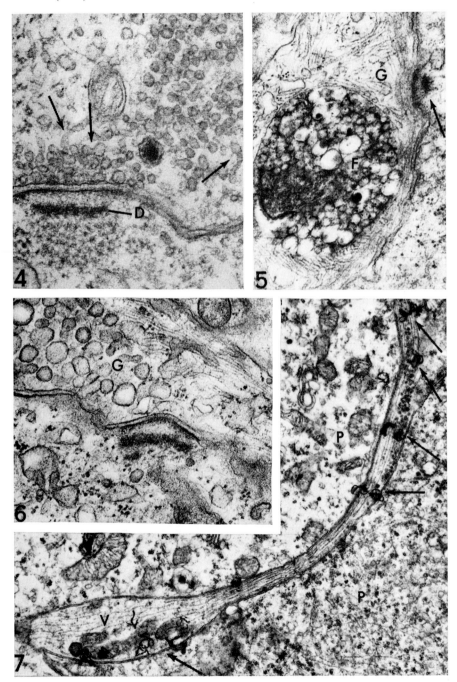

It was the merit of Wolfe *et al.* (1962) to have shown that the radioautographic method is suitable for the localization of certain water-soluble compounds, such as [³H]noradrenaline, provided they are bound to storage structures, in this case the SGV. These authors' observations were fully confirmed by our results on several organs of the rat (epiphysis, vas deferens, ureter and perivascular innervation) (Fig. 8). A substantial labelling of the nerve fibres containing SGV is obtained almost instanteously after an injection of [³H]noradrenaline; a moderate decrease follows, which is obvious in the tissues taken off 30 min after the injection; the amount of silver grains then remains nearly constant for up to 6 h.

4 h after an injection of reserpine, 5 mg/kg i.p., there is almost no labelling on nerve fibres. The dense core of the SGV has almost completely disappeared, and only rarely are silver grains found on the nerve fibres, which provides evidence that the negative result of the radioautography is not due to a failure of the technique (Taxi and Droz, 1966b).

It is to be noticed that nerve fibres devoid of vesicular structures may also be labelled, at least in certain circumstances. For instance, such pictures were observed in the nerve bundles of the nictitating membrane of the cat, *in vitro* incubated with [³H]noradrenaline (Taxi, 1967b).

The properties of the peripheral sympathetic fibres were also investigated with the radioautographic method for several other compounds of the catecholamine group ([³H]dopamine, [³H]adrenaline, [³H]normetanephrine, [³H]metaraminol) and two of the indolealkylamine group ([³H]5-hydroxytryptophan = [³H]5-HTP, and [³H]5-hydroxytryptamine = [³H]serotonin = [³H]5-HT).

The injection of [³H]dopamine or [³H]adrenaline resulted in a rich labelling of the nerve fibres containing SGV in the epiphysis (Figs. 7, 9) and vas deferens (Taxi and Droz, 1967b). With [³H]DOPA, only a weak labelling was obtained. It seems probable that this last result is due to the low doses we used (about 0.5 mg/kg), whereas in pharmacological experiments 20 mg/kg and more were usually injected (Andén *et al.*, 1966).

Fig. 4. Sympathetic ganglion of the frog. ($\times$ 72 000.) Typical aspect of a subsynaptic dense layer (D), with another cytoplasmic differentiation deeper in the cytoplasm of the ganglionic neuron, which appear as a cluster of small tubular structures. Different forms of vesicles, sometimes related to a tubular system (arrows) are seen in the presynaptic area.

Fig. 5. (from Sotelo, 1968) Sympathetic ganglion of the frog. ($\times$ 34 200.) 7 days after the section of the rami communicantes, preganglionic fibres are involved in a degenerative process (F). The synaptic contact is disrupted and the glial cytoplasm (G) has taken the initial place of the presynaptic area, but the postsynaptic differentiations, including the subsynaptic dense layer (arrow), are still normal.

Fig. 6. (from Sotelo, 1968) Sympathetic ganglion of the frog. ($\times$ 38 200.) 12 days after the section of the rami communicantes, the preganglionic fibres have completely disappeared, but the postsynaptic differentiations remain apparently unchanged. G, glia.

Fig. 7. Epiphysis of a rat injected with [³H]adrenaline. ($\times$ 18 000.) Silver grains are localized on a nerve fibre showing a varicosity (V); they are superimposed on amounts of small granulated vesicles (arrows). P, pinealocytes.

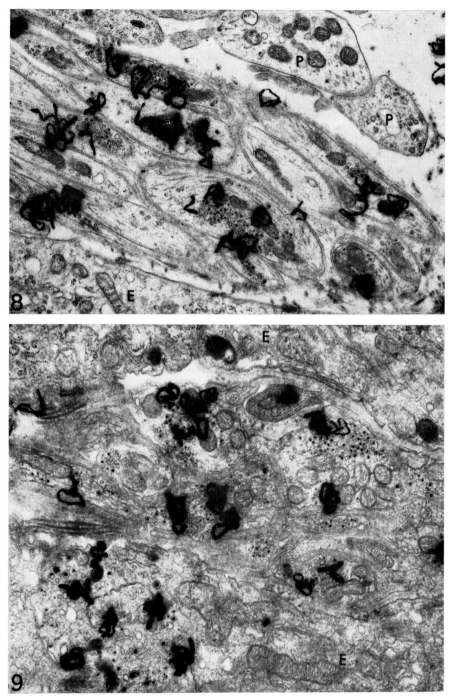

Fig. 8. Part of a nerve bundle in the epiphysis of a rat injected with [³H]noradrenaline. (× 24 000.)
There is a striking concordance between the localization of silver grains and the clusters of small
granulated vesicles. E, pinealocytes; p, pinealocytes processes.
Fig. 9. A nerve bundle in the epiphysis of a rat injected with [³H]dopamine. (× 25 100.) The nerve
fibres containing small granulated vesicles are well labelled. E, pinealocytes.

fibres, when the dense core of the SGV has disappeared under the action of reserpine (Fig. 10) (Taxi and Droz, 1968). Unfortunately, the size of the silver grains in the present state of the emulsion technique does not allow us to recognize to what cytoplasmic structure the [³H]noradrenaline is bound.

These observations agree with the idea of a reserpine-resistant uptake put forward by Hamberger *et al.* (1964). In a recent investigation, Hamberger (1967) emphasized the effect of an MAO inhibitor on the process. With our technique, we also observed that any labelling is impossible to obtain in reserpine-treated rats in the absence of an MAO inhibitor. A possible interpretation is that an extravesicular pool of [³H]noradrenaline is especially exposed to MAO effects, a conclusion already drawn by Van Orden *et al.* (1967) on the basis of other methods. The results obtained suggest that this pool is much smaller than the intravesicular one linked to the dense cores.

In agreement with many biochemical data (see review in Iversen's book, 1967), there is much cytochemical evidence that the uptake and storage are not specific to the physiological transmitter, but they apply for a number of compounds more or less chemically related to it, the so-called "false transmitters". It is difficult to estimate the possible interference of the compounds we studied with the transmitter in normal physiological conditions; except for adrenaline, it seems that these compounds are not normally present in the blood in significant amounts.

In spite of this relative lack of specificity of the uptake and storage processes, different types of nerve fibre seem clearly defined in consideration of their ability to accumulate certain substances. For instance, preganglionic endings in the superior cervical ganglion, known as cholinergic, were never labelled in our preparations. A noteworthy example of another type is provided by certain nerve fibres of the mollusc *Aplysia californica**. In the heart of this animal, certain nerve fibres and presynaptic endings of neuromuscular junctions quickly accumulate [³H]serotonin (Fig. 12). As [³H]serotonin is scarcely stored at all by vertebrate sympathetic nerve fibres under normal conditions (see above), this property defines a new type of (probably) serotoninergic nerve fibres. This conclusion is in agreement with biochemical and physiological results pointing to the probable existence of serotoninergic fibres in the *Mollusca*, especially *Aplysia* (Welsh and Moorhead, 1960; Chase *et al.*, 1968).

Fig. 10. Part of a nerve bundle in the epiphysis of a rat treated with reserpine and pheniprazine before an injection of [³H]noradrenaline. (× 24 000.) Even though the vesicles have no dense core (arrows), a moderate labelling is seen on the nerve fibres.

Fig. 11. Part of a nerve bundle in the epiphysis of a rat treated with pheniprazine and then injected with [³H]serotonin. (× 32 800.) A limited labelling appears on the nerve fibres.

Fig. 12. A nerve bundle in the heart of a mollusc, *Aplysia californica*. (× 46 000.) A nerve fibre containing a small number of empty vesicles is strongly labelled after 30 min of incubation in a bath containing [³H]serotonin (100 μC of serotonin, specific activity 6 C/mmol, in 3 ml seawater). H, heart muscle in transverse section; G, glial cells.

---

* This material was kindly given to us by Dr. Tauc.

References p. 17–20

(2) Storage and dense-core vesicles

The SGV usually provides a good morphological criterion for identifying the nor-adrenergic fibres in the peripheral autonomic nervous system of vertebrates. Un-fortunately, there is a source of uncertainty in that, according to the animal species and even in different tissues of the same animal, the dense core of the SGV may be more or less intensely stained or even not stained at all. This observation has been reported by several authors (Merrillees *et al.*, 1963; Taxi, 1965; Tranzer and Thoenen, 1967; Tranzer *et al.*, 1969).

In order to obtain more reliable fixation of the dense cores, Richardson (1966) recommended the fixation by potassium permanganate at high concentration, Tranzer and Thoenen (1967) by glutaraldehyde followed by osmium tetroxide, and Tranzer *et al.* (1969) described a new way of fixation using glutaraldehyde followed by potassium dichromate.

In so far as the dense core may represent the catecholamine in the vesicle, we tried various fixatives in order to obtain the best preservation of [³H]noradrenaline *in situ*, which can be estimated by the number of silver grains found superimposed on the nerve fibres. In the epiphysis and vas deferens of rats injected with [³H]noradrenaline, there is no clear difference in the numbers of silver grains present on nerve fibre sections between the preparations fixed by osmium tetroxide and those fixed according to Tranzer and Thoenen (1967). In the tissues fixed by potassium permanganate, the dense cores of the SGV are better preserved; only few of the vesicles remain empty, the majority being filled almost completely by a dense material. However, the number of silver grains in these preparations is obviously smaller than after the two other fixatives above-mentioned have been used. A statistical study after osmium tetroxide and potassium permanganate fixations fully confirms this impression (Taxi, 1968).

The interpretation of this unexpected result seemed to us to be that the potassium permanganate, probably owing to its high oxidative power, destroys either the [³H]-noradrenaline itself or at least the binding between the noradrenaline and a storage structure. According to the known properties of the potassium permanganate as a fixative, it might be accepted that the dense core represents a lipoprotein storage structure. This conclusion agrees with a hypothesis of Stjärne (1964) based on his extensive biochemical studies of the storage structures.

In the course of this meeting, Tranzer (1968) suggested to us another interpretation: the dense core seen after the permanganate fixation might be only a precipitation of Mn or MnO_2 from $KMnO_4$ reduced by the noradrenaline stored in the vesicle. The [³H]noradrenaline would be destroyed in the course of the reduction, and the tritium washed out in the fixative. Thus the dense cores seen after permanganate fixation would be different in nature of the dense core seen after the osmium or glutaraldehyde fixation, which would be the catecholamine itself. Nevertheless the presence of a Mn-dense core would be related to the initial presence of noradrenaline in the vesicle. Only new experiments will make us better able to interpret the nature of the dense core seen after the use of potassium permanganate.

Another use of the radioautographic method, related to the uncertainties of the

SGV fixations, was the tentative labelling of the noradrenergic fibres in the intestine. In this organ, from our experience, the SGV are rather difficult to recognize, either because of the usual failure of the staining of the dense core for unknown reasons or because the vesicles are really different in some respects from other noradrenergic SGV.

After an injection of [^{3}H]noradrenaline, a limited number of nerve fibres and pre-synaptic areas of interneuronal synapses is labelled in Auerbach's and Meissner's plexuses. We were so fortunate as to obtain two serial sections of the same presynaptic ending, both richly labelled (see the figure in Taxi and Droz, 1968); this observation allows us definitively to exclude that the labelling seen was a random phenomenon and brings new and convincing evidence for the existence of interneuronal adrenergic synapses in the plexuses of the intestine, a conclusion already reached by several workers using the fluorescence method (Norberg, 1964, 1967; Hollands and Vanov, 1965; Jacobowitz, 1965; Gabella and Costa, 1967).

All the labelled fibres in the intestine plexuses contain vesicles which appear empty or filled with a slightly dense material, but by no means typical SGV (Taxi, 1967a,b; Taxi and Droz, 1968). This seems inconsistent with the widespread and perhaps too simple hypothesis according to which there is a strict correlation between the presence of noradrenaline and that of dense cores in the vesicles. In several materials this correlation is good, as Van Orden et al. (1966) demonstrated in the rat vas deferens, and the radioautographic studies confirm. But on account of the results reported in this paper, it does not seem likely that a radioautographic reaction so intense as that obtained in the plexuses of the intestine can be attributed to an extravesicular pool. A better interpretation might be that the vesicles in this organ, especially their storage structures, have special staining properties. This situation resembles to a certain extent that found in certain regions of the central nervous system, for instance in the locus coeruleus (Descarries and Droz, 1968). In this material, presynaptic endings exhibit a rich labelling superimposed on nerve fibres containing apparently empty vesicles.

REFERENCES

ANDÉN, N. E., JUKES, M. G., LUNDBERG, A., AND VYKLICKY, L., (1966); The effect of DOPA on the spinal cord. 1. Influence on transmission from primary afferents; 2. A pharmacological analysis. *Acta physiol. scand.*, **67**, 373–386.

BIRKS, R. I., (1965); The fine structure of motor nerve endings at frog myoneural junctions. *Ann. N.Y. Acad Sci.*, **135**, 8–19.

BONDAREFF, W., AND GORDON, B., (1966); Submicroscopic localization of norepinephrine in sympathetic nerves of rat pineal body. *J. Pharmacol. exp. Ther.*, **153**, 42–47.

BURGEN, A. S. V., AND IVERSEN, L. L., (1965); The inhibition of noradrenaline uptake by sympathomimetic amines in the rat isolated heart. *Brit. J. Pharmacol. Chemother.*, **25**, 34–49.

CHASE, T. N., BREESE, G. R., CARPENTER, D. O., SCHANBERG, S. M., AND KOPIN, I. J., (1968); Stimulation-induced release of serotonin. *Advanc. Pharmacol.*, **6A**, 351–364.

CLEMENTI, F., MANTEGAZZA, P., AND BOTTURI, M., (1966); A pharmacologic and morphologic study on the nature of the dense-core granules present in the presynaptic endings of sympathetic ganglia. *Int. J. Neuropharmacol.*, **5**, 281–285.

COUTEAUX, R., (1947); Contribution à l'étude de la synapse myoneurale. *Rev. canad. Biol.*, **6**, 563–711.

COUTEAUX, R., (1961); Principaux critères morphologiques et cytochimiques utilisables aujourd'hui pour définir les divers types de synapses. *Actualités neurophysiol.*, **3ème série**, 145–173.

DE ROBERTIS, E., AND BENNETT, H. S., (1954); Submicroscopic vesicular component in the synapse. *Fed. Proc.*, **13**, 35.

DE ROBERTIS, E., AND PELLEGRINO DE IRALDI, A., (1961); Plurivesicular secretory processes and nerve endings in the pineal gland of the rat. *J. biophys. biochem. Cytol.*, **10**, 361–372.

DE ROBERTIS, E., PELLEGRINO DE IRALDI, A., DE LOREZ ARNAÏZ, R., AND SALGANICOFF, L., (1962); Cholinergic and non-cholinergic nerve endings in rat brain. I. Isolation and subcellular distribution of acetylcholine and acetylcholinesterase. *J. Neurochem.*, **9**, 23–25.

DESCARRIES, L., AND DROZ, B., (1968); Incorporation de noradrénaline-^{3}H(NA-^{3}H) dans le système nerveux central du rat adulte. Étude radioautographique en microscopie électronique. *C.R. Acad. Sci. (Paris)*, **266**, 2480–2482.

ELFVIN, L. G., (1963); The ultrastructure of the superior cervical sympathetic ganglion of the cat. *J. Ultrastruct. Res.*, **8**, 403–440, 441–476.

GABELLA, G., AND COSTA, M., (1967); Le fibre adrenergiche nel canale alimentare. *G. Accad. Med. Torino*, **130**, 12 p.

FOSTER, M., AND SHERRINGTON, C. S., (1897); *A Textbook of Physiology*, MacMillan, London.

GERSHON, M. D., AND ROSS, L. L., (1966); Radioisotopic studies of the binding, exchange and distribution of 5-hydroxytryptamine synthesized from its radioactive precursor. *J. Physiol. (Lond.)*, **186**, 451–476.

GERSHON, M. D., DRAKONTIDES, A. B., AND ROSS, L. L., (1965); Serotonin: synthesis and release from the myenteric plexus of the mouse intestine. *Science*, **149**, 197–199.

GRAY, E. G., (1966); Problems of interpreting the fine structure of vertebrate and invertebrate synapses. *Int. Rev. gen. exp. Zool.*, **2**, 139–170.

GRAY, E. G., AND GUILLERY, R. W., (1966); Synaptic morphology in the normal and degenerating nervous system. *Int. Rev. Cytol.*, **19**, 111–182.

GRILLO, M. A., (1966); Electron microscopy of sympathetic tissues. *Pharmacol. Rev.*, **18**, 387–399.

GRILLO, M. A., AND PALAY, S. L., (1962); Granule-containing vesicles in the autonomic nervous system, in S. S. BREESE (Ed.), *Proc. Vth Int. Congr. Electr. Micr.*, Philadelphia, New York, Academic Press, p. 2, U 1.

HAMBERGER, B., (1967); Reserpine-resistant uptake of catecholamines in isolated tissues of the rat. *Acta physiol. scand.*, suppl. **295**.

HAMBERGER, B., MALMFORS, T., NORBERG, K. A., AND SACHS, C., (1964); Uptake and accumulation of catecholamines in peripheral adrenergic neurons of reserpinized animals, studied with a histochemical method. *Biochem. Pharmacol.*, **13**, 841–844.

HOLLANDS, B. C. S., AND VANOV, S., (1965); Localization of catecholamines in visceral organs and ganglia of the rat, guinea-pig and rabbit. *Brit. J. Pharmacol.*, **25**, 307–316.

IVERSEN, L. L., (1967); *The Uptake and Storage of Noradrenaline in Sympathetic Nerves.* Cambridge University Press, Cambridge.

JACOBOWITZ, D., (1965) Histochemical studies of the autonomic innervation of the gut. *J. Pharmacol. exp. Ther.*, **149**, 358–364.

KAPPELER, K., AND MAYOR, D., (1967); The accumulation of noradrenaline in constricted sympathetic nerves as studied by fluorescence and electron microscopy. *Proc. Roy. Soc., B*, **167**, 282–292.

MANOLOV, S., (1967); Recherches sur la morphologie des vésicules synaptiques des synapses de la moëlle épinière du chat. *C.R. Acad. bulgare Sci.*, **20**, 493–495.

MERRILLEES, N. C., BURNSTOCK, G., AND HOLMAN, M. E., (1963); Correlation of fine structure and physiology of the innervation of smooth muscle in the guinea pig vas deferens. *J. Cell Biol.*, **19**, 529–550.

NORBERG, K. A., (1964); Adrenergic innervation of the intestinal wall studied by fluorescence microscopy. *Int. J. Neuropharmacol.*, **3**, 379–382.

NORBERG, K. A., (1967); Transmitter histochemistry of the sympathetic adrenergic nervous system. *Brain Res.*, **5**, 125–170.

PALADE, G. E., AND PALAY, S. L., (1954); Electron microscope observations of interneuronal and neuromuscular synapses. *Anat. Rec.*, **118**, 335–336.

PALAY, S. L., (1956); Synapses in the central nervous system. *J. biophys. biochem. Cytol.*, **2**, 193–202.

PALAY, S. L., (1958); The morphology of synapses in the central nervous system. *Exp. Cell Res.*, Suppl. **5**, 275–293.

PALAY, S. L., (1967); Principles of cellular organization in the nervous system. In G. C. QUARTON,

TH. MELCHENUCK AND F. O. SCHMITT (Eds.), *The Neurosciences*, The Rockefeller University Press, New York.

PELLEGRINO DE IRALDI, A., AND DE ROBERTIS, E., (1961); Action of reserpine on the submicroscopic morphology of the pineal gland. *Experientia (Basel)*, **17** ,122–123.

PELLEGRINO DE IRALDI, A., AND DE ROBERTIS, E., (1968); The neurotubular system of the axon and the origin of granulated and non-granulated vesicles in regenerating nerves. *Z. Zellforsch.*, **87**, 330–344.

PELLEGRINO DE IRALDI, A., ZIEHER, L. M., AND DE ROBERTIS, E., (1965); Ultrastructure and pharmacological studies of nerve endings in pineal organ. In J. ARIËNS KAPPERS AND J. P. SCHADÉ (Eds.), *Structure and Function of the Epiphysis Cerebri (Progress in Brain Research*, Vol. 10), Elsevier, Amsterdam, pp. 389–421.

RICHARDSON, K. G., (1962); The fine structure of autonomic nerve endings in smooth muscle of the rat vas deferens. *J. Anat. (Lond.)*, **96**, 427–442.

RICHARDSON, K. G., (1964); The fine structure of the albino rabbit iris, with special reference to the identification of adrenergic and cholinergic nerves and nerve endings in its intrinsic muscles. *Amer. J. Anat.*, **114**, 173–205.

RICHARDSON, K. G., (1966); Electron microscope identification of autonomic nerve endings. *Nature (Lond.)*, **210**, 756.

SOTELO, C., (1968); Permanence of postsynaptic specializations in the frog sympathetic ganglion cells after denervation. *Exp. Brain Res.*, **6**, 294–305.

SOTELO, C., AND TAXI, J., (1968); Unpublished observations on frog spinal cord.

STJÄRNE, L., (1964); Studies of catecholamine uptake, storage and release mechanisms. *Acta physiol. scand.*, **62**, suppl. 228.

TAXI, J., (1961); Étude de l'ultrastructure des zones synaptiques dans les ganglions sympathiques de Grenouille. *C.R. Acad. Sci. (Paris)*, **252**, 174–176.

TAXI, J., (1962); Étude au microscope électronique de synapses ganglionnaires chez quelques vertébrés. *IVth Intern. Congr. Neuropathol. Munich*, Vol. 2, Springer, Berlin, pp. 197–203.

TAXI, J., (1965); Contribution à l'étude des connexions des neurones moteurs du système nerveux autonome. *Ann. Sci. Nat. Zool.*, [12] **7**, 413–674.

TAXI, J., (1967a); Observations on the ultrastructure of the ganglionic neurons and synapses of the frog *Rana esculenta* L. In H. HYDÉN, (Ed.), *The Neuron*, Elsevier, Amsterdam, pp. 221–254.

TAXI, J., (1967b); Identification des fibres nerveuses adrénergiques dans quelques muscles lisses de mammifères par la méthode autoradiographique utilisée en microscopie électronique. *Bull. Ass. Anat. 52ème Reunion, Paris-Orsay*, pp. 1132–1139.

TAXI, J., (1968); Sur la fixation et la signification du contenu dense des vésicules des fibres adrénergiques étudiées au microscope électronique. *C.R. Acad. bulg. Sci.*, in the press.

TAXI, J., AND DROZ, B., (1966a); Étude de l'incorporation de noradrénaline-³H (NA-³H) et de 5-hydroxytryptophane-³H (5-HTP-³H) dans les fibres nerveuses du canal déférent et de l'intestin. *C.R. Acad. Sci. (Paris)*, **263**, 1237–1240.

TAXI, J., AND DROZ, B., (1966b); Étude de l'incorporation de noradrénaline-³H (NA-³H) et de 5-hydroxytryptophane-³H (5-HTP-³H) dans l' épiphyse et dans le ganglion cervical supérieur. *C. R. Acad. Sci. (Paris)*, **263**, 1326–1329.

TAXI, J., AND DROZ, B., (1967a); Localisation d'amines biogènes dans le système neurovégétatif périphérique (Étude radioautographique en microscopie électronique après injection de noradrenaline-³H et de 5-hydroxytryptophane-³H). In F. STUTINSKY (Ed.), *Neurosecretion*, Springer, Berlin, pp. 191–202.

TAXI, J., AND DROZ, B., (1967b); Détection radioautographique des amines biogènes dans le système neurovégétatif. *J. Microscopie*, **6**, 84a.

TAXI, J., AND DROZ, B., (1968); Radioautographic studies of the accumulation of some biogenic amines in the autonomic nervous system. In S. BARONDES (Ed.), *Dynamics of the Neuron*, Academic Press, New York.

TILNEY, L. G., AND PORTER, K. B., (1967); Studies on the microtubules in Helozoa. II. *J. Cell Biol.*, **34**, 327–343.

TRANZER, J. P., (1968); Personal communication.

TRANZER, J. P., AND THOENEN, H., (1967); Significance of "empty vesicles" in post-ganglionic sympathetic nerve terminals. *Experientia (Basel)*, **23**, 123–124.

TRANZER, J. P., THOENEN, H., SNIPES, R. L., AND RICHARDS, J. G., (1969); Recent developments on the ultrastructural aspects of adrenergic nerve endings in various experimental conditions. In

K. Akert and P. G. Waser (Eds.), *Mechanisms of Synaptic Transmission (Progress in Brain Research*, Vol. 31) Elsevier, Amsterdam, pp. 33–46.

Uchizono, K., (1965); Characteristics of excitatory and inhibitory synapses in the central nervous system of the cat. *Nature (Lond.)*, **207**, 642–643.

Van Orden III, L. S., Bensch, K. G., and Giarman, N. J., (1967); Histochemical and functional relationships of catecholamines in adrenergic nerve endings. II. Extravesicular norepinephrine. *J. Pharmacol. exp. Ther.*, **155**, 428–439.

Van Orden III, L. S., Bloom, F. E., Barnett, R. J., and Giarman, N. J., (1966); Histochemical and functional relationships of catecholamines in adrenergic nerve endings. I. Participation of granular vesicles. *J. Pharmacol. exp. Ther.*, **154**, 185–199.

Welsh, J. H., and Moorhead, M., (1960); The quantitative distribution of 5-hydroxytryptamine in the invertebrates, especially in their nervous systems. *J. Neurochem.*, **6**, 146–169.

Whittaker, V. P., (1960); The binding of neurohormones by subcellular particles of brain tissues. Proc. 4th Int. Neurochem. Symp., in S. Kety and J. Eccles (Eds.), *Regional Neurochemistry*, pp. 259–263.

Whittaker, V. P., (1965); The application of subcellular fractionation techniques to the study of brain function. *Progr. Biophys.*, **15**, 39–96.

Wolfe, D. E., Potter, L. T., Richardson, K. C., and Axelrod, J., (1962); Localizing tritiated norepinephrine in sympathetic axons by electron microscopic autoradiography. *Science*, **138**, 440–442.

The Uptake, Storage, Release and Metabolism of Noradrenaline in Sympathetic Nerves

J. AXELROD AND I. J. KOPIN

Laboratory of Clinical Science, National Institute of Mental Health, Bethesda, Md. (U.S.A.)

Since the discovery of noradrenaline as the neurotransmitter of sympathetic nerves in mammals (Von Euler, 1948), there has been a considerable increase in our knowledge concerning the biochemistry of this catecholamine. For the past decade our laboratory has been involved in studies of the uptake, storage, release, formation and metabolism of noradrenaline. This report will describe some of these investigations.

BIOCHEMISTRY OF THE SYMPATHETIC NERVE ENDINGS

The main approach to studying the biochemistry of adrenergic neurones was the use of adrenergic drugs and radioactive catecholamines. In the initial experiments, [³H]-catecholamines (Axelrod et al., 1959; Whitby et al., 1961) of high specific activity were administered intravenously to animals and the accumulation of the radioactive catecholamine in various tissues was examined. To stimulate the sudden discharge of noradrenaline into the circulation, cats were given a tracer dose of [³H]noradrenaline intravenously and killed 2 min after the injection. At this time the [³H]noradrenaline was taken up and distributed unequally among the tissues. The highest levels were present in the heart, spleen and salivary gland. Little of the radioactive catecholamine was found in the brain. The same experiment was repeated but the tissues were examined 2 h after the injection, long after the physiological effects had disappeared. The concentration of noradrenaline by this time had declined in most tissues, but the amount of the catecholamine in tissues with a considerable sympathetic nerve innervation (heart, spleen, salivary gland) had remained high. The results suggested that the circulating noradrenaline was taken up and retained in certain tissues. The site of uptake and binding of the catecholamine appeared to be the sympathetic neurone.

To examine the possibility of uptake by the sympathetic nerves, the superior cervical ganglia of the cats or rats were removed unilaterally; and 5 days later (when the nerve had degenerated), [³H]noradrenaline was administered intravenously (Hertting et al., 1961; Fischer et al., 1965b). Two minutes after the intravenous administration of [³H]noradrenaline the denervated salivary gland contained half as much of the radioactive catecholamine as the innervated gland. The disappearance of the [³H]noradrenaline from the denervated side was very rapid. After 2 h only about 10% remained in the denervated side but 70% of the initial [³H]noradrenaline was

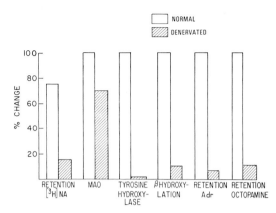

Fig. 1. The retention and metabolism of noradrenaline and other sympathomimetic amines in the denervated rat salivary gland. Adult-rat salivary glands were denervated by removing the superior cervical ganglia bilaterally, and the various experiments were carried out 5 days later. NA is noradrenaline, Adr is adrenaline, and MAO is monoamine oxidase.

retained in the innervated side (Fig. 1). These observations clearly demonstrated that the circulating noradrenaline was taken up and retained in the sympathetic nerve. Similar results were obtained when other organs such as the heart (Potter *et al.*, 1965) and spleen were denervated.

The enzymes involved in the formation of noradrenaline, tyrosine hydroxylase (Sedvall and Kopin, 1967a) and dopamine-β-hydroxylase (Fischer *et al.*, 1964) were also demonstrated to be present in the sympathetic nerve by denervation experiments (Fig. 1). When the rat salivary gland was denervated the conversion of tyrosine to dopa was completely abolished. In addition chemical sympathectomy of rats with 6-hydroxydopamine resulted in the complete disappearance of tyrosine hydroxylase in tissues (Mueller *et al.*, 1969).

The final step in the formation of noradrenaline involves the β-hydroxylation of dopamine by the enzyme dopamine-β-oxidase (Levin and Kaufman, 1961). This enzyme can also β-hydroxylate other amines such as tyramine. [^{3}H]Tyramine was injected in rats in which the superior cervical ganglia was removed unilaterally. Almost all of the labeled amine found on the intact side was β-hydroxylated tyrosine (octopamine) while little octopamine was found in the denervated side (Fischer *et al.*, 1964). This indicated that the sympathetic nerves of the salivary gland not only contained the β-hydroxylase enzyme but also were able to retain octopamine. Adrenaline was also taken up and selectively bound in the sympathetic nerve (Fig. 1).

Noradrenaline is metabolized *via* two major metabolic pathways, deamination by monoamine oxidase and *O*-methylation by catechol-*O*-methyltransferase (Axelrod, 1959). To examine whether these enzymes were present in sympathetic nerves the superior cervical ganglia were removed unilaterally and the activity of these enzymes was measured in the innervated and denervated sides. Sympathetic denervation caused a 30% fall in monoamine oxidase (MAO) activity in the salivary gland (Fig. 1) and a 50% fall in the pineal and iris (Snyder *et al.*, 1965; Waltman and Sears, 1964).

There was little change in catechol-O-methyltransferase activity. Because of the partial fall of MAO after denervation this enzyme appeared to be localized both within the neurone and outside the neurone while catechol-O-methyltransferase was present mainly outside the neurone.

SUBCELLULAR LOCALIZATION OF NORADRENALINE IN THE SYMPATHETIC NERVE

Radioactive noradrenaline served as a useful tool to study the subcellular localization of noradrenaline in the sympathetic neurone. It was previously shown that endogenous noradrenaline is localized in a particulate component within the splenic nerves (Von Euler and Hillarp, 1956). Electron-microscopic studies also showed the presence of granulated vesicles about 50 mμ wide with an electron-dense core in preterminal axoplasm of many autonomic axons (Wolfe et al., 1962). Since our studies showed that [^{3}H]noradrenaline was taken up and bound in sympathetic nerves, this provided an opportunity to examine whether these dense-core granules were the site of storage of noradrenaline. 30 min after an injection of radioactive noradrenaline, the pineal glands of rats (an organ rich in sympathetic fibers) were fixed with osmium tetroxide, prepared for radioautography and examined in an electron microscope. There was a striking localization of photographic grains in areas overlying nonmyelinated axons which contained granulated vesicles in the immediate vicinity of grain aggregation. These observations again indicated that the sympathetic nerves concentrated noradrenaline and that the catecholamine was stored in the dense-core vesicles within the nerves.

The noradrenaline storage vesicles in the heart were labeled and separated by density-gradient procedures, and their properties were studied (Potter and Axelrod, 1963b). Rats were given [^{3}H]noradrenaline, and after 1 h the hearts were removed and homogenized in isotonic sucrose. The various subcellular fractions were separated by a continuous sucrose gradient, and the endogenous and radioactive noradrenaline measurements were determined in each fraction. The predominant peak of both radioactive and endogenous noradrenaline coincided with a microsomal band. A similar distribution was obtained with other sympathetically innervated tissues including the salivary gland, pineal gland and vas deferens. These microsomal particles were then separated, and their properties were studied. The particles were found to contain dopamine-β-oxidase activity, indicating that noradrenaline can be formed from dopamine within the storage granules. Monoamine oxidase was also present in heart granules in considerable amounts (De Champlain et al., 1968). Adenosine triphosphate (ATP) was found in the particles in the same molar ratio to noradrenaline, as has been previously described in adrenal chromaffin granules (Hillarp et al., 1955); and this might serve to form a storage complex with the noradrenaline. The microsomal particles were also capable to taking up noradrenaline by a temperature-dependent process.

It can be concluded from these studies that the synthesis of noradrenaline from tyrosine takes place mainly within the sympathetic nerves as follows: The tyrosine

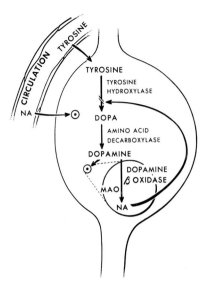

Fig. 2. The biosynthesis of noradrenaline in the sympathetic nerve. NA is noradrenaline; MAO is monoamine oxidase.

enters the axonal membrane by a concentrating mechanism, and it is then hydroxylated to dopa by the enzyme tyrosine hydroxylase. The dopa is then decarboxylated in the axoplasm by the widespread and nonspecific enzyme L-aromatic amino acid decarboxylase. The resulting dopamine then enters the granulated storage vesicle where it is β-hydroxylated to noradrenaline which is retained within the vesicle until it is released. Noradrenaline can also be taken up by the axonal membrane. The uptake is presumably accomplished by an active transport requiring sodium and potassium ions (Iversen and Kravitz, 1966). The uptake of noradrenaline across the neuronal membrane is saturable and stereospecific (Iversen, 1967). When noradrenaline reaches the axoplasm it is taken up and stored in the granulated vesicle. The level of noradrenaline in the nerve is maintained by a negative feedback mechanism (see below). Elevation of noradrenaline in the axoplasm causes an inhibition of conversion of tyrosine to dopa by tyrosine hydroxylase. The biosynthesis steps in the synthesis of noradrenaline within the sympathetic nerve terminal are shown in Fig. 2.

STORAGE, RELEASE AND INACTIVATION OF NORADRENALINE AT THE SYMPATHETIC NERVE TERMINALS

The uptake and binding of [³H]noradrenaline by granulated vesicles of the sympathetic nerves serves as a rapid and effective means for the temporary inactivation of the catecholamine. The relative importance of binding and metabolism of noradrenaline was obtained by examining the total fate of the catecholamine in the isolated perfused heart (Kopin et al., 1962). Isolated hearts were perfused with [³H]noradrenaline, and [³H]noradrenaline and its metabolites were examined 12 min after the infusion was ended. About 10% of the infused [³H]noradrenaline was retained by the heart while about 4% was present as combined metabolites. The O-methylated metabolite normetanephrine accounted for most of the transformation products. Thus inactivation by binding seems to predominate over inactivation by metabolism. In support of this is the observation that physiological effects of injected noradrenaline are rapidly terminated even after both monoamine oxidase and catechol-O-methyltransferase are inhibited (Crout, 1961).

The storage of noradrenaline in the sympathetic neurone requires an optimal electrolyte milieu. When rats are put on a high sodium chloride intake together with the salt-retaining steroid DOCA for several weeks, the ability to retain both endogenous noradrenaline and the radioactive catecholamine in the storage vesicle is reduced (Krakoff et al., 1967). This results from a leakiness of noradrenaline from the intraneuronal storage site, and this might be related to the elevation of blood pressure.

Since the neurotransmitter in the sympathetic nerves can be labeled, its fate after release was studied (Hertting and Axelrod, 1961). [³H]Noradrenaline was administered to cats, and several hours later the spleen had taken up considerable quantities of the labeled amine. The splenic nerve was stimulated, and [³H]noradrenaline and its metabolites were assayed in the venous outflow before and after nerve stimulation. There was a marked increase in the concentration of noradrenaline in the efferent outflow. Small amounts of the O-methylated metabolite were also discharged after nerve stimulation, but no evidence for the discharge of deaminated metabolites was obtained. These and other experiments described above demonstrated that the

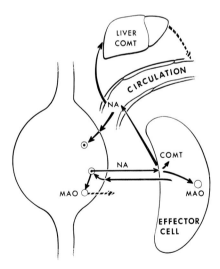

Fig. 3. The fate of noradrenaline in sympathetic nerve and tissues. NA is noradrenaline, COMT is catechol-O-methyltransferase, and MAO is monoamine oxidase. Dotted line represents metabolized noradrenaline.

neurotransmitter noradrenaline undergoes a complex fate after its discharge from the nerve. A fraction is removed by diffusion into the blood stream; a small amount is metabolized locally by O-methylation; the major fraction is taken up again by the nerves and bound again (Fig. 3).

The importance of reuptake of noradrenaline into sympathetic nerves as a mechanism of inactivation has been obtained by an experiment similar to that described above (Rosell *et al.*, 1963). The sympathetic nerves of the dog skeletal muscle were perfused with blood containing [³H]noradrenaline. A small amount of [³H]noradrenaline was discharged from the venous blood under resting conditions. During stimulation of the vasomotor nerve there was a delay in the outflow of [³H]noradrenaline. Just before stimulation stopped there was a sharp increase in the outflow of the catecholamine followed by a gradual decline to the prestimulatory level. After treatment with phenoxybenzamine, a drug that blocks the reuptake of noradrenaline, stimulation of the sympathetic nerves caused an immediate and greater rise in noradrenaline. This noradrenaline released from the sympathetic nerves causes a constriction which then traps the hormone in the vascular bed. This allows the discharged noradrenaline to return to the sympathetic nerves in the same manner as exogenously administered noradrenaline.

Noradrenaline is continuously released from the sympathetic nerve granule into the axoplasm. Upon release the major fraction is inactivated within the neurone by deamination by monoamine oxidase (Kopin, 1964). The noradrenaline released from the nerve after stimulation is metabolized by catechol-O-methyltransferase (Eisenfeld *et al.*, 1967b) in the effector cell. If the noradrenaline passes into the circulation it is mainly metabolized by liver catechol-O-methyltransferase (Fig. 3).

The bound stores of noradrenaline can be tagged with a tracer dose of the catecholamine and the rate of release from sympathetic nerves studied. Interruption of nerve impulse by either decentralization of the sympathetic nerves or the administration of ganglionic blocking agents will slow the release of noradrenaline (Hertting *et al.*, 1962). Many drugs such as sympathomimetic amines, reserpine and guanethidine increase the release of the catecholamines. Abnormal physiological conditions such as hypophysectomy, thyroidectomy, adrenalectomy and stress will also increase the release of catecholamines from the sympathetic neurone (Landsberg and Axelrod, 1968). The noradrenaline that is released by tyramine reaches the effector cell in a physiologically active form and is then metabolized mainly by catechol-O-methyltransferase (Kopin and Gordon, 1962). The noradrenaline released by reserpine is inactivated within the nerve by monoamine oxidase and then leaves the nerve as a physiologically inactive metabolic product.

CONTROL OF NORADRENALINE METABOLISM IN SYMPATHETIC NERVES

The rate of noradrenaline synthesis varies with the rate of utilization of the catecholamine. When nerve impulses to one salivary gland were interrupted by unilateral removal of a portion of the cervical sympathetic chain while the opposite nerve was stimulated, a fivefold increase in the conversion of intravenously administered [¹⁴C]-

TABLE I

EFFECT OF SYMPATHETIC NERVE IMPULSES ON NORADRENALINE SYNTHESIS AND TYROSINE
HYDROXYLASE ACTIVITY IN THE RAT SALIVARY GLAND

| | Noradrenaline formed in vivo from | | In vitro assay of tyrosine hydroxylase[a] |
	[14C]Tyrosine (counts/min)	[3H]Dopa (counts/min)	
Decentralized	68	410	3190
Stimulated	358	396	3170

[a] Tyrosine hydroxylase is expressed as counts/min [14C]dopa formed from [14C]tyrosine by an aliquot of homogenate of the salivary glands.

tyrosine to [14C]noradrenaline was found in the stimulated salivary gland (Sedvall and Kopin, 1967b) (Table I). In these experiments there was no difference in the rate of conversion of [3H]dopa to [3H]noradrenaline. These results indicate that noradrenaline synthesis was accelerated in the stimulated salivary gland by an increase in the hydroxylation of tyrosine. Similar results have been obtained by Gordon *et al.* (1966) in the rat heart. Tyrosine hydroxylase has been suggested as the rate-limiting enzyme in noradrenaline synthesis (Nagatsu *et al.*, 1964), and acceleration of synthesis would be expected to be apparent in conversion of tyrosine to dopa. When the levels of tyrosine hydroxylase in the stimulated salivary gland were measured (Sedvall and Kopin, 1967a), there was no difference between the stimulated and decentralized sides (Table I). This indicates that acceleration was not a consequence of synthesis of more tyrosine hydroxylase and must have been due to removal of feedback inhibition by the cytoplasmic catecholamines (Fig. 2).

There is considerable evidence that the entire neural store of noradrenaline is not involved in feedback control of tyrosine hydroxylation. The striking acceleration of noradrenaline synthesis which was found when the sympathetic nerves were stimulated was not accompanied by a change in total tissue levels of the catecholamine. Furthermore, several procedures which result in noradrenaline depletion are not associated with a significant increase in noradrenaline synthesis (Weise and Kopin, 1967). Following depletion of the stores of noradrenaline with reserpine, a marked decrease in excretion of the major metabolite of noradrenaline, 3-methoxy-4-hydroxyphenylglycol (MHPG), was found (Kopin and Weise, 1968). This indicates that noradrenaline synthesis is decreased when the stores of the catecholamine were almost completely depleted by the drug. The excretion of homovanillic acid, the major metabolite of dopamine, was markedly elevated and appeared to compensate for the decrease in MHPG excretion. Apparently dopamine formation (and tyrosine hydroxylation) continue at the normal rate after reserpine administration. Dopamine cannot be taken up by the storage vesicle, the site of the β-hydroxylating enzyme; and this conversion to noradrenaline is reduced. Dopamine is then deaminated by monoamine oxidase and methylated by catechol-*O*-methyltransferase to homovanillic acid.

Shortly after administration of an amine which displaces noradrenaline from its storage sites (*e.g.* metaraminol or octopamine), there is a decrease in noradrenaline formation from [^{14}C]tyrosine as well as from [^{3}H]dopa. There appears to be a block of both tyrosine hydroxylation and conversion of dopamine to noradrenaline. Neither metaraminol nor octopamine directly inhibits tyrosine hydroxylase or dopamine-β-oxidase so that these substances must act indirectly. Once noradrenaline has been displaced by the administration of amine, the rate of tyrosine hydroxylation returns to normal; but there is still some block in conversion of [^{3}H]dopa to noradrenaline, presumably by interference of dopamine entry into the vesicles. If the substance replacing the catecholamine is rapidly destroyed (*e.g.* octopamine is metabolized by MAO), then an increase in noradrenaline formation from [^{14}C]-tyrosine occurs with replenishment of the noradrenaline stores. These observations and the effect of nerve stimulation-induced release of noradrenaline on tyrosine hydroxylation are most easily explained if intraneuronal cytoplasmic catecholamine levels are responsible for the feedback inhibition of tyrosine hydroxylase.

Noradrenaline is stored in sympathetic nerves in a heterogenous fashion. Following administration of labeled noradrenaline, the decrease in its specific activity in various tissues was found to be multiphasic and the specific activity of noradrenaline which was easily released by tyrosine was different from that which remained in the heart (Potter and Axelrod, 1963a). Such findings indicate that there are more than one store of noradrenaline in the sympathetic neurone. When spleens of cats were perfused with Krebs–Ringer solution containing radioactive tyrosine, labeled noradrenaline was formed and released during nerve stimulation. The specific activity of the noradrenaline released after about 5 min of stimulation was about 9 times as high as that found in the spleen (Kopin *et al.*, 1968). The newly synthesized noradrenaline apparently enters both a reserve and an available store. Because of the relatively small size of the available store, its specific activity is much higher than that of the reserve store (Fig. 4). Newly formed noradrenaline seems to be more

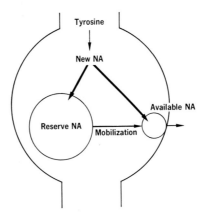

Fig. 4. Selective release of newly synthesized noradrenaline. NA is noradrenaline. NA which is released by nerve stimulation comes from a small immediately "available" store. Both newly synthesized NA and NA mobilized from the reserve stores are used to replenish the NA in the available store. While new NA can also enter the reserve store, new NA is a greater fraction of the smaller available store.

important in replenishing the available store than mobilization of the reserve store. This is consistent with the observation (Kopin *et al.*, 1968) that inhibition of synthesis markedly reduced the amount of neurotransmitter noradrenaline released during continuous nerve stimulation.

The processes for synthesis, storage and release of noradrenaline are not entirely specific. Structurally related compounds can be formed and stored in sympathetic nerve endings and are released during nerve stimulation. Such false adrenergic transmitters vary in their potency and are generally less active than the physiological transmitter. Thus their presence in nerves may interfere with adrenergic function. Following administration of [^{3}H]tyramine, [^{3}H]α-methyltyramine, [^{3}H]*m*-tyramine or [^{3}H]α-methyltyramine (Fischer *et al.*, 1965a), labeled compounds were released from isolated perfused cat spleens during nerve stimulation. Only β-hydroxylated metabolites of these amines were released. Catechols without β-hydroxyl groups, dopamine and α-methyldopamine, were also discharged. The β-hydroxyl group or the catechol group was required for retention of phenylethylamine derivatives in the subcellular particles which bind noradrenaline (Musacchio *et al.*, 1965). There appears to be striking correlation of vesicular binding and release by nerve stimulation: Only those amines which are bound are released. After MAO inhibition, octopamine, a false adrenergic transmitter, accumulates in the sympathetic nerves and is released by nerve stimulation. The substitution of this inactive amine for the physiological transmitter may account for the diminished sympathetic responsiveness which develops after chronic MAO inhibition (Kopin *et al.*, 1965).

EXTRANEURAL UPTAKE OF NORADRENALINE

Although most of the noradrenaline in tissues is present within the sympathetic nerves, there is a pool of the catecholamine outside the nerve. In denervated tissues there is a small uptake of noradrenaline extraneurally (Fischer *et al.*, 1965a). Other studies have also indicated that when spleens and denervated nictitating membrane are perfused with noradrenaline there is a binding of the catecholamine to spleen arteriole smooth muscle (Gillespie and Hamilton, 1966) and the nictitating membrane (Draskoczy and Trendelenburg, 1968). To further examine the nature of this extra-neural uptake process, isolated rats hearts were perfused with noradrenaline in the presence of cocaine (Eisenfeld *et al.*, 1967b). It was previously shown that cocaine blocks the uptake of [^{3}H]noradrenaline into sympathetic nerves (Whitby *et al.*, 1960). When uptake into the neurone is blocked by cocaine there was a small extra-neural accumulation of noradrenaline in the heart. In addition, the *O*-methylated metabolite normetanephrine and deaminated metabolites were also present. When adrenergic blocking agents were added to the perfusing media, there was a marked inhibition of noradrenaline uptake extraneurally. The α-blocking agents were more potent than β-blocking agents (Table II). Adrenergic blocking agents also reduced the formation of metabolites of noradrenaline. To further establish whether the inhibition of uptake was extraneural, immunosympathectomized rat hearts (which were completely devoid of sympathetic nerves) were perfused with [^{3}H]noradrenaline in the

TABLE II

EFFECT OF DRUGS ON THE EXTRANEURAL UPTAKE OF NORADRENALINE IN THE RAT HEART

	Accumulation of [^3H]noradrenaline (% of control value)	
	Intraneural	Extraneural
Nylidrin	4	14
Metanephrine	38	27
Synephrine	14	29
Normetanephrine	61	36
Methoxyamine	97	58
Metaraminol	0	100
Phenoxybenzamine ($10^{-6}\,M$)	45	50
Dichlorisoproterenol ($10^{-4}\,M$)	—	40
Pyrogallol	—	500
Pheniprazine	—	100

Rat hearts were perfused with [^3H]noradrenaline in the presence and absence of cocaine and drugs ($10^{-4}\,M$). Cocaine serves to block the intraneural uptake of noradrenaline.

presence of phenoxybenzamine. Again there was a considerable reduction in the uptake of noradrenaline and the formation of its metabolites. Similar results were obtained with the uptake of noradrenaline into smooth muscles of spleen arterioles (Gillespie and Hamilton, 1966). All of these results indicate a transport mechanism for uptake of noradrenaline into extraneural cells. Since adrenergic blocking agents interfere with this transport it is likely that these extraneural cells are effector cells. It is also possible that the extraneural transport mechanism either regulates access of the neurotransmitter to the receptor, or it may be part of the receptor mechanism itself.

The molecular specificity of the uptake of compounds by sympathetic nerves and the effector cells are different (Eisenfeld et al., 1967b). Metaraminol is taken up selectively by the neuronal axon but not by the effector cell, while isoproterenol is taken up by the extraneural cell but not the sympathetic nerve. Both α- and β-adrenergic blocking agents inhibit the extraneural uptake of isoproterenol. A number of sympathomimetic amines were examined for their ability to block extraneural and intraneural uptake of noradrenaline (Table II). A marked reduction in the uptake of noradrenaline extraneurally was found with nylidrin, normetanephrine, metanephrine, synephrine and isoxsuprine. A dissociation in the blocking action of drugs on the intra- and extraneural uptake of noradrenaline was observed. Metaraminol markedly inhibited the neuronal uptake of noradrenaline but had no effect on extraneural uptake. Normetanephrine and methoxyamines, on the other hand, had a greater inhibiting effect on extraneural uptake of noradrenaline. Normetanephrine is a normal metabolite of the neurotransmitter. When it is produced locally it might serve to reduce the entry of excessive amounts of noradrenaline to extraneural intracellular sites where the adrenergic receptors are localized. Thus the metabolite might have some control over the entry of the neurotransmitter to effector cells.

Catechol-*O*-methyltransferase and monoamine oxidase inhibitors were examined for their effects on the metabolism and retention of extraneural noradrenaline. When catechol-*O*-methyltransferase inhibitors (pyrogallol or tropolone) were added to the perfusion medium there were no *O*-methylated products in the heart but the concentration of noradrenaline and deaminated products increased several fold. MAO inhibitors (pargyline, pheniprazine) completely blocked the formation of deaminated products; but in contrast to catechol-*O*-methyltransferase inhibitors, they had no effect on the concentration of noradrenaline. The selective elevation of noradrenaline by catechol-*O*-methyltransferase inhibitors might be the result of the differences in the subcellular localization of the two noradrenaline-metabolizing enzymes, catechol-*O*-methyltransferase being in closer juxtaposition to the extraneural noradrenaline binding site than monoamine oxidase (Fig. 3). It is also possible that *O*-methylation serves as a mechanism for the rapid removal of noradrenaline from the extraneural pool.

REFERENCES

AXELROD, J., (1959); Metabolism of epinephrine and other sympathomimetic amines. *Physiol. Rev.*, **39**, 751–776.

AXELROD, J., WEIL-MALHERBE, H., AND TOMCHICK, R., (1959); The physiological disposition of H^3-epinephrine and its metabolite metanephrine. *J. Pharmacol. exp. Ther.*, **127**, 251–256.

CROUT, J. R., (1961); Effect of inhibiting both catechol-*O*-methyltransferase and monoamine oxidase on cardiovascular responses to norepinephrine. *Proc. Soc. exp. Biol. Med. (N.Y.)*, **108**, 482–484.

DE CHAMPLAIN, J., AXELROD, J., KRAKOFF, L. R., AND MUELLER, R. A., (1968); Microsomal localization of monoamine oxidase in the heart and salivary gland. *Fed. Proc.*, **27**, 399.

DRASKOCZY, P. R., AND TRENDELENBURG, U., (1968); Extraneural uptake of D,L-H^3-norepinephrine in the isolated nictitating membrane of the cat. *Fed. Proc.*, **27**, 467.

EISENFELD, A. J., AXELROD, J., AND KRAKOFF, L. R., (1967a); Inhibition of the extraneural accumulation and metabolism of norepinephrine by adrenergic blocking agents. *J. Pharmacol. exp. Ther.*, **156**, 107–113.

EISENFELD, A. J., LANDSBERG, L., AND AXELROD, J., (1967b); Effect of drugs on the accumulation of extraneuronal norepinephrine in the rat heart. *J. Pharmacol. exp. Ther.*, **158**, 378–385.

EULER, U. S. VON, (1948); Identification of the sympathomimetic ergone in adrenergic nerves of cattle with laevo-noradrenaline. *Acta physiol. scand.*, **16**, 63–74.

EULER, U. S. VON, AND HILLARP, N. A., (1956); Evidence for the presence of noradrenaline in submicroscopic structures of adrenergic axons. *Nature (Lond.)*, **177**, 44–45.

FISCHER, J. E., HORST, W. D., AND KOPIN, I. J., (1965a); β-Hydroxylated sympathomimetic amines as false neurotransmitters. *Brit. J. Pharmacol.*, **24**, 477–484.

FISCHER, J. E., KOPIN, I. J., AND AXELROD, J., (1965b); Evidence for extraneuronal binding of norepinephrine. *J. Pharmacol. exp. Ther.*, **147**, 181–185.

FISCHER, J. E., MUSACCHIO, J., KOPIN, I. J., AND AXELROD, J., (1964); Effects of denervation on the uptake and β-hydroxylation of tyramine in the rat salivary gland. *Life Sci.*, **3**, 413–419.

GILLESPIE, J. S., AND HAMILTON, D. N. H., (1966); Binding of noradrenaline to smooth muscle cells in the spleen, *Nature (Lond.)*, **212**, 524–525.

GORDON, R., REID, J. V. O., SJOERDSMA, A., AND UDENFRIEND, S., (1966); Increased synthesis of norepinephrine in the rat heart on electrical stimulation of the stellate ganglia. *Molec. Pharmacol.*, **2**, 610–613.

HERTTING, G., AND AXELROD, J., (1961); Fate of tritiated noradrenaline at the sympathetic nerve endings. *Nature (Lond.)*, **192**, 172–173.

HERTTING, G., AXELROD, J., KOPIN, I. J., AND WHITBY, L. G., (1961); Lack of uptake of catecholamines after chronic denervation of sympathetic nerves. *Nature (Lond.)*, **189**, 66.

HERTTING, G., AXELROD, J., AND PATRICK, R. W., (1962); Action of bretylium and guanethidine on the uptake and release of H^3-noradrenaline. *Brit. J. Pharmacol.*, **18**, 161–166.

HILLARP, N. A., HOGBERG, B., AND WILSON, B., (1955); Adenosine triphosphate in the adrenal medulla of the cow. *Nature (Lond.)*, **176**, 1032–1033.

IVERSEN, L. L., (1963); The uptake of noradrenaline by the isolated perfused rat heart. *Brit. J. Pharmacol.*, **21**, 523–537.

IVERSEN, L. L., AND KRAVITZ, E. H., (1966); Sodium dependence of transmitter uptake at adrenergic nerve terminals. *Molec. Pharmacol.*, **2**, 360–362.

KOPIN, I. J., (1964); Storage and metabolism of catecholamines: The role of monoamine oxidase. *Pharmacol. Rev.*, **16**, 179–191.

KOPIN, I. J., BREESE, G. R., KRAUSS, K. R., AND WEISE, V. K., (1968); Selective release of newly synthesized norepinephrine from the cat spleen during sympathetic nerve stimulation. *J. Pharmacol. exp. Ther.*, **161**, 271–278.

KOPIN, I. J., FISCHER, J. E., MUSACCHIO, J. M., HORST, W. D., AND WEISE, V. K., (1965); False neurochemical transmitters and the mechanism of sympathetic blockade by monoamine oxidase inhibitors. *J. Pharmacol. exp. Ther.*, **147**, 186–193.

KOPIN, I. J., AND GORDON, E. K., (1962); Metabolism of norepinephrine-H^3 released by tyramine and reserpine. *J. Pharmacol. exp. Ther.*, **138**, 351–359.

KOPIN, I. J., HERTTING, G., AND GORDON, E. K., (1962); Fate of H^3-norepinephrine in the isolated perfused rat heart. *J. Pharmacol. exp. Ther.*, **138**, 34–40.

KOPIN, I. J., AND WEISE, V. K., (1968); Effect of reserpine and metaraminol on excretion of homovanillic acid and 3-methoxy-4-hydroxyphenylglycol in the rat. *Biochem. Pharmacol.*, **17**, 1461–1464.

KRAKOFF, L. R., DE CHAMPLAIN, J., AND AXELROD, J., (1967); Abnormal storage of norepinephrine in experimental hypertension in the rat. *Circulation Res.*, **21**, 583–597.

LANDSBERG, L., AND AXELROD, J., (1968); Influence of pituitary, thyroid and adrenal hormones on norepinephrine turnover and metabolism in the rat heart. *Circulation Res.*, **22**, 559–571.

LEVIN, E. Y., AND KAUFMAN, S., (1961); Studies on the enzyme catalyzing the conversion of 3,4-dihydroxyphenylethylamine to norepinephrine. *J. biol. Chem.*, **236**, 2043–2049.

MUELLER, R. A., THOENEN, H., AND AXELROD, J., (1969); Adrenal tyrosine hydroxylase: compensatory increase in activity after chemical sympathectomy. *Science*, in the press.

MUSACCHIO, J. M., KOPIN, I. J., AND WEISE, V. K., (1965); Subcellular distribution of some sympathomimetic amines and their β-hydroxylated derivatives in the rat heart. *J. Pharmacol. exp. Ther.*, **148**, 22–28.

NAGATSU, T., LEVITT, H., AND UDENFRIEND, S., (1964); The initial step in norepinephrine biosynthesis. *J. biol. Chem.*, **239**, 2910–2917.

POTTER, L. T., AND AXELROD, J., (1963a); Studies on the storage of norepinephrine and the effect of drugs. *J. Pharmacol. exp. Ther.*, **140**, 199–206.

POTTER, L. T., AND AXELROD, J., (1963b); Properties of a norepinephrine storage particle of the rat heart. *J. Pharmacol. exp. Ther.*, **142**, 299–305.

POTTER, L. T., COOPER, T., WILLMAN, V. L., AND WOLFE, D. E., (1965); Synthesis, binding, release and metabolism of norepinephrine in normal and transplanted dog hearts. *Circulation Res.*, **16**, 468–481.

ROSELL, S., KOPIN, I. J., AND AXELROD, J., (1963); Fate of H^3-noradrenaline in skeletal muscle before and following sympathetic stimulation. *Amer. J. Physiol.*, **205**, 317–321.

SEDVALL, G. C., AND KOPIN, I. J., (1967a); Influence of sympathetic denervation and nerve impulse activity of tyrosine hydroxylase in the rat submaxillary gland. *Biochem. Pharmacol.*, **16**, 39–46.

SEDVALL, G. C., AND KOPIN, I. J., (1967b); Acceleration of norepinephrine synthesis in the rat submaxillary gland *in vivo* during sympathetic nerve stimulation. *Life Sci.*, **6**, 45–51.

SNYDER, S. H., FISCHER, J. E., AND AXELROD, J., (1965); Evidence for the presence of monoamine oxidase in sympathetic nerve endings. *Biochem. Pharmacol.*, **14**, 363–365.

WALTMAN, S., AND SEARS, M., (1964); Catechol-*O*-methyltransferase and monoamine oxidase activity in ocular tissue of albino rabbits. *Invest. Ophthal.*, **3**, 601–605.

WEISE, V. K., SEDVALL, G. C., AND KOPIN, I. J., (1967); False transmitter accumulation *versus* catecholamine synthesis and storage in rat brain and heart. *Fed. Proc.*, **26**, 463.

WHITBY, L. G., AXELROD, J., AND WEIL-MALHERBE, H., (1961); The fate of H^3-norepinephrine in animals. *J. Pharmacol. exp. Ther.*, **132**, 193–201.

WHITBY, L. G., HERTTING, G., AND AXELROD, J., (1960); Effect of cocaine on the disposition of noradrenaline labelled with tritium. *Nature (Lond.)*, **187**, 604–605.

WOLFE, D. E., POTTER, L. T., RICHARDSON, K. C., AND AXELROD, J., (1962); Localizing tritiated norepinephrine in sympathetic axons by electron microscopic autoradiography. *Science*, **138**, 440–442.

Recent Developments on the Ultrastructural Aspect of Adrenergic Nerve Endings in Various Experimental Conditions

J. P. TRANZER, H. THOENEN, R. L. SNIPES AND J. G. RICHARDS

Department of Experimental Medicine, F. Hoffmann-La Roche & Co. Ltd., Basle (Switzerland)

INTRODUCTION

Electron-microscopic radioautography in correlation with pharmacological experiments has brought forth strong evidence that the electron dense core in the vesicles of the terminal part of postganglionic adrenergic nerves represents the chemical neuro-transmitter noradrenaline (NA) (Wolfe *et al.*, 1962; Bloom and Barrnett, 1966). The possibility of a direct, visual localization of this neuro-transmitter with a high degree of resolution opened a new field of investigation in the physiology and pharmacology of the adrenergic nervous system.

In this paper we will briefly review some of our recent work which deals mainly with the precise and direct ultrastructural localization of neuro-transmitter substances in the vesiculated part of postganglionic adrenergic nerves in various organs of the cat and rat. Only preliminary results on the central nervous system will be reported. Particular attention was paid neither to the exact relationship and proximity of the nerve endings to the smooth muscle cells, nor to the precise identification of the vesiculated nerve endings as terminal, preterminal or en passage*. In these respects the pertinent work of Taxi (1964), Thaemert (1966) and Merrillees (1968) should be consulted.

(1) PROBLEMS CONCERNING THE PRECISE LOCALIZATION OF THE CHEMICAL NEURO-TRANSMITTER IN THE VESICLES OF THE ADRENERGIC NERVES BY ELECTRON MICROSCOPY

Adrenergic, vesiculated nerve endings, as seen with the electron microscope, contain both small dense-core vesicles and small empty-looking vesicles measuring about 500 Å units in diameter. This dual population of vesicles is usually observed when the tissues have been prepared for electron microscopy by conventional methods, *i.e.*, a single fixation with osmium tetroxide (Fig. 1a). The dense core of the vesicles most

---

* The term vesiculated nerve endings serves, therefore, to include observations made on all three types throughout this paper.

References p. 45–46

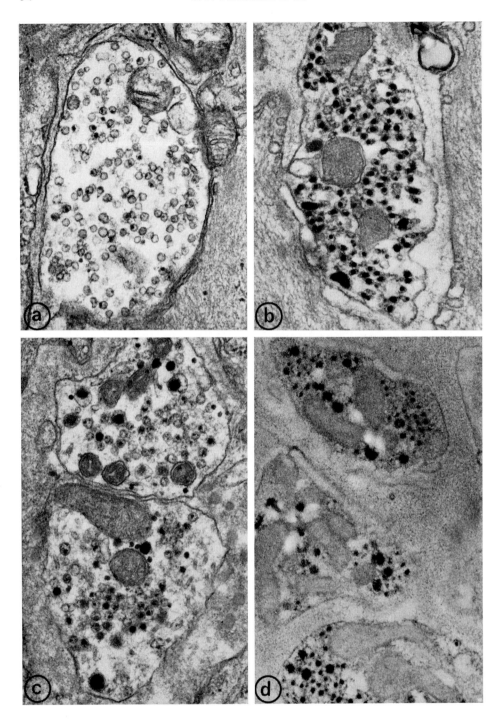

probably represents the physiological transmitter noradrenaline (NA). This is based on the fact that all the small vesicles appear empty after pre-treatment of the animals with drugs producing a depletion of NA, such as reserpine or α-methylmetatyrosine (α-MMT). On the other hand, however, cholinergic nerve endings contain a homogenous population of small empty vesicles which are probably the storage site of acetylcholine (ACh) (De Robertis and Bennett, 1955; Whittaker et al., 1964).

Burn and Rand postulated that the empty vesicles in adrenergic nerve endings might contain ACh and thus represent the morphological correlate of a cholinergic link in postganglionic sympathetic transmission (Burn and Rand, 1959; Burn, 1963).

We attempted to verify the validity of this interpretation by experiments which can be summarized as follows:

(a) The proportion of dense core to empty vesicles in the adrenergic nerve endings within a single animal varied both from tissue to tissue and within the same tissue sample, and was strongly dependent upon the method of fixation (Tranzer and Thoenen, 1967a; Tranzer and Snipes, 1968). Thus, osmium tetroxide fixation yielded fewer dense-core vesicles than did a double fixation in glutaraldehyde and osmium tetroxide.

(b) After pre-incubation of tissue slices in solutions containing high concentrations of NA, a much greater proportion of the vesicles in the adrenergic nerve endings contained a dense core, whereas the vesicles of cholinergic nerves remained empty. To verify that the nerves with exclusively empty vesicles were cholinergic and those with dense-core vesicles adrenergic, the corresponding organs were alternatively subjected to a sympathetic or parasympathetic denervation (Thoenen et al., 1966; Tranzer and Thoenen, 1967a).

From these results we conclude that all the vesicles of the adrenergic nerve endings have the potential to take up and store the neuro-transmitter NA. Our results thus speak strongly against the interpretation of Burn and Rand that empty vesicles in adrenergic nerves can be considered as a morphological correlate of the postulated cholinergic link in postganglionic sympathetic transmission.

Nevertheless the problem of the presence of empty vesicles in normal adrenergic nerve endings remains. Our results, as well as those of others, strongly suggest that the empty vesicles in these nerves are the result of a poor preservation of the NA during fixation (Richardson, 1966; Tranzer and Thoenen, 1967a). For this reason, and in the hope of achieving a better preservation of NA, which in turn would allow new and more precise studies in this field, we re-investigated the fine structural aspect of such nerve endings under various conditions of fixation using the vas deferens of the rat as a test tissue.

Fig. 1. Influence of various fixation techniques on the ultrastructural appearance of the dense core in adrenergic vesiculated nerve endings. (a) and (b) from rat vas deferens; (c) and (d) from cat iris: (a) Osmium tetroxide fixation alone; (b) triple fixation sequence in glutaraldehyde–p-formaldehyde, dichromate and osmium tetroxide. Note the difference in the aspect of the dense cores of the vesicles. (c) Double fixation in glutaraldehyde and osmium tetroxide; (d) fixation in glutaraldehyde followed by a dichromate treatment without osmium tetroxide post-fixation. The dichromate treatment in (d) is a specific cytochemical test for biogenic amines and indicates that the large as well as the small dense-core vesicles store biogenic amines. ($\times$ 40 500)

We found that with a triple fixation sequence of glutaraldehyde–*p*-formaldehyde, dichromate and osmium tetroxide employed in well-defined conditions, virtually all the vesicles of the adrenergic nerve endings in the rat vas deferens contained an electron dense core, in other words the physiological neuro-transmitter NA (Tranzer and Snipes, 1968) (Fig. 1b). It thus became evident that the technique of processing the tissues for electron microscopy, especially the fixation, is of prime importance for the interpretation of the physiological significance of ultrastructural findings.

At least three main reasons may account for the difficulty of retaining the adrenergic neuro-transmitter(s) in their proper location:

(*1*) The neuro-transmitters are small and highly water-soluble molecules.

(*2*) The neuro-transmitters exist in their storage organelles and perhaps at other sites in a labile state, such that they are readily liberated by depolarization of the nerve-cell membrane which occurs physiologically upon arrival of an electrical impulse at the nerve endings. A similar depolarization may occur during manipulation and processing of the tissues for electron microscopy especially during fixation.

(*3*) Little is known about the physico-chemical state of the neuro-transmitter in the vesicles. The retention of the amine may be primarily dependent upon a stable configuration of the vesicular and/or nerve membrane. During fixation the membrane permeability may be altered and the amine may escape before some capturing agent can retain it in its proper location.

(2) AMINE CONTENT OF THE LARGE DENSE-CORE VESICLES

In addition to the small vesicles of 400–600 Å units in diameter, there exist in the vesiculated endings of the autonomic nerves larger vesicles which always contain a dense core (Fig. 1c). They measure 700–1200 Å units (mean 900-Å units) in diameter. According to the Grillo and Palay (1962) classification of vesicles they belong to type I. Because of the presence of the dense core the following questions arise: (*a*) do they store amines like the small vesicles; (*b*) do they contain other osmiophilic, electron-dense substances not related to amines, or (*c*) do they content both?

It must be emphasized that these large dense-core (LDC) vesicles exist not only in adrenergic but also in cholinergic nerves.

After treatment with reserpine or α-MMT all the small vesicles appear empty, whereas the osmiophilic content of the LDC vesicles persists. Since after these treat-ments the NA content of the tissues approached zero, various authors concluded that the LDC vesicles most probably do not store NA (Van Orden *et al.*, 1966; Bondareff and Gordon, 1966; Hökfelt, 1966). From these experiments it is evident that the LDC vesicles contain an electron-dense material of unknown nature which is not related to NA. There still remains the question whether or not the LDC vesicles contain NA in addition. For this reason we re-investigated this problem using the cytochemical technique of Wood and Barrnett (1964) which has been shown to be specific for biogenic amines in the adrenal medulla. The method consists of a modified chromaffin reaction, performed in well defined conditions and adapted to electron microscopy. Our own results confirm the high specificity of this cytochemical reaction with one exception, the melanine pigment granules. However, the amine-storage organelles can be influenced by various pharmacological manipulations, while the melanine granules remain unaffected.

Using this cytochemical technique, investigations on iris and vas deferens of cats (Tranzer and Thoenen, 1968b) led to the following conclusions: the LDC vesicles of the adrenergic nerve endings contain biogenic amines, most probably NA, whereas the LDC vesicles of the cholinergic nerves do not contain these amines. After aldehyde fixation followed by the dichromate treatment without osmium tetroxide post-fixation, electron-dense centers of at least two different sizes appear in adrenergic nerve endings (Fig. 1d). Vesicles could only be recognized by their dense cores since the membranes were poorly stained by this technique. These dense centers could easily be equated by their size and number to the dense cores of the small and the LDC vesicles of adrenergic nerves seen in thin sections from material prepared by the usual methods for electron microscopy. With this specific cytochemical technique no such centers were observed in the cholinergic nerves.

After pre-treatment of the animals with reserpine or with α-MMT no dense centers of any type could be detected in either adrenergic or cholinergic nerves by the use of the dichromate technique. An additional, but more indirect evidence that the LDC vesicles of adrenergic but not cholinergic nerves are capable of storing amines, has been obtained by administration of a synthetic "false" transmitter, 5-hydroxy-dopamine (refer to section 3).

In summary, the results of these investigations strongly indicate that in adrenergic vesiculated nerve endings biogenic amines are not only stored in the small but also in the LDC vesicles. It remains to be elucidated whether the amine in the latter vesicles is NA or another related amine. In addition nothing is as yet known concerning the function of these LDC vesicles.

(3) ELECTRON-MICROSCOPIC LOCALIZATION OF "FALSE" TRANSMITTERS IN ADRENERGIC NERVES

The direct and precise localization of "false" adrenergic transmitters with the electron microscope requires as a pre-requisite that they are rendered insoluble and electron-dense during the processing of the tissues for electron microscopy.

We attempted to localize with the electron microscope 5-hydroxydopamine, a synthetic phenethylamine and 5-hydroxytryptamine, an indolamine, in storage sites of adrenergic nerves. Both of these compounds become insoluble and electron-dense by routine fixation in glutaraldehyde and osmium tetroxide for electron microscopy.

(a) 5-Hydroxydopamine (5-HO-DA)*

In a previous study it has been shown that pre-treatment of cats with 5-hydroxy-dopa leads to a marked depletion of NA in various sympathetically innervated organs of the cat. The NA depletion is accompanied by an accumulation of 5-HO-DA and

---

* 3, 4, 5-Trihydroxyphenylethylamine.

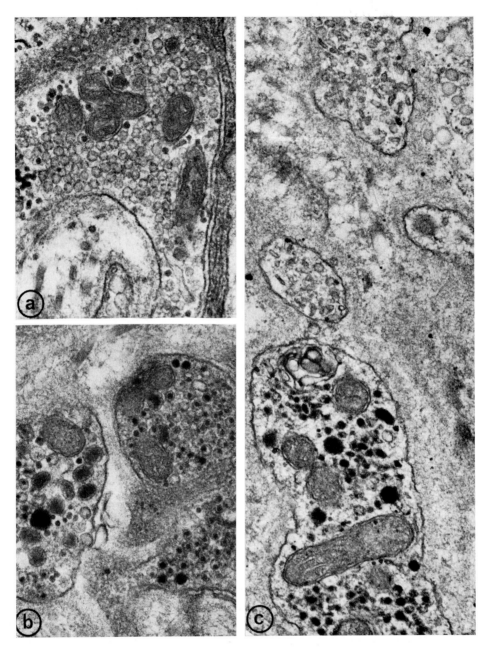

Fig. 2. Localization of "false" adrenergic transmitters. Iris of cat pre-treated with α-MMT. (a) Control, incubated in Krebs–Henseleit solution alone, shows that the small vesicles of the nerve processes appear empty. After incubation in a similar solution but containing either 5-HT (b) or 5-HO-DA (c) the vesicles of the adrenergic nerve endings contained numerous granulated vesicles. Note also in (c) the cholinergic nerve endings which contain only empty looking vesicles. ($\times$ 49 500)

its β-hydroxylated and/or O-methylated metabolites which are liberated as "false" transmitters by sympathetic nerve stimulation (Thoenen et al., 1967). Thus it seemed of interest to observe whether the replacement of NA by 5-HO-DA and its possible metabolites, was accompanied by fine structural changes. After injection of cats with 5-HO-DA the NA content of various organs including iris, vas deferens and spleen dropped to less than 10% of controls. The electron-microscopic examination of these tissues revealed that the adrenergic nerve endings contained numerous dense-core vesicles (Tranzer and Thoenen, 1967b) (Fig. 2c). Virtually all the vesicles of the adrenergic nerves contained a dense core which filled the vesicles almost completely. The LDC as well as the small dense-core vesicles contained the electron-dense material. Occasionally small cytoplasmic structures, most probably belonging to the endoplasmic reticulum, also contained dense material. In contrast, the cholinergic nerves remained unchanged, i.e., they still contained only empty small vesicles and LDC vesicles of medium density. All other cellular or subcellular structures examined did not show any changes. Pre-treatment of animals with reserpine preceding the administration of 5-HO-DA prevented the accumulation of the dense material in the vesicles of adrenergic nerves.

From these results we concluded that the dense core in the vesicles of the adrenergic nerves represents 5-HO-DA and its eventual metabolites.

Also, it has recently been shown that 5-HO-DA is strongly taken up and concentrated in vesicles of the perivascular endings of the autonomic nerves in the rat pineal gland (Richards and Tranzer, 1969). Bondareff (1966) has shown that another "false" transmitter, α-methylnoradrenaline, can be localized by electron microscopy in these nerves.

In addition to these observations pertaining directly to the localization of the "false" transmitter, other features of interest were noticed from these experiments regarding the general problems of demonstrating amines at the ultrastructural level. Thus in the studies with 5-HO-DA the fact that all the vesicles of the adrenergic nerves were filled with an electron-dense core, brought additional evidence to the major points discussed earlier in this paper, i.e., that all the vesicles of the adrenergic nerves, the small as well as the LDC vesicles are able to take up and to store amines. In spite of its non-physiological nature this amine seems to be a most interesting marker for aminergic nerves and their amine storage sites.

In contrast to the foregoing results concerning the vesiculated nerve endings we were unable to detect with the electron microscope both physiological and "false" transmitters in the perikaryon of adrenergic neurons even after incubation of sympathetic ganglia slices in solutions containing high amounts of these amines (unpublished results). This seems to indicate that the amines detected in these perikaryons by means of the fluorescent technique (Hamberger et al., 1963) may be present in a state which we are presently unable to demonstrate by electron microscopy, for example, diffusely distributed rather than concentrated in vesicles. This assumption is further supported by studies concerning the subcellular distribution of NA in sympathetic ganglia which revealed that in contrast to the nerve endings, the main part of the NA was localized in the soluble and not in the microsomal fraction (Fischer and Snyder, 1965).

References p. 45–46

(b) 5-Hydroxytryptamine (5-HT)

There exist both radioautographic and biochemical evidence that 5-HT can be accumulated and stored in adrenergic nerves and that this indolamine can also act as a "false" transmitter (Taxi and Droz, 1966; Thoa *et al.*, 1967; Eccleston *et al.*, 1968). The recent successful fine structural localization of 5-HT in specific organelles of blood platelets (Tranzer *et al.*, 1966, 1968) encouraged us to attempt a direct and precise localization of this "false" transmitter at the ultrastructural level in adrenergic nerves (Snipes *et al.*, 1968).

Iris and vas deferens of cats pre-treated with α-MMT were incubated in solutions containing 5-HT. The NA content of these tissues was less than 10% of that of non-treated animals. The examination of thin sections with the electron microscope revealed numerous dense-core vesicles exclusively in the adrenergic, vesiculated nerve endings (Fig. 2b). Control samples of the same animals incubated in the same solutions in the absence of 5-HT revealed only empty vesicles (Fig. 2a). Thus, the observed electron-dense core in the vesicles of adrenergic nerves from those tissues incubated in 5-HT represents the accumulated 5-HT. Consequently the "false" adrenergic transmitters are not restricted to the group of phenethylamines, but can be found also in the group of indolamines.

In conclusion, "false" transmitters can be localized precisely with the electron microscope in the vesicles of the adrenergic nerves providing they can be fixed and made electron opaque in a proper way. Besides their pharmacological interest, some "false" transmitters appear to be excellent tracers for adrenergic nerve fibres and for the ultrastructural amine-storage sites.

(4) ACTION OF 6-HYDROXYDOPAMINE* (6-HO-DA) ON AUTONOMIC NERVES

6-Hydroxydopamine, another synthetic isomer of NA, has been reported to provoke an efficient and long lasting NA-depletion in various sympathetically innervated organs of different species (Porter *et al.*, 1963, 1965; Laverty *et al.*, 1965). Two different hypotheses have previously been proposed in an attempt to explain the effects of this drug. (*a*) Stoichiometric replacement of NA by 6-HO-DA and/or its metabolites (Porter *et al.*, 1965). (*b*) Irreversible damage of the NA-storage sites (Porter *et al.*, 1963; Laverty *et al.*, 1965).

We investigated the action of this drug on adrenergic nerves of various organs of cats and rats (Tranzer and Thoenen, 1968a; Thoenen and Tranzer, 1968) by electron microscopy, in the hope that such a study would help to elucidate the action of 6-HO-DA.

Three days after injection of 6-HO-DA, which reduced the NA content in all organs studied to less than 10%, the electron-microscopic investigations revealed a degeneration of virtually all the adrenergic nerve endings in various tissues including iris, vas deferens, spleen capsule and right heart auricle. They appeared in various stages of degeneration ranging from a slight injury to complete lysis of the nerve

---

* 2, 4, 5-Trihydroxyphenylethylamine.

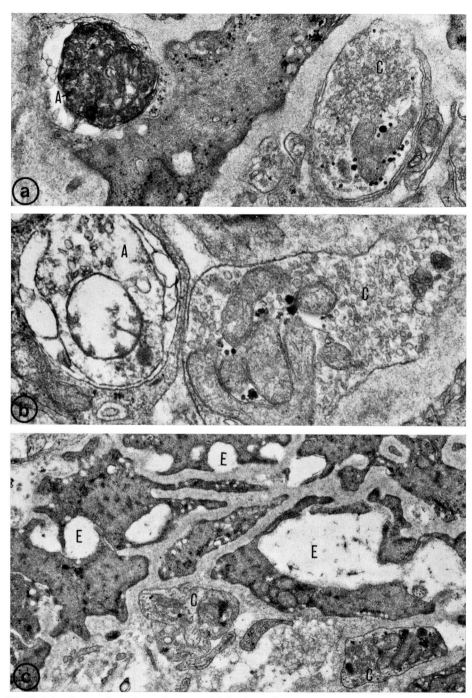

Fig. 3. Iris of a cat three days after several injections of 6-HO-DA. Note that in (a) and (b) the vesiculated adrenergic nerve endings (A) are in various stages of degeneration. In (c) no such nerve endings are visible; rather there exist many empty spaces (E), often in close contact with smooth muscle cells, which may represent completely lysed adrenergic nerve profiles. The cholinergic nerve endings (C) appear normal. (a) × 31 500; (b) × 40 500; (c) × 16 200.

(Fig. 3). Some of the nerves contained still-recognizable, characteristic, ultrastructural components. Others which were more altered could only be recognized by their topographical localization between smooth muscle cells and by the surrounding Schwann cells. In many instances the Schwann cell appeared to engulf the injured nerve. The plasma membrane of the nerve was hardly discernible from that of the Schwann cell, so that it appeared as if the Schwann cell was in the process of digesting the injured nerve ending. These results correlate with observations made after surgical sympathectomy (Van Orden *et al.*, 1967).

In organs such as iris and vas deferens where adrenergic and cholinergic nerves are often in close proximity, it became evident that only the adrenergic nerves were injured whereas the cholinergic nerves appeared completely normal. In addition no other cellular or subcellular elements appeared to be altered.

In consequence, it seems that, under these experimental conditions, 6-HO-DA produces a selective degeneration of the terminal parts of the adrenergic nerve axons.

A study of the perikaryons of the injured nerve axons in the corresponding ganglions did not reveal any fine morphological changes. However, since a non-detectable ultramorphological change does not necessarily imply a lack of injury we preferred to extend our observations in order to obtain additional evidence on the integrity of the perikaryon by the study of the regeneration capacity of the axons. Tissues were examined 3–4 months after treatment of the animals with 6-HO-DA and it was found that numerous nerve endings with granulated vesicles were again present in the iris, vas deferens and spleen capsule. The NA content determined in these organs had risen and approached again the values obtained from control animals.

The mechanism by which 6-HO-DA leads to a selective destruction of adrenergic nerve endings is not yet completely understood. It has been discussed in detail previously (Thoenen and Tranzer, 1968).

In conclusion, 6-HO-DA acts in a completely different way from that of all other known related amines. Despite the fact that there exist considerable organ and species differences, the specific, but reversible degeneration of the terminal part of the adrenergic neuron of sympathetic nerves provides a new and interesting tool for chemical sympathectomy.

(5) FINE STRUCTURAL LOCALIZATION OF BIOGENIC AMINES IN THE CENTRAL NERVOUS SYSTEM

Although the fluorescent technique of Falk has proven useful for the localization of biogenic amines in neurons of specialized areas of the brain at the light-microscope level, little is known about the ultrastructural localization of these amines. Techniques combining radioautography with electron microscopy were up to now the most fruitful in this respect. Unfortunately because of a lack of resolution (limited to 1000–3000 Å units) inherent to this technique the amines could not be clearly related to single vesicles in the nerves or to any other ultrastructural components. A recent pertinent review on this topic has been published by Bloom and Giarman (1968). Radioautographic studies revealed that after injection of labelled amines or of their

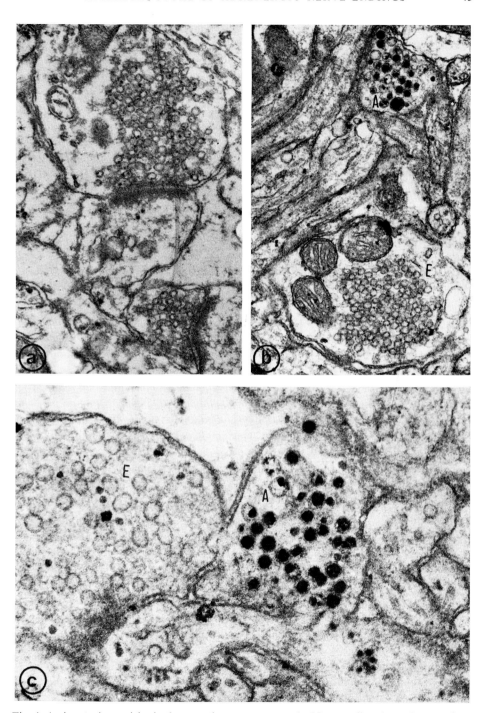

Fig. 4. Amine-storing vesicles in the central nervous system. (a) Nerve endings in nucleus caudatus of a rabbit. The tiny dense cores in the vesicles of the pre-synaptic nerve endings are not related to biogenic amines. ($\times$ 40 500), (b) and (c) Vesiculated nerve endings in hypothalamus of a rat after intraventricular injection of 5-HO-DA. Some nerves contain empty-looking synaptic vesicles only (E) whereas others contain dense-core synaptic vesicles (A). The dense core in these vesicles represents 5-HO-DA. (b) $\times$ 40 500; (c) $\times$ 83 700.

precursors, the silver grains were overlying neurons containing large dense-core vesicles measuring 800–1200 Å units in diameter. However, it is now established that these vesicles contain osmiophilic material other than that representative of biogenic amines. A recent critical report failed to find a change in electron opacity in these large dense-core vesicles after various pharmacological manipulations (Bloom and Aghajanian, 1968). Nevertheless, with a specific cytochemical method, Wood (1966) has shown that, in the hypothalamus of the hamster, some of these large dense-core vesicles may contain biogenic amines.

Whereas fine structural studies of the peripheral autonomic nervous system have identified dense-core vesicles, 400–600 Å units in diameter, as the main storage organelles of NA, efforts to visualize the same type of small granular vesicles as the amine-storage site in the central nervous system have failed in most laboratories. Recently Hökfelt (1967a,b,c) reported the presence of small dense-core vesicles in the brain of rats with the use of potassium permanganate as fixative. Small granular vesicles were observed in some nerve terminals in areas which are known from biochemical and from fluorescent light-microscopical investigations to contain appreciable amounts of amines. Unfortunately this fixation technique yields a very poor general preservation of most ultrastructures and is thus of limited value (Pease, 1964).

We also found that the small synaptic vesicles of numerous nerve terminals in areas of the brain rich in amines often contain a tiny dense core even after conventional fixation of the brain by glutaraldehyde and osmium tetroxide (Fig. 4a). We were, however, unable to influence these granules by various pharmacological treatments nor to demonstrate by specific cytochemical techniques that the dense core was related to biogenic amines. In consequence it was concluded that these dense cores do not represent biogenic amines but rather another compound of unknown nature. Indeed the mere presence of a dense core in vesicles of a nerve ending is not sufficient evidence for its biogenic amine nature. Only by means of additional cytochemical and/or pharmacological manipulations can such conclusions be drawn with certitude.

Since 5-HO-DA has proven to be a useful and a specific marker for the vesicles of adrenergic nerves in the periphery, experiments to locate aminergic nerves in the central nervous system (CNS) were undertaken. At this time only preliminary results from the rat brain are available. After intraventricular injection of 5-HO-DA or after incubation of brain slices in 5-HO-DA containing solutions the tissues were fixed in glutaraldehyde and osmium tetroxide and processed routinely for electron microscopy. The results, illustrated in Figs. 4b and 4c, show that some neurons of the hypothalamus and nucleus caudatus take up and store 5-HO-DA into their small, synaptic vesicles. Most of the synaptic vesicles of these nerve terminals contained a dense core which filled the vesicle almost to capacity whereas the remaining and majority of neurons contained only empty synaptic vesicles. In brain tissue of re-serpine-treated animals also incubated in 5-HO-DA containing solutions, no such dense cores could be found in any synaptic vesicles. At the present time little is known about the specificity of the tracer. Further investigations are necessary to decide if all nerves storing catecholamines and/or indolamines are traced by 5-HO-DA.

Nevertheless, these preliminary observations clearly show that the small vesicles of some nerves of the CNS are able to take up and to store amines in a way similar to that in the adrenergic nerves of the periphery. Hence, the question arises why difficulty exists in demonstrating the endogenous amines in the vesicles of the nerves of the CNS by electron microscopy. As pointed out earlier one main reason most probably is of a technical nature, *i.e.*, the correct fixation of the amines.

REFERENCES

BLOOM, F. E., AND AGHAJANIAN, G. K., (1968); An electron microscopic analysis of large granular synaptic vesicles of the brain in relation to monoamine content. *J. Pharmacol. exp. Therap.*, **159**, 261–273.

BLOOM, F. E., AND BARRNETT, R. J., (1966); Fine structural localization of noradrenaline in vesicles of autonomic nerve endings. *Nature (Lond.)*, **210**, 599–601.

BLOOM, F. E., AND GIARMAN, N. J., (1968); Physiologic and pharmacologic considerations of biogenic amines in the nervous system. *Ann. Rev. Pharmacol.*, **8**, 229–258.

BONDAREFF, W., (1966); Localization of α-methylnorepinephrine in sympathetic nerve fibers of the pineal body. *Exp. Neurol.*, **16**, 131–135.

BONDAREFF, W., AND GORDON, B., (1966); Submicroscopic localization of norepinephrine in sympathetic nerves of rat pineal. *J. Pharmacol. exp. Therap.*, **153**, 42–47.

BURN, J. H., (1963); The release of norepinephrine from the sympathetic postganglionic fibre. *Bull. Johns Hopkins Hosp.*, **112**, 167–182.

BURN, J. H., AND RAND, M. J., (1959); Sympathetic postganglionic mechanism. *Nature (Lond.)*, **184**, 163–165.

DE ROBERTIS, E., AND BENNETT, H. S., (1955); Some features of the submicroscopic morphology of synapses in frog and earthworm. *J. biophys. biochem. Cytol.*, **1**, 47–58.

ECCLESTON, D., THOA, N. B., AND AXELROD, J., (1968); Inhibition by drugs of the accumulation *in vitro* of 5-hydroxytryptamine in guinea-pig vas deferens. *Nature (Lond.)*, **217**, 846–847.

FISCHER J. E., AND SNYDER, S., (1965); Disposition of norepinephrine-H^3 in sympathetic ganglia. *J. Pharmacol. exp. Therap.*, **150**, 190–195.

GRILLO, M. A., AND PALAY, S. L., (1962); in BREESE, S. S. (Ed.), *Granule-Containing Vesicles in the Autonomic Nervous System*. Vth Intern. Congr. Electron Microscopy, Philadelphia, Vol. 2, p. U-1, Academic Press, New York.

HAMBERGER, B., NORBERG, K.-A., AND SJÖQVIST, F., (1963); Cellular localization of monoamines in sympathetic ganglia of the cat. A preliminary report. *Life Sci.*, **9**, 659–661.

HÖKFELT, T., (1966); The effect of reserpine on the intraneuronal vesicles of the rat vas deferens. *Experientia (Basel)*, **22**, 56.

HÖKFELT, T., (1967a); Electron microscopic studies on brain slices from regions rich in catecholamine nerve terminals. *Acta physiol. scand.*, **69**, 119–120.

HÖKFELT, T., (1967b); On the ultrastructural localization of noradrenaline in the central nervous system of the rat. *Z. Zellforsch.*, **79**, 110–117.

HÖKFELT, T., (1967c); The possible ultrastructural identification of tubero-infundibular dopamine-containing nerve endings in the median eminence of the rat. *Brain Res.*, **5**, 121–123.

LAVERTY, R., SHARMAN, D. F., AND VOGT, M., (1965); Action of 2,4,5-trihydroxyphenylethylamine on the storage and release of noradrenaline. *Brit. J. Pharmacol.*, **24**, 549–560.

MERRILLEES, N. C. R., (1968); The nervous environment of individual smooth muscle cells of the guinea pig vas deferens. *J. Cell Biol.*, **37**, 794–817.

PEASE, D. C., (1964); *Histological Techniques for Electron Microscopy*. Academic Press, New York, pp. 63–67.

PORTER, C. C., TOTARO, J. A., AND BURCIN, A., (1965); The relationship between radioactivity and norepinephrine concentrations in the brains and hearts of mice following administration of labelled methyldopa or 6-hydroxydopamine. *J. Pharmacol. exp. Therap.*, **150**, 17–22.

PORTER, C. C., TOTARO, J. A., AND STONE, C. A., (1963); Effect of 6-hydroxydopamine and some other compounds on the concentration of NE in the hearts of mice. *J. Pharmacol. exp. Therap.*, **140**, 308–316.

RICHARDS, J. G., AND TRANZER, J. P., (1969); Electron microscopic localization of 5-hydroxydopamine, a "false" adrenergic neurotransmitter, in the autonomic nerve endings of the rat pineal gland. *Experientia (Basel)*, **25**, 53–54.

RICHARDSON, K. C., (1966); Electron microscopic identification of autonomic nerve endings. *Nature (Lond.)*, **210**, 756.

SNIPES, R. L., THOENEN, H., AND TRANZER, J. P., (1968); Fine structural localization of exogenous 5-HT in vesicles of adrenergic nerve terminals. *Experientia (Basel)*, **24**, 1026–1027.

TAXI, J., (1964); Étude, au microscope électronique, de l'innervation du muscle lisse intestinal, comparée à celle de quelques autres muscles lisses de mammifères. *Arch. Biol. (Liège)*, **75**, 301–328.

TAXI, J., AND DROZ, B., (1966); Étude de l'incorporation de noradrénaline-^{3}H (NA-^{3}H) et de 5-hydroxytryptophane-^{3}H (5-HTP-^{3}H) dans les fibres nerveuses du canal déférent et de l'intestin. *C. R. Acad. Sci. (Paris)*, **263**, 1237–1240.

THAEMERT, J. C., (1966); Ultrastructural interrelationships of nerve processes and smooth muscle cells in three dimensions. *J. Cell Biol.*, **28**, 37–49.

THOA, N. B., AXELROD, J., AND ECCLESTON, D., (1967); Uptake and release of C^{14}-serotonin in the nor-adrenergic neurones of the guinea pig vas deferens. *Pharmacologist*, **9**, 251.

THOENEN, H., HAEFELY, W., GEY, K. F., AND HÜRLIMANN, H., (1967); Diminished effect of sympathetic nerve stimulation in cats pretreated with 5-hydroxydopa; formation and liberation of false adrenergic transmitters. *Arch. exp. Path. Pharmak.*, **259**, 17–33.

THOENEN, H., AND TRANZER, J. P., (1968); Chemical sympathectomy by selective destruction of adrenergic nerve endings with 6-hydroxydopamine. *Arch. exp. Path. Pharmak.*, **261**, 271–288.

THOENEN, H., TRANZER, J. P., HÜRLIMANN, A., AND HAEFELY, W., (1966); Untersuchungen zur Frage eines cholinergischen Gliedes in der postganglionären sympathischen Transmission. *Helv. physiol. pharmacol. Acta*, **24**, 229–246.

TRANZER, J. P., DA PRADA, M., AND PLETSCHER, A., (1966); Ultrastructural localization of 5-hydroxytryptamine in blood platelets. *Nature (Lond.)*, **212**, 1574–1575.

TRANZER, J. P., DA PRADA, M., AND PLETSCHER, A., (1968); Electron microscopic study of the storage site of 5-hydroxytryptamine in blood platelets. *Advanc. Pharmacol.*, **6A**, 125–128.

TRANZER, J. P., AND SNIPES, R. L., (1968); Fine structural localization of noradrenaline in sympathetic nerve terminals: A critical study on the influence of fixation. *Proceedings of the 4th European Regional Conference on Electron Microscopy, Rome*, **2**, 519–520.

TRANZER, J. P., AND THOENEN, H., (1967a); Significance of "empty vesicles" in postganglionic sympathetic nerve terminals. *Experientia (Basel)*, **23**, 123–124.

TRANZER, J. P., AND THOENEN, H., (1967b); Electronmicroscopic localization of 5-hydroxydopamine (3,4,5-trihydroxy-phenyl-ethylamine), a new "false" sympathetic transmitter. *Experientia (Basel)*, **23**, 743–745.

TRANZER, J. P., AND THOENEN, H., (1968a); An electron microscopic study of selective, acute degeneration of sympathetic nerve terminals after administration of 6-hydroxydopamine. *Experientia (Basel)*, **24**, 155–156.

TRANZER, J. P., AND THOENEN, H., (1968b); Various types of amine-storing vesicles in peripheral adrenergic nerve terminals. *Experientia (Basel)*, **24**, 484–486.

VAN ORDEN, L. S., BENSCH, K. G., LANGER, S. Z., AND TRENDELENBURG, U., (1967); Histochemical and fine structural aspects of the onset of denervation supersensitivity in the nictitating membrane of the spinal cat. *J. Pharmacol. exp. Therap.*, **157**, 274–283.

VAN ORDEN, L. S., BLOOM, F. E., BARRNETT, R. J., AND GIARMAN, N. J., (1966); Histochemical and functional relationships of catecholamines in adrenergic nerve endings. I. Participation of granular vesicles. *J. Pharmacol. exp. Therap.*, **154**, 185–199.

WHITTAKER, V. P., MICHAELSON, I. A., AND KIRKLAND, R. J. A., (1964); The separation of synaptic vesicles from nerve-ending particles ("synaptosomes"). *Biochem. J.*, **90**, 293–303.

WOLFE, D. E., POTTER, L. T., RICHARDSON, K. C., AND AXELROD, J., (1962); Localizing tritiated norepinephrine in sympathetic axons by electron microscopic autoradiography. *Science*, **138**, 440–442.

WOOD, J. G., (1966); Electron microscopic localization of amines in central nervous tissue. *Nature (Lond.)*, **209**, 1131–1133.

WOOD, J. G., AND BARRNETT, R. J., (1964); Histochemical demonstration of norepinephrine at a fine structural level. *J. Histochem. Cytochem.*, **12**, 197–209.

Transfer and Storage of Biogenic Monoamines in Subcellular Organelles of Blood Platelets

A. PLETSCHER, M. DA PRADA AND J. P. TRANZER

Research Department, F. Hoffmann-La Roche & Co. Ltd., Basle (Switzerland)

The transfer and storage of 5-hydroxytryptamine (5HT) in blood platelets and of norepinephrine in sympathetic nerve endings show striking similarities. In both systems, the amines are taken up by at least two mechanisms which seem to be located in the outer membrane and within the cell respectively. The membrane system seems to depend on metabolic energy, whereas the mechanism of the intracellular storage of the amines is not exactly known (Carlsson, 1966; Pletscher, 1968). Recently, it has been demonstrated that the platelets like the sympathetic nerve endings contain specific intracellular organelles which, owing to their monoamine content, are osmiophilic and can be visualized by electron microscopy (Bak *et al.*, 1967; Tranzer *et al.*, 1966). These organelles could be isolated in pure form by density-gradient centrifugation of platelet homogenates and were shown to contain the major part of the intracellular 5HT, adenosine triphosphate (ATP) and histamine. On incubation of the isolated organelles in plasma or synthetic media at 37°, liberation of endogenous 5HT, ATP and histamine occurs proportionally to the time of incubation. Furthermore, the organelles accumulate ^{14}C-5HT from the incubation medium against a considerable concentration gradient. This accumulation is strongly inhibited by reserpine and less by imipramine which acts mainly on the transport of 5HT through the platelet membrane (Da Prada and Pletscher, 1968; Da Prada *et al.*, 1967).

In the present experiments, isolated 5HT organelles of blood platelets of rabbits have been taken as a model for further studying the mechanism of the intracellular transfer and storage of aromatic monoamines. Special attention was given to the question whether the accumulation of 5HT in the organelles occurs as a consequence of mere passive diffusion (exchange with endogenous 5HT) or whether a more specific mechanism is involved.

(1) 5HT CONCENTRATION OF THE ORGANELLES

The concentration (g/ml) of 5HT within the organelles is difficult to determine since the volume of the organelles per platelet cannot be measured accurately. The volume has been estimated in two ways. The first method (I) uses a special tube for the density-gradient centrifugation of the platelet homogenates. The bottom of this tube narrows into a small cylindrical prolongation with a diameter of 0.8 mm and a length of 5 mm.

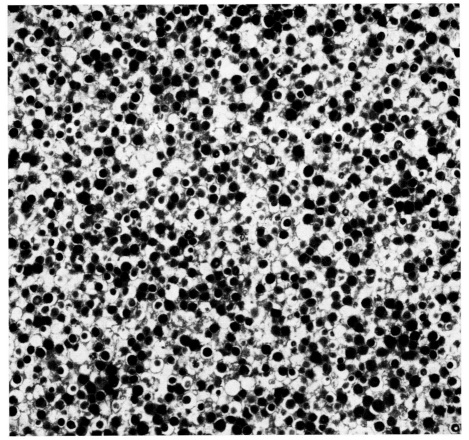

Fig. 1. 5-Hydroxytryptamine (5HT) organelles isolated from rabbit platelets by density-gradient centrifugation according to method I. ($\times$ 16 200)

The dense 5HT-organelles sediment in this prolongation forming a small cylinder the height of which can be measured. Estimations based on the electron-microscopic appearance of this sediment indicate that the osmiophilic material (consisting of 5HT) occupies at the most 1/3 of the total volume, the rest being empty (intra-vesicular space and empty organelles) (Fig. 1). The 5HT content of the sediment column can be measured by biochemical procedures as previously described (Bogdanski *et al.*, 1956). Method II uses the electron microscope for estimating the average diameter as well as the number of organelles within the intact platelets. This enables the volume of the organelles per platelet to be calculated, since the shape of the organelles seems to be spherical. From the volume of the organelles as well as the content of 5HT per platelet, the concentration of the amine in the organelles can be calculated, assuming that the 5HT is exclusively located within the organelles.

The results of these measurements (Table I) indicate that the 5HT concentrations evaluated by the two methods are different. Method I possibly yields too low results sinse some of the 5HT may have been lost during the procedure of isolating the or-

TABLE I

SOME PHYSICO-CHEMICAL PROPERTIES OF 5-HYDROXYTRYPTAMINE (5HT) ORGANELLES
OF RABBIT PLATELETS

The values obtained by method I have been corrected for the estimated intravesicular space and
empty vesicles

Average diameter		1800 Å
5HT concentration (g/ml × 100)	*Method I*	22 ± 2
	Method II	~ 45
5HT molecules per organelle (average)		$2\text{--}5 \cdot 10^6$
Average density		1.27 ± 0.01

ganelles. The values obtained by method II are probably too high since some of the platelet 5HT might be located outside the 5HT organelles. Taking these sources of error into account, the concentration of 5HT in the organelles may be estimated to be at least 20%. Assuming that 5HT is freely dissolved within the organelles, the osmotic pressure exerted by this amine alone would be 2–3 times that of plasma. Since the organelles also contain relatively large amounts of ATP and histamine besides 5HT, the osmotic pressure would be still higher (4–6 times that of plasma) if all these constituents were dissolved in free form. The high density of the 5HT organelles (Table I) which corresponds with the density of a 55% saccharose solution is in agreement with the estimated high intravesicular content of 5HT and ATP.

These considerations as well as the low solubility of 5HT under physiological conditions (less than 1% at pH 7.4 and 37°) lead to the conclusion that the amine is probably not present in free form in the intravesicular fluid. It might occur in a special form, *e.g.* as crystals, soluble complexes or bound to protein. A major degree of protein binding is, however, unlikely since, according to results from this laboratory the 5HT organelles contain about 3–4 times less protein than 5HT on a weight basis. In order to study whether there are crystalline structures within the organelles, fractions of pure organelles were submitted to X-ray diffractometry*. The result was negative since no interference lines appeared. Therefore, the possibility must be considered that 5HT is stored within the organelles in form of a soluble complex. Previous authors have suggested that the platelet 5HT may be bound to ATP (see Pletscher, 1968). Existence and nature of such a complex remain to be further investigated.

---

* Performed by Dr. W. Oberhänsli, Physical Department, F. Hoffmann-La Roche & Co. Ltd., Basle.

References p. 52

TABLE II

UPTAKE OF RADIOACTIVE AMINES BY ISOLATED 5-HYDROXYTRYPTAMINE (5HT)
ORGANELLES INCUBATED IN PLASMA AT 37° FOR 30 min

Concentration of amines in incubation fluid 0.57 μM. The values represent averages with S.E. and are expressed in % of the ^{14}C-5HT taken up by the organelles in the same experiment. Absolute uptake of ^{14}C-5HT in mμg/μg endogenous 5HT: 0.91 $\pm$ 0.08 (14 experiments).

Amine	Uptake
5-Hydroxytryptamine	100 $\pm$ 9
Tryptamine	10 $\pm$ 2
Dopamine	68 $\pm$ 2
Tyramine	13 $\pm$ 2
Histamine	2 $\pm$ 1

(2) DIFFERENTIAL UPTAKE OF VARIOUS MONOAMINES

The mechanism of the uptake of 5HT by the organelles (see above) is not clear. Therefore, isolated organelles were incubated in plasma at 37° for 30 min with labelled aromatic monoamines other than 5HT (final concentration 0.57 μM), and thereafter the amount of radioactive amines taken up by the organelles was determined (Da Prada and Pletscher, 1969).

Table II shows that the various monoamines behave quite differently from each other. The uptake of 5HT is most marked, whereas that of histamine, tryptamine and tyramine is very low; dopamine enters the organelles in amounts lying in between. These differences are also seen with higher concentrations of the amines (5.7 and 57 μM) as well as after shorter periods of incubation (5 and 15 min).

Some structural features of the amines might determine their uptake by the organelles. An OH-group in *m*-position on the phenyl ring seems to be of importance since 5HT and dopamine enter the organelles to a higher extent than tryptamine and tyramine respectively. On the other hand, preliminary experiments show that additional OH-groups may again diminish the uptake. Thus, epinephrine and norepinephrine (OH-group in 2-position in the side-chain) as well as 5-hydroxydopamine enter the organelles less readily than dopamine.

These studies indicate that the organelles seem to be able to discriminate between various monoamines concerning their uptake. The marked differences in this uptake cannot therefore be explained by mere passive diffusion in a non-structured medium, since the thermic movements at a given temperature depend mainly on the molecular size which is not very different for the various amines tested.

(3) ROLE OF METABOLIC ENERGY

The finding that certain amines, especially 5HT, are accumulated more markedly than others as well as the high ATP content of the organelles might indicate the participation of specific, active (*i.e.* energy-dependent) processes. Therefore, the

TABLE III

EFFECT OF OUABAIN AND INCUBATION MEDIUM ON THE UPTAKE OF [^{14}C]5-HYDROXY-
TRYPTAMINE (5HT) OF ISOLATED 5HT ORGANELLES INCUBATED FOR 30 min AT 37°

The values represent averages with S.E. of 2 experiments and are expressed in percent of the ^{14}C-5HT
taken up by organelles in normal plasma. Absolute uptake of 5HT by organelles incubated in plasma
(per experiment): 9.5 ± 0.1 mμg.

Medium	Supplement	^{14}C-5HT uptake
Plasma	None	100 ± 1
Plasma	Ouabain 10^{-4} M	99 ± 2
Plasma	Ouabain 10^{-3} M	96 ± 2
Synthetic[a]	Glucose	180 ± 8
Synthetic[a]	No glucose	175 ± 17

[a] Tyrode buffer devoid of CaCl$_2$ and sugars, but added EDTA 0.80 g/l.

influence of ouabain, glucose and metabolic inhibitors on the uptake of ^{14}C-HT by isolated organelles has been investigated. It may be seen from Table III that ouabain in concentrations as high as 10^{-3} M does not inhibit the uptake of ^{14}C-5HT. In other systems (*e.g.* of electrolytes) the glucoside is thought to interfere with the "transport ATP-ase" (Czáky, 1965), and ouabain (10^{-5} M and less) also markedly diminishes the entry of 5HT into intact platelets (*e.g.* of guinea pigs and man) (Pletscher *et al.*, 1967; Weissbach *et al.*, 1960). Participation of an ATP-dependent transport mechanism for 5HT in the organelles therefore seems unlikely. The presence of metabolic enzymes (*e.g.* of carbohydrate metabolism) in pure fractions of 5HT organelles (devoid of mitochondria, microsomes and platelet supernatant) is improbable. In fact, absence of metabolic substrates such as glucose does not diminish the transfer of 5HT into isolated organelles (compare tyrode with and without glucose as well as tyrode and plasma, Table III), and, according to preliminary results, metabolic inhibitors (monoiodo-acetate and NaF) do not inhibit the 5HT uptake either. In consequence, there is no evidence up to now that the transfer of 5HT into the organelles is dependent on metabolic energy.

In conclusion, the discriminating properties of isolated 5HT organelles concerning the uptake of aromatic monoamines seem not to be connected with a mechanism dependent on metabolic energy. They are rather due to physico-chemical qualities of the amines and the organelles which may influence the extra-intravesicular distribution of the amines, their penetration through the membrane of the organelles, their binding to intravesicular constituents, etc. These physico-chemical properties may be of importance especially for the formation of complexes between the amines and ATP within the organelles.

SUMMARY

In isolated 5-hydroxytryptamine (5HT) organelles, the 5HT content is very high in relation to the relatively low solubility of the amine under physiological conditions. Furthermore, the organelles possess discriminating properties with regard to the uptake of various monoamines. 5HT and dopamine enter the organelles more readily than tryptamine, tyramine and histamine. The uptake of 5HT is not influenced by glucose, ouabain and metabolic inhibitors. In conclusion, the discriminating ability of the organelles is probably mainly due to physico-chemical properties which might, for instance, be involved in the formation of complexes between amines and intra-vesicular constituents.

REFERENCES

BAK, I. J., HASSLER, R., MAY, B., AND WESTERMANN, E., (1967); Morphological and biochemical studies on the storage of serotonin and histamine in blood platelets of the rabbit. *Life Sci.*, **6**, 1133–1146.

BOGDANSKI, D. F., PLETSCHER, A., BRODIE, B. B., AND UDENFRIEND, S., (1956); Identification and assay of serotonin in brain. *J. Pharmacol. exp. Ther.*, **117**, 82–88.

CARLSSON, A., (1966); Pharmacological depletion of catecholamine stores. *Pharmacol. Rev.*, **18**, 541–549.

CZÁKY, T. Z., (1965); Ttansport through biological membranes. *Ann. Rev. Physiol.*, **27**, 415–450.

DA PRADA, M., AND PLETSCHER, A., (1968); Isolated 5-hydroxytryptamine organelles of rabbit blood platelets: Physiological properties and drug-induced changes. *Brit. J. Pharmacol.*, in the press.

DA PRADA, M., AND PLETSCHER, A., (1969); Differential uptake of biogenic amines by isolated 5-hydroxytryptamine organelles of blood platelets. *Life Sci.*, in the press.

DA PRADA, M., PLETSCHER, A., TRANZER, J. P., AND KNUCHEL, H., (1967); Subcellular localisation of 5-hydroxytryptamine and histamine in blood platelets. *Nature (Lond.)*, **216**, 1315–1317.

PLETSCHER, A., BURKARD, W. P., TRANZER, J. P., AND GEY, K. F., (1967); Two sites of 5-hydroxytryptamine uptake in blood platelets. *Life Sci.*, **6**, 273–280.

PLETSCHER, A., (1968); Metabolism, transfer and storage of 5-hydroxytryptamine in blood platelets. *Brit. J. Pharmacol.*, **32**, 1–16.

TRANZER, J. P., DA PRADA, M., AND PLETSCHER, A., (1966); Ultrastructural localization of 5-hydroxytryptamine in blood platelets. *Nature (Lond.)*, **212**, 1574–1575.

WEISSBACH, H., REDFIELD, B. G., AND TITUS, E., (1960); Effect of cardiac glycosides and inorganic ions on binding of serotonin by platelets. *Nature (Lond.)*, **185**, 99–100.

Pharmacology of Synaptic Monoamine Transmission

A. CARLSSON

Department of Pharmacology, University of Göteborg (Sweden)

The topic I have been asked to talk about is rather broad and cannot possibly be covered in half an hour. I have chosen to tell you briefly about a number of investigations carried out or going on in our laboratory. One of them deals with the mechanism of transmitter release by the nerve impulse, the others with the role of the monoamines of the central nervous system.

ROLE OF THE AMINE GRANULES

The intraneuronal distribution of noradrenaline (NA) in the peripheral adrenergic neuron and of brain monoamines are very similar. The amine occurs in nearly all parts of the neuron, though in much higher concentration in the so-called varicosities of the terminal system than elsewhere. The reason for this is in all probability the accumulation in these structures of amine storage granules, which in the electron microscope can be made to stand out as dense-cored vesicles. In the adrenergic neuron the number of such granules per varicosity is about 1000 and the number of NA molecules per granule is about 15 000 (Dahlström and Häggendal, 1966a; Dahlström *et al.*, 1966). The granules appear to be synthesized in the cell bodies and transported at a rate of several mm per hour down the axon to the varicosities (Dahlström, 1965, 1966; Dahlström *et al.*, 1965; Dahlström and Häggendal, 1966b). This can be demonstrated by measuring the accumulation of NA proximal to a nerve ligation. There is considerable evidence that the amine granules are essential for the neurohumoural transmission mechanism. The evidence is mainly derived from experiments with reserpine, which blocks a specific ATP-dependent amine-incorporating mechanism of the granules. This leads to depletion of the transmitter, which is no longer available for release by the nerve impulse. Loading of the cytoplasm outside the granules with NA does not restore function (Andén *et al.*, 1969).

These observations, demonstrating the essential and specific role of the amine granules for the transmission mechanism, might seem to be in line with the concept of quantal release formulated by Katz (1962; *cf.* also Eccles, 1964). According to Katz, each quantum or packet of acetylcholine molecules released at one time would correspond to the content of one vesicle. In other words, the vesicle is assumed to empty its whole content of transmitter, possibly through negative pinocytosis. Similar evidence for quantal release from adrenergic nerve endings has been presented (Burnstock and Holman, 1966).

However, actual measurements of the release of NA at nerve stimulation do not support this concept. In these experiments the NA released into the blood stream from cat skeletal muscle was carefully collected, and every possible precaution was taken to keep the losses under control. The number of adrenergic varicosities in the muscle being known, the release of NA per nerve impulse per varicosity could be calculated to be 400 molecules, corresponding to only 3% of the calculated NA content in one single amine granule. Thus only a fraction of the content of one granule is released by the nerve impulse (Folkow and Häggendal, 1967; Folkow et al., 1967).

There are two main possibilities to explain the essential role of the amine granules in the release mechanism. The nerve impulse may directly or indirectly influence the granule to give off a fraction of its content into the synaptic cleft. That being so the granule in question must be assumed to be in very close contact or even fused together with the cell membrane. Alternatively, the nerve impulse may cause release of a hypothetical transmitter pool attached to specific sites of the cell membrane. Reloading of these sites could then be achieved specifically by the amine granules. Here, too, a close contact between granule and cell membrane has to be postulated. Both alternatives appear to be compatible with the concept of "quantal release".

The amine granules are capable of exerting their function even when the store is practically depleted, provided that their uptake mechanism is intact. There is evidence that the transmitter store of the granules consists of a small immediately available pool and a large reserve pool (For review, see Andén et al., 1969).

CENTRAL MONOAMINE TRANSMISSION

One of the most important problems in the monoamine field is no doubt the role of these neurohumours in the normal function of the central nervous system and in mental and other brain disorder. Needless to say, in order to answer this question it is absolutely essential to know the exact localization of these amines in the brain and spinal cord. In this field considerable progress has been made, mainly thanks to the new histochemical fluorescence technique of Hillarp, Falck and coworkers. By these techniques, in combination with electron microscopy and biochemical analyses, it has been shown that the occurrence and distribution of central NA, dopamine (DA) and 5-hydroxytryptamine (5-HT) is remarkably similar to that of NA in the peripheral nervous system. Thus these amines are accumulated in nerve-ending varicosities which appear to make synaptic contact with dendrites or nerve-cell bodies. Within the varicosities the main part of the amine appears to be stored in dense-cored vesicles (Carlsson et al., 1962; Dahlström and Fuxe, 1964; Fuxe, 1965; Ungerstedt, unpublished). The main monoamine-carrying neuronal pathways have been mapped out. In general they originate in the lower brain stem, while their terminal nets are widely distributed in various parts of the brain and spinal cord (Carlsson et al., 1964; Dahlström and Fuxe, 1965; Andén et al., 1966c). The relatively detailed knowledge thus obtained forms an excellent starting-point for functional studies.

For a discussion of the criteria for a central monoamine neurotransmission I have to refer to our recent review (Andén et al., 1969). Suffice it to say here that the weight of evidence supports the view that NA, DA and 5-HT do indeed serve as neurohumoural transmitters in the central nervous system.

EXPERIMENTAL MODELS FOR STUDYING CENTRAL MONOAMINE NEUROTRANSMISSION

Certain neuronal pathways have proved particularly suitable for analyzing central monoaminergic mechanisms, namely, the bulbospinal NA and 5-HT and the nigro-neostriatal DA tracts.

After transection of the spinal cord the monoamine pathways, which are all bulbospinal, should receive no nerve impulses below the lesion. The turnover of NA and 5-HT, below but not above the lesion, is very much reduced. It would thus appear that the monoamine turnover is very closely linked to impulse flow centrally, just as has been found in the peripheral adrenergic system. This resting state of the monoamine tracts can be converted to an active one by using different pharmacological tools, which serve to increase the concentration of monoamines at the synaptic cleft. After injection of DOPA, for example, decarboxylation seems to occur mainly in the monoamine-carrying nerve terminals, resulting in the accumulation of DA and subsequently NA intraneuronally. If the accumulation is sufficiently large, overflow will occur, and postsynaptic receptors will be activated. This will lead to functional changes, which have been analyzed electrophysiologically. The most striking effect is an increased flexor reflex activity. A similar action, though clearly different in certain respects, is brought about by 5-HT overflow (through 5-hydroxytryptophan) (Carlsson et al., 1963; Andén et al., 1964a, 1966d,e,f; Jankowska et al., 1966, 1967a,b).

The nigro-neostriatal DA neurons are investigated after unilateral lesions of these neurons. This hardly results in any disturbance of movement in the rat. However, if the remaining nigro-neostriatal pathway is influenced asymmetry develops, and the direction of turning movements depends on whether an increase or decrease of DA is brought about at the receptor sites. Thus DOPA or nialamide plus reserpine cause the animals to rotate to the side of the lesion, reserpine, haloperidol and chlorpromazine to the opposite side (Andén et al., 1966b).

MODE OF ACTION OF PSYCHOTROPIC DRUGS

Using these models as well as observations on gross behaviour and conditioned reactions it has been possible to obtain an insight into the mode of action of several centrally acting drugs (Table I). Certain agents appear to activate the receptors directly, since they retain their activity after depletion of the transmitter store by reserpine plus an inhibitor of transmitter synthesis. This is true of apomorphine, which seems to be a specific DA-receptor activating agent (Ernst, 1967; Andén et al., 1967b), and LSD, which seems to activate central 5-HT receptors selectively (Andén et al., 1968). Amphetamine appears to act only indirectly by releasing DA and NA

TABLE I

MODE OF ACTION OF SOME CENTRALLY ACTING DRUGS

Agent	System acted upon	Mechanism
NA } (*via* DOPA)	NA (DA ?)	Receptor activation
DA }	DA (NA ?)	Receptor activation
5-HT (*via* 5-HTP)	5-HT	Receptor activation
Apomorphine	DA	Receptor activation
LSD	5-HT	Receptor activation
Amphetamine	DA, NA	Release of DA and NA
Chlorpromazine	DA, NA	Receptor blockade
Haloperidol	DA, NA	Receptor blockade
Phenoxybenzamine	NA	Receptor blockade
Reserpine	DA, NA, 5-HT	Transmitter depletion
Desipramine	NA (5-HT)	Blockade of recapture
Imipramine, chlorimipramine	5-HT (NA)	Blockade of recapture

(Weissman *et al.*, 1966; Hanson, 1966; Carlsson *et al.*, 1966). The neuroleptics chlor-promazine and haloperidol appear to block DA and NA receptors, whereas phenoxy-benzamine blocks NA receptors only (Andén *et al.*, 1966e, 1967a). It thus seems clear that central DA, NA and 5-HT receptors are different.

Antidepressive drugs of the imipramine group appear to act by blocking the cell membrane's pump mechanism by means of which the transmitter released into the synaptic cleft is transported back into the nerve terminal. Blockade of this mechanism will enhance and prolong the accumulation of transmitter at the synaptic cleft. Interestingly, the structural requirements of the different amine pumps do not appear to be identical. The pump mechanism of DA neurons appears to be resistant to all drugs of the imipramine group. Desipramine and protriptyline seem to act mainly on the amine pump of the NA neurons, whereas imipramine, chlorimipramine and amitriptyline appear to have their strongest action on the pump mechanism of 5-HT neurons. When these data are compared with observations on qualitative differences in clinical efficacy, it may be suggested that the ability of antidepressive drugs to elevate the mood of the depressed patient is related to an action on 5-HT neurons, whereas their ability to stimulate drive is related to an action on NA neurons (Carlsson *et al.*, 1966, 1968, 1969a,b).

FEEDBACK CONTROL OF SYNAPTIC ACTIVITY

An interesting correlation has been found between receptor activation or inhibition by drugs and the effect of these drugs on monoamine turnover. It appears that receptor blockade is specifically accompanied by stimulation of the turnover of the mono-amine in question, while receptor activation and retarded turnover occur together. Thus haloperidol and chlorpromazine block DA and NA receptors and stimulate DA and NA turnover; phenoxybenzamine blocks NA receptors and stimulates NA turnover (Carlsson and Lindqvist, 1963; Andén *et al.*, 1964b, 1966a; Corrodi *et al.*,

1967). Apomorphine stimulates DA receptors and slows DA turnover, while LSD has corresponding actions on the 5-HT system. Imipramine will increase the concentration of 5-HT at receptor sites by blocking recapture and inhibits 5-HT turnover (Corrodi and Fuxe, 1968). The conclusion appears inescapable that a causal relationship exists between the activity of the postsynaptic receptor and the turnover of the presynaptic transmitter. Since the latter appears to be controlled by the impulse flow in the presynaptic fibre, it is tempting to suggest that the impulse flow is under the influence of a feedback mechanism, brought into play by changes in receptor activity.

CONCLUDING REMARKS

There are several important groups of centrally acting drugs that have been shown to exert at least some of their actions by interfering with monoamine-carrying neuronal systems. These drugs have proved to be useful tools for elucidating the functions of the central monoamine systems. We have reasons to believe, for example, that the characteristic syndrome of mental changes and motor and endocrine disturbances caused by reserpine is largely due to a general monoamine depletion in the brain. The remarkably similar, though in certain respects different, syndrome caused by the phenothiazine and butyrophenone neuroleptics is probably brought about by blockade of central catecholamine receptors. The syndromes induced by these and other psychotropic drugs may well serve as models for brain disorders. For example, the parkinsonian syndrome frequently encountered in patients treated with neuroleptics is probably related to an interference with the nigro-neostriatal DA system — depletion of DA after administration of reserpine, blockade of DA receptors after phenothiazines or butyrophenones. This pharmacological model formed the basis for the discovery that the DA content of the nigro-neostriatal system is very much reduced in clinical cases of parkinsonism and for the successful treatment of this disease with L-DOPA (see Costa et al., 1966; Cotzias et al., 1968).

There are good reasons for believing that the continued investigation of the monoamine-carrying systems of the central nervous system will lead to further important progress in our understanding of normal and disordered brain function and to the discovery of new therapeutic principles.

REFERENCES

ANDÉN, N.-E., JUKES, M. G. M., AND LUNDBERG, A., (1964a); Spinal reflexes and monoamine liberation. *Nature (Lond.)*, **202**, 1222–1223.

ANDÉN, N.-E., Roos, B.-E., AND WERDINIUS, B., (1964b); Effects of chlorpromazine, haloperidol and reserpine on the levels of phenolic acids in rabbit corpus striatum. *Life Sci.*, **3**, 149–158.

ANDÉN, N.-E., DAHLSTRÖM, A., FUXE, K., AND HÖKFELT, T., (1966a); The effect of haloperidol and chlorpromazine on the amine levels of central monoamine neurons. *Acta physiol. scand.*, **68**, 419–420.

ANDÉN, N.-E., DAHLSTRÖM, A., FUXE, K., AND LARSSON, K., (1966b), Functional role of the nigro-neostriatal dopamine neurons. *Acta pharmacol. (Kbh.)*, **24**, 263–274,

ANDÉN, N.-E., DAHLSTRÖM, A., FUXE, K., LARSSON, K., OLSON, L., AND UNGERSTEDT, U, (1966c); Ascending monoamine neurons to the telencephalon and diencephalon. *Acta physiol. scand.*, **67**, 313–326.

ANDÉN, N.-E., JUKES, M. G. M., LUNDBERG, A., AND VYKLICKY, L., (1966d); The effect of DOPA on the spinal cord. 1. Influence on transmission from primary afferents. *Acta physiol. scand.*, **67**, 373–386.

ANDÉN, N.-E., JUKES, M. G. M., AND LUNDBERG, A., (1966e); The effect of DOPA on the spinal cord. 2. A pharmacological analysis. *Acta physiol. scand.*, **67**, 387–396.

ANDÉN, N.-E., JUKES, M. G. M., LUNDBERG, A., AND VYKLICKY, L., (1966f); The effect of DOPA on the spinal cord. 3. Reciprocal organization of pathways transmitting excitatory action to alpha motoneurones of flexors and extensors. *Acta physiol. scand.*, **68**, 322–336.

ANDÉN, N.-E., CORRODI, H., FUXE, K., AND HÖKFELT, T., (1967a); Increased impulse flow in bulbospinal noradrenaline neurons produced by catecholamine receptor blocking agents. *European J. Pharmacol.*, **2**, 59–64.

ANDÉN, N.-E., RUBENSON, A., FUXE, K., AND HÖKFELT, T., (1967b); Evidence for dopamine receptor stimulation by apomorphine. *J. Pharm. Pharmacol.*, **19**, 627–629.

ANDÉN, N.-E., CORRODI, H., FUXE, K., AND HÖKFELT, T., (1968); Evidence for a central 5-hydroxytryptamine receptor stimulation by lysergic acid diethylamide. *Brit. J. Pharmacol.*, **34**, 1–7.

ANDÉN, N.-E., CARLSSON, A., AND HÄGGENDAL, J., (1969); Adrenergic mechanisms. *Ann. Rev. Pharmacol.*, in the press.

BURNSTOCK, G., AND HOLMAN, M. E., (1966); Junction potentials at adrenergic synapses. *Pharmacol. Rev.*, **18**, 481–493.

CARLSSON, A., AND LINDQVIST, M., (1963); Effect of chlorpromazine or haloperidol on formation of 3-methoxytyramine and normetanephrine in mouse brain. *Acta pharmacol. (Kbh.)*, **20**, 140–144.

CARLSSON, A., FALCK, B., AND HILLARP, N.-Å., (1962); Cellular localization of brain monoamines. *Acta physiol. scand.*, **56**, Suppl. 196.

CARLSSON, A., MAGNUSSON, T., AND ROSENGREN, E., (1963); 5-Hydroxytryptamine of the spinal cord normally and after transection. *Experientia (Basel)*, **19**, 359.

CARLSSON, A., FALCK, B., FUXE, K., AND HILLARP, N.-Å., (1964); Cellular localization of monoamines in the spinal cord. *Acta physiol. scand.*, **60**, 112–119.

CARLSSON, A., FUXE, K., HAMBERGER, B., AND LINDQVIST, M., (1966); Biochemical and histochemical studies on the effects of imipramine-like drugs and (+)-amphetamine on central and peripheral catecholamine neurons. *Acta physiol. scand.*, **67**, 481–497.

CARLSSON, A., FUXE, K., AND UNGERSTEDT, U., (1968); The effect of imipramine on central 5-hydroxytryptamine neurons. *J. Pharm. Pharmacol.*, **20**, 150–151.

CARLSSON, A., CORRODI, H., FUXE, K., AND HÖKFELT, T., (1969a); Effect of some anti-depressant drugs on the depletion of intraneuronal brain catecholamine stores caused by 4,α-dimethyl meta-tyramine. *Europ. J. Pharmacol.*, in the press.

CARLSSON, A., CORRODI, H., FUXE, K., AND HÖKFELT, T., (1969b); Effect of anti-depressant drugs on the depletion of intraneuronal brain 5-hydroxytryptamine stores caused by 4-methyl-α-ethyl-metatyramine. *Europ. J. Pharmacol.*, in the press.

COSTA, E., COTÉ, L. J., AND YAHR, M. D., (Eds.), (1966); *Biochemistry and Pharmacology of the Basal Ganglia.* Raven Press, Hewlett, N.Y., 238 pp.

COTZIAS, G. C., PAPAVASILIOU, P. S., AND GELLENE, R., (1968); Modification of Parkinsonism: Chronic treatment with L-Dopa. *New Engl. J. Med.*, in the press.

CORRODI, H., AND FUXE, K., (1968); The effect of imipramine on central monoamine neurons. *J. Pharm. Pharmacol.*, **20**, 230–231.

CORRODI, H., FUXE, K., AND HÖKFELT, T., (1967); The effect of neuroleptics on the activity of central catecholamine neurons. *Life Sci.*, **6**, 767–774.

DAHLSTRÖM, A., (1965); Observations on the accumulation of noradrenaline in the proximal and distal parts of peripheral adrenergic nerves after compression. *J. Anat. (Lond.)*, **99**, 677–689.

DAHLSTRÖM, A., (1966); The intraneuronal distribution of noradrenaline and the transport and life-span of amine storage granules in the sympathetic adrenergic neuron, *Thesis*, Karolinska Institutet, Stockholm.

DAHLSTRÖM, A., AND FUXE, K., (1964); Evidence for the existence of monoamine-containing neurons in the central nervous system. I. Demonstration of monoamines in the cell bodies of brain stem neurons. *Acta physiol. scand.*, **62**, Suppl. 232.

DAHLSTRÖM, A., AND FUXE, K., (1965); Evidence for the existence of monoamine-containing neurons in the central nervous system. II. Experimentally induced changes in the intraneuronal amine levels in bulbospinal neuron systems. *Acta physiol. scand.*, **64**, Suppl. 247, 5–36.

DAHLSTRÖM, A., AND HÄGGENDAL, J., (1966a); Some quantitative studies on the noradrenaline content in the cell bodies and terminals of a sympathetic adrenergic neuron system. *Acta physiol. scand.*, **67**, 271–277.

DAHLSTRÖM, A., AND HÄGGENDAL, J., (1966b); Studies on the transport and life-span of amine storage granules in a peripheral adrenergic neuron system. *Acta physiol. scand.*, **67**, 278–288.

DAHLSTRÖM, A., FUXE, K., AND HILLARP, N.-Å., (1965); Site of action of reserpine. *Acta pharmacol. (Kbh.)*, **22**, 277–292.

DAHLSTRÖM, A., HÄGGENDAL, J., AND HÖKFELT, T., (1966); The noradrenaline content of the nerve terminal varicosities of sympathetic adrenergic neurons in the rat. *Acta physiol. scand.*, **67**, 289–294.

ECCLES, J. C., (1964); *The Physiology of Synapses*. Springer, Berlin. 316 pp.

ERNST, A. M., (1967); Mode of action of apomorphine and dexamphetamine on gnawing compulsion in rats. *Psychopharmacologia (Berl.)*, **10**, 316–323.

FOLKOW, B., AND HÄGGENDAL, J., (1967); Quantitative studies on the transmitter release at adrenergic nerve endings. *Acta physiol. scand.*, **70**, 453–454.

FOLKOW, B., HÄGGENDAL, J., AND LISANDER, B., (1967); Extent of release and elimination of noradrenaline at peripheral adrenergic nerve terminals. *Acta physiol. scand.*, **72**, Suppl. 307.

FUXE, K., (1965); Evidence for the existence of monoamine neurons in the central nervous system. IV. Distribution of monoamine nerve terminals in the central nervous system. *Acta physiol. scand.*, **64**, Suppl. 247, 37–85.

HANSON, L. C. F., (1966); Evidence that the central action of amphetamine is mediated *via* catecholamines. *Psychopharmacologia (Berl.)*, **9**, 78–80.

JANKOWSKA, E., LUND, S., AND LUNDBERG, A., (1966); The effect of DOPA on the spinal cord. 4. Depolarization evoked in the central terminals of contralateral Ia afferent terminals by volleys in the flexor reflex afferents. *Acta physiol. scand.*, **68**, 337–341.

JANKOWSKA, E., JUKES, M. G. M., LUND, S., AND LUNDBERG, A., (1967a); The effect of DOPA on the spinal cord. 5. Reciprocal organization of pathways transmitting excitatory action to alpha motoneurones of flexors and extensors. *Acta physiol. scand.*, **70**, 369–388.

JANKOWSKA, E., JUKES, M. G. M., LUND, S., AND LUNDBERG, A., (1967b); The effect of DOPA on the spinal cord. 6. Half-center organization of interneurones transmitting effects from the flexor reflex afferents. *Acta physiol. scand.*, **70**, 389–402.

KATZ, B., (1962); The transmission of impulses from nerve to muscle and the subcellular unit of synaptic action. *Proc. roy. Soc. B*, **155**, 455–479.

UNGERSTEDT, U., unpublished observations.

WEISSMAN, A., KOE, B. K., AND THENEN, S. S., (1966); Antiamphetamine effects following inhibition of tyrosine hydroxylase. *J. Pharmacol. exp. Ther.*, **151**, 339–352.

Effects of Catecholamines in the Cat Superior Cervical Ganglion and Their Postulated Rôle as Physiological Modulators of Ganglionic Transmission

W. E. HAEFELY

Department of Experimental Medicine, F. Hoffmann-La Roche and Co. Ltd., Basle (Switzerland)

Interest in the effects of catecholamines on synaptic transmission in autonomic ganglia was aroused 30 years ago when Marrazzi (1939a, b) discovered the inhibitory action of adrenaline in the cat superior cervical ganglion. Marrazzi's studies were carried out at a time when prominent neurophysiologists considered synaptic transmission to be an essentially electrical phenomenon which could possibly be modulated by neuro-humoral factors in the sense of facilitation or inhibition. During the last few years the effects of catecholamines on ganglionic synaptic transmission have again been intensively studied. One of the reasons for this was the discovery of neuron systems in the brain and spinal cord using most probably the catecholamines noradrenaline and dopamine as neurotransmitters (Andén *et al.*, 1966). Although the direct application of these suspected transmitters to single neurons in the central nervous system has become an established method, the autonomic ganglion cells with their monosynaptic connections, their simple input–output relations and easy accessibility remain favoured models for studying synaptic mechanisms. Besides acting as a model synapse the sympathetic ganglion was suspected to be the very site of a physiological action of catecholamines when a new class of drugs — inhibitors of monoamine oxidase — was found to lower arterial blood pressure in man and animals. A hypothetical explanation for the unexpected effect of these drugs has been advanced by Costa *et al.* (1961) who suggested an increase of catecholamines in sympathetic ganglia and their continuous release on ganglion cells with consequent depression of synaptic transmission. From studies on isolated sympathetic ganglia of the rabbit and frog it has been inferred that catecholamines could be involved in the generation of slow synaptic potentials (Eccles and Libet, 1961; Tosaka *et al.*, 1968).

Some results of recent experiments together with findings described in the literature pertinent to this problem will be discussed.

(1) THE EFFECTS OF CATECHOLAMINES ON GANGLIONIC TRANSMISSION AND ON DRUG-INDUCED EXCITATION OF GANGLION CELLS

The literature on the ganglionic effects of catecholamines contains many controversial findings, most of which may be explained by the different techniques used. Ganglionic transmission has been studied by measuring the response of adrenergically innervated effector organs — such as the nictitating membrane — to pre-ganglionic nerve impulses. The ganglion was either normally supplied with blood or perfused with artificial media of somewhat varying ionic composition. In electrophysiological investigations either action potentials in post-ganglionic nerves or changes in the potential difference between the ganglionic surface and an inactive cut end of a post-ganglionic nerve, the so-called ganglionic potentials (Eccles, 1935a) are recorded. Ganglia *in situ* or isolated from the animal are frequently used. Intracellular recordings from ganglionic cells have been obtained successfully only from isolated ganglia of the rabbit and the frog. Impalement of the cells by the microelectrode is difficult owing to the small size of the cells and the resistant connective tissue surrounding them. With leads from the ganglionic surface one records extracellular potential changes from a large population of cells — possibly not only from ganglion cells. A comparison with the absolute potentials measured with the intracellular microelectrode shows that the potentials led off from the ganglionic surface are a fairly true mirror image of the mean relative changes of the polarization of a mass of ganglion cells when rapid changes are studied. Slow changes of the polarization of ganglion cells, *e.g.* induced by drugs, seem to be relatively too prominent as compared with the rapid changes such as the spike of the action potential.

The superior cervical ganglion receives its pre-ganglionic input by the cervical sympathetic trunk which can be easily prepared for stimulation. The output is more complex, there being usually 6–10 post-ganglionic branches of different size and direction (Fig. 1). In the experiments described in this report some of them were

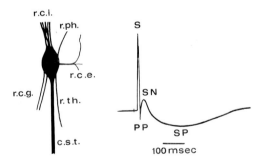

Fig. 1. Left: Schematic drawing of the superior cervical ganglion of the cat with its main post-ganglionic branches. c.s.t. cervical sympathetic trunk; r.th. ramus thyreoideus; r.c.g. rami communicantes grisei to the upper cervical spinal nerves; r.c.e. ramus caroticus externus; r.ph. ramus laryngopharyngicus; r.c.i. ramus caroticus internus. Right: Schematic ganglionic potential; S spike potential; PP positive phase of the spike; SN slow negative wave (after-negativity); SP slow positive wave (after-positivity).

prepared for antidromic stimulation or monophasic recording of the post-ganglionic action potentials. Drugs were injected through a needle fixed in the common carotid artery, the external carotid artery being ligated. The potential recorded from the ganglionic surface in response to a pre-ganglionic volley (Fig. 1) is of a rapid initial negativity, consisting of 1–4 spikes dependent on the stimulus strength and the distance of the stimulating electrodes from the ganglion. The spike is followed (usually separated by a positive phase of the spike of uncertain origin) by two slow waves (Eccles, 1935a). The slow negative wave (or after-negativity) mainly represents the residual synaptic potential; the positive slow wave (or after-positivity) seems to be a true hyperpolarizing after-potential.

The *post-ganglionic spike amplitude* was regularly decreased in a dose-dependent manner by noradrenaline injected towards the ganglion (Fig. 2). The threshold dose

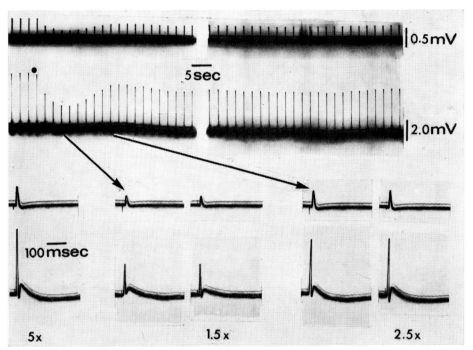

Fig. 2. Effect of noradrenaline (10 nanomoles) on postganglionic (upper line) and ganglionic (lower line) action potentials. A control response as well as the 4th and the 10th potentials after injection are shown also at a higher beam speed. The two responses after noradrenaline are compared with those to submaximal stimulation in the absence of noradrenaline. The figures below the corresponding potentials indicate stimulus strength in threshold units.

was usually 1 nanomole. The maximal depression obtainable when using supramaximal volleys was never more than 60%. The effect set in 2–3 sec after the injection and lasted up to several minutes depending on the dose. Similar results were obtained by Matthews (1956), Pardo *et al.* (1963) and Weir and McLennan (1963). Matthews (1956) and McIsaak (1966) found that adrenaline depressed ganglionic transmission less at higher frequencies of stimulation. The same may be expected to be the case with noradrenaline. Isoproterenol in equimolar doses had either no effect on postganglionic spike amplitudes or slightly increased them (Fig. 3). The increase when present was very small and never more than 20%. It occurred in a given ganglion in response to both submaximal and supramaximal volleys. The facilitation was

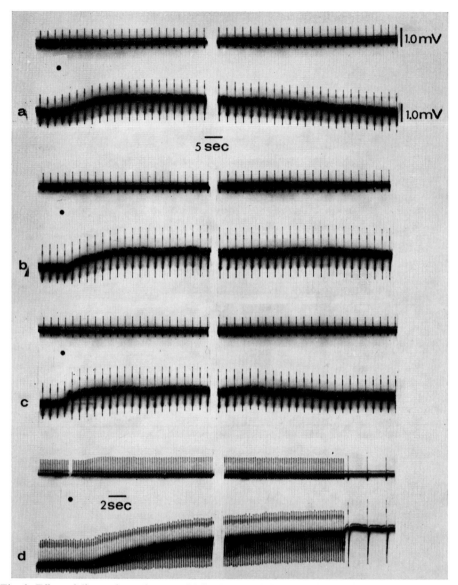

Fig. 3. Effect of (from above downwards) isoproterenol 3 nanomoles (a), isoproterenol 10 nanomoles (b), and nicotine 3 nanomoles (c), on post-ganglionic and ganglionic potentials elicited by
supramaximal volleys at a frequency of 0.5/sec. Bottom record (d) shows the effect of isoproterenol
10 nanomoles, when the frequency of stimulation was 5/sec.

greater at higher frequencies of stimulation (Fig. 3) confirming results obtained by
Matthews (1956). Maximal facilitation did not occur before about 30 sec after the injection but lasted up to 20 min depending on the dose. From the pharmacological
point of view it is important to note that inhibition by noradrenaline and facilitation
by isoproterenol could be blocked by the α-adrenergic receptor blocker dihydroergotamine and the β-adrenergic receptor blocker propranolol respectively. De

Groat and Volle (1966a) observed that after blockade of α-adrenergic receptors noradrenaline could produce facilitation of ganglionic transmission, but with less than one tenth the potency of adrenaline. It seems, therefore, that the β-adrenergic receptors involved in ganglionic facilitation are more similar to the type of β-adrenergic receptors mediating vasodilatation than to that mediating the positive chronotropic and inotropic effects on the heart. De Groat and Volle (1966a) have shown that the ganglionic effects of adrenaline — as can be expected from its actions on peripheral autonomic effectors — are composed of both inhibitory α- and facilitatory β-adrenergic actions. Either of these components may be obtained in a pure form by using α- or β-adrenergic receptor blocking agents. The choice of a specific adrenolytic is important; conclusions drawn *e.g.* with dibenamine (Eccles and Libet, 1961) are likely to be erroneous as this substance seems to block acetylcholine receptors as well (Konzett, 1950).

Of the ganglionic potentials studied the noradrenaline-induced depression of the *ganglionic spike amplitude* was unequivocal (Fig. 2) and in line with earlier reports by Matthews (1956), De Groat and Volle (1966a) and McIsaak (1966). The increase by isoproterenol was inconsistent and small (Fig. 3). I did not observe increases as large as those observed by De Groat and Volle (1966a). Post-ganglionic spike amplitudes were sometimes increased without a concomitant increase of the ganglionic spike, resembling findings after low doses of nicotine. The *ganglionic steady potential* was found to become more positive — indicating hyperpolarization of the ganglion — following some 90% of the noradrenaline injections, although this hyperpolarization was usually very small (De Groat and Volle, 1966a). In my own experiments no more than half the noradrenaline injections depressing ganglionic transmission produced a measurable hyperpolarization. Furthermore, even when present, hyperpolarization showed no correlation with the degree of depression of ganglionic transmission from increasing doses of noradrenaline. This lack of dose-dependence can also be seen in the figures of De Groat and Volle (1966a). Noradrenaline was observed to produce hyperpolarization in chronically denervated ganglia. Hence, this is a direct effect on post-synaptic membranes and is not due — as one could have expected — to the inhibition of the spontaneous release of acetylcholine from presynaptic endings. Isoproterenol behaved quite differently as it regularly depolarized the ganglion (Fig. 3). As already described by De Groat and Volle (1966a) depolarization developed slowly and was of long duration. It was dose-dependent both in amplitude and duration and attained its maximum with about 10 nanomoles.

De Groat and Volle (1966a) described characteristic changes of the *ganglionic slow potentials* after the injection of catecholamines, namely an apparent increase of the slow after-negativity and an apparent decrease of the slow after-positivity following noradrenaline and inverse changes after isoproterenol. The ganglionic slow potentials are dependent on the spike amplitude, the ganglionic polarization at the moment of their generation and may affect one another's amplitude and form. These facts have to be considered when studying drug effects on them. In several experiments the stimulus strength was reduced until the post-ganglionic spike amplitude was identical with that observed with supramaximal pulses at the maximum of depression obtained with noradrenaline (Fig. 2). No differences in the slow potentials could be observed except in ganglia responding to noradrenaline with hyperpolarization. The changes in slow potentials produced by noradrenaline could then be duplicated by applying a submaximal volley at a suitable interval after a conditioning supramaximal one so that the action potential started at a comparable state of polarization. One may conclude, therefore, that noradrenaline does not affect the mechanisms responsible for the production of slow potentials. The effect of isoprotere-

TABLE I

EFFECTS OF NORADRENALINE AND ISOPROTERENOL IN THE CAT SUPERIOR CERVICAL GANGLION

1–3: own unpublished results; 4–8: results of De Groat and Volle, 1966b

	Noradrenaline	*Blocked by DHET*[a]	*Isoproterenol*	*Blocked by propranolol*
1. Orthodromic post-ganglionic action potential	decrease	+	inconsistent slight increase	+
2. Ganglionic action potential				
spike amplitude	decrease	+	inconsistent increase	+
slow negative wave	inconsistent slight apparent increase	+	apparent decrease	+
slow positive wave	inconsistent slight apparent decrease	+	apparent increase	+
3. Ganglionic surface potential	no change or slight hyperpolarization	+	low-amplitude depolarization	+
4. Nicotine				
depolarization	no effect		decrease	+
firing	no effect		no effect	
5. Acetylcholine				
D-potential	increase	+	decrease	+
H-potential	decrease	+	increase	+
LD-potential	increase	+	conversion to hyper-polarization	+
ER	no effect	+	no effect	+
LR	inconsistent increase	+	unmasked or increased	+
6. Anticholinesterase-firing (atropine-sensitive, dependent on intact pre-synaptic endings)	decrease	+	increase	+
7. Oxotremorine and methacholine firing (atropine-sensitive, independent of presynaptic endings)	decrease	+	increase	+
8. KCl				
depolarization	increase		decrease	
firing			decrease	

[a] Dihydroergotamine.

nol is not quite so clear. The qualitative changes of the slow potentials are as expected in a depolarized ganglion, but it was observed, especially after higher doses, that the peak of the after-positivity following isoproterenol did not reach the preinjection level (Fig. 3). This would point to a specific interaction with the production of the after-positivity and would be consistent with the postulated decrease of potassium permeability of the membrane by isoproterenol (De Groat and Volle, 1966b) on the one hand and with the increase of the permeability to this cation or its increased active uptake by the neuron as the basis of the slow positive wave on the other hand.

The effects of noradrenaline and isoproterenol as observed in my own experiments are summarized in Table I which also gives a survey of the findings by De Groat and Volle (1966b) on the effects of these amines on ganglionic stimulants. The most important finding of these authors was that the firing produced by excitation of nicotinic receptors on the ganglion cells either by nicotine or acetylcholine was not reduced, but that the firing induced by stimulation of muscarinic receptors was inhibited by noradrenaline and unmasked or increased by isoproterenol. Furthermore, the latter reduced depolarization as well as firing induced by potassium.

De Groat and Volle (1966a) upheld the view that the inhibition of ganglionic transmission by noradrenaline was largely due to its hyperpolarizing action on ganglion cells. Lundberg (1952) had declined this interpretation on the basis of experiments with adrenaline. In my opinion, the overwhelming evidence is in favour of a presynaptic site of the action of noradrenaline: (a) Fig. 4 (taken from one animal)

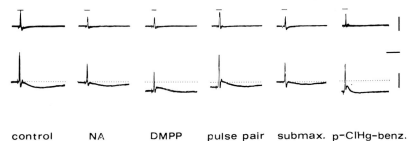

control   NA   DMPP   pulse pair   submax.   p–ClHg–benz.

Fig. 4. Post-ganglionic (above) and corresponding ganglionic (below) potentials in response to supramaximal (except the 5th potential) pre-ganglionic volleys. From left to right: Control response; at the maximum of ganglionic depression by noradrenaline 10 nanomoles; during the second (hyperpolarizing) phase of ganglionic inhibition following 1,1-dimethyl-4-phenylpiperazinium iodide (DMPP) 10 nanomoles; test volley 200 msec after a conditioning volley evoked by an identical stimulus strength; response to a submaximal pre-ganglionic volley; at the maximum of depression by p-chloromercuribenzoate 3 μmoles. Calibration: 0.5 mV (upper line) and 2.0 mV (lower line), 100 msec.

shows that noradrenaline, although producing only a minute hyperpolarization, depressed post-ganglionic spike amplitudes more than 1,1-dimethyl-4-phenylpiperazinium iodide (DMPP) during its hyperpolarizing second phase of transmission block (Haefely et al., 1967), p-chloromercuribenzoate (Volle, 1967) or the slow positive wave of a preceding conditioning volley (Eccles, 1935b). Conversely, the post-ganglionic and ganglionic potentials after noradrenaline can be imitated reasonably well by reducing the strength of stimulation. (b) Inhibition of transmission by varying doses of noradrenaline was not correlated with the degree of hyperpolarization. (c) Stimulation of nicotinic receptors was not found to be altered by noradrenaline (De Groat and Volle, 1966b). The depression by noradrenaline of the firing induced through muscarinic receptors is unlikely to be involved in transmission block, since these receptors do not seem to be of importance in the transmission of single volleys and as scopolamine did not antagonize the inhibitory effect of noradrenaline. (d) Paton and Thompson (1953) and Birks and MacIntosh (1961) found a reduced output of acetylcholine from the perfused ganglion under the influence of adrenaline. Noradrenaline inhibits the release of acetylcholine from post-ganglionic cholinergic fibres (Vizi, 1967).

The mechanism by which noradrenaline can reduce the release of acetylcholine is completely obscure. It is tempting to speculate on a depolarization of the presynaptic endings, but the reverse effect on the post-synaptic membrane together with the finding of Goffart and Holmes (1962) that noradrenaline increases the membrane potential of isolated A and C fibres is against this view. The facilitatory action of isoproterenol may plausibly be explained by the low-amplitude depolarization of ganglion cells. De Groat and Volle (1966b) found evidence for a reduced potassium permeability of the membrane following isoproterenol. Unmasking and increase of firing due to muscarinic receptor activation is found after the low-amplitude depolarization produced by isoproterenol and that following repetitive orthodromic stimulation. One could speculate, therefore, that facilitation of ganglionic transmission by isoproterenol was in some way connected with muscarinic receptors. However, in preliminary experiments neither facilitation nor depolarization induced by isoproterenol was prevented by prior application of scopolamine.

(2) ON POSTULATED SYNAPTIC ACTIONS OF CATECHOLAMINES RELEASED WITHIN THE GANGLION BY ORTHODROMIC VOLLEYS

The inhibitory effect on ganglionic transmission of noradrenaline reaching the ganglion by its blood supply and the presence of considerable amounts of this amine in the ganglion led to speculations about its involvement in normal ganglionic transmission. Hypothetically, pre-ganglionic impulses may liberate noradrenaline within the ganglion by one or more of the mechanisms indicated schematically in Fig. 5. (a) Accessory ganglia of varying size can be observed by the naked eye and under the dissecting microscope within the cervical sympathetic trunk in about 5% of the cats; scattered ganglion cells would not be detected. Stimulation of the cervical sympathetic trunk could, therefore, excite post-ganglionic adrenergic fibres forming synapses with ganglion cells. Alternatively, vasoconstrictor fibres originating in the superior cervical ganglion could liberate noradrenaline within or outside the ganglion and the overflowing transmitter could reach the ganglion cells from the blood circulating through the ganglion. Evidence of a similar remote effect of endogenous noradrenaline from vessels has been found in the nictitating membrane and the spleen (Haefely et al., 1964). (b) Pre-ganglionic cholinergic fibres may excite chromaffin cells and thereby release catecholamines onto ganglion cells. Chromaffin cells have been found

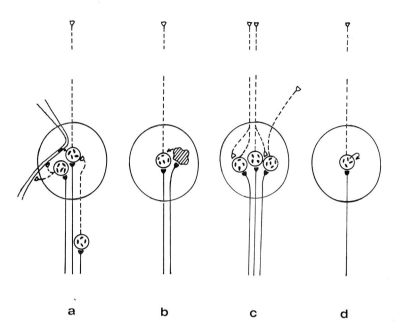

Fig. 5. Hypothetical ways by which noradrenaline could be released within the ganglion by pre-ganglionic stimulation (see text). Post-ganglionic adrenergic axons are indicated by broken lines.

in the superior cervical ganglion of the rat and in abdominal ganglia of various species (De Ribaupierre *et al.*, 1966; Norberg, 1967). (*c*) Post-ganglionic axons may have collaterals forming synapses with neighbouring ganglion cells. This possibility is especially interesting, since the inhibitory action of noradrenaline would permit a recurrent inhibition without the need of an inhibitory interneuron. (*d*) Finally, it must not be overlooked that synaptic excitation of the ganglion cell could possibly lead to a leakage of noradrenaline from the cell body which contains the amine as shown histochemically (Norberg, 1967) and structures resembling synaptic vesicles in the electron microscope, although these have not been shown to contain the neurotransmitter. Lissák (1939) could release an adrenaline-like substance from the isolated ganglion by antidromic stimulation. Reinert (1962) concluded that antidromic stimulation of the perfused superior cervical ganglion of the cat released noradrenaline from the ganglion cells into the perfusion fluid, but the figures given in his paper hardly support this view. Although the mechanisms involved in the release of noradrenaline from the nerve terminals have been elucidated up to a certain point, we still do not know whether or not the neurotransmitter is released only from the endings and not from the cell body and proximal axon where it is also present, and if so, why the amine behaves differently in the proximal parts of the neuron and at its endings.

Experiments to test the above-mentioned possibilities were conducted on normal untreated cats, on animals treated with reserpine 3 mg/kg intraperitoneally 16 h before the experiment in order to deplete almost completely the ganglion of its noradrenaline content (Muscholl and Vogt, 1958) and on cats treated twice daily over 5 days with 3 mg/kg of the monoamine oxidase inhibitor pheniprazine, as a result of which the ganglionic noradrenaline content should have almost doubled (Sanan and Vogt, 1962). The results can be summarized briefly: (*a*) Amplitude, form and time course of orthodromic ganglionic spikes and slow potentials to single pre-ganglionic impulses did not differ in the 3 groups of animals used. Dihydroergotamine did not produce any changes of these parameters in either group. Hence, ganglionic nor-adrenaline is unlikely to play any rôle in the transmission of single volleys. (*b*) In all 3 groups trains of pre-ganglionic impulses at a frequency of 50/sec and 5 or 10 sec duration produced identical post-tetanic facilitation of orthodromic post-ganglionic test responses which were accompanied by the characteristic post-tetanic hyper-polarization of the ganglion and the well-known changes of ganglionic spike amplitude and of the slow potentials. Dihydroergotamine, which blocked the effect of injected noradrenaline, had no effect on either of these post-tetanic phenomena. It may therefore be concluded that trains of high-frequency volleys do not release nor-adrenaline in amounts sufficient to affect synaptic transmission. (*c*) The sensitivity of ganglia to injected noradrenaline and isoproterenol was identical in all 3 groups. If inhibition of monoamine oxidase caused a continuous background action of nor-adrenaline, the sensitivity to this amine and to isoproterenol might be expected to differ from that of normal ganglia and from those depleted of the amine. (*d*) Anti-dromic repetitive stimulation of one postganglionic branch or nerve strand never reduced orthodromic test responses in any other branch or nerve strand. The existence of recurrent inhibition between different cell groups seems therefore very unlikely.

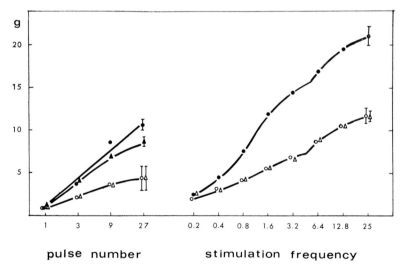

Fig. 6. Responses of the nictitating membranes of spinal cats to supramaximal pre- and post-gan-glionic stimulation with either single pulses and trains of 3, 9 and 27 pulses at 1.6/sec or repetitively at frequencies from 0.2/sec to 25/sec. Closed symbols: Untreated control cats. Open symbols: Cats treated over 5 days with twice daily subcutaneous injections of pheniprazine 3 mg/kg. ●, un-treated pre-ganglionic; ▲, untreated post-ganglionic; ○, pheniprazine pre-ganglionic; △, phen-iprazine post-ganglionic.

(e) Since with electrophysiological methods it is almost impossible to detect a slight inhibition of ganglionic transmission in a group of pretreated animals as compared with a control group, 6 cats treated with the monoamine oxidase inhibitor pheniprazine over 5 days were set up as spinal preparations and the responses of the nictitating membranes to pre- and post-ganglionic stimulation compared with those of the group of untreated controls. From Fig. 6 it can be seen that the responses of the nictitating membranes to longer trains of stimuli at a low frequency and to repetitive stimulation at increasing frequencies were markedly reduced. The change of the dose–response curve for noradrenaline makes it probable that the effect of the amine was antagonized in a non-competitive manner. The more important finding in this connection, however, is the identical reduction of responses to pre- and post-ganglionic stimulation. Hence, treatment with an inhibitor of monoamine oxidase known to increase markedly the noradrenaline content of the cat superior cervical ganglion did not induce any detectable impairment of ganglionic transmission.

The experimental findings reported, some of which confirm earlier results of other authors, are strong evidence against a physiological modulating rôle of noradrenaline released within the superior cervical ganglion of the cat in response to pre-ganglionic stimulation. Morphological findings in the superior cervical ganglion of other species and in other sympathetic ganglia of the cat make it not unlikely that the conclusions drawn from the cat superior cervical ganglion may not hold true for synapses of other autonomic ganglia.

SUMMARY

The effects of noradrenaline and isoproterenol on transmission in the superior cervical ganglion of the cat are described. It is concluded that noradrenaline depresses ganglionic transmission mainly by an action on pre-synaptic structures, most probably by reducing the release of acetylcholine. Isoproterenol produces facilitation by depolarization of the ganglion. The effects of the catecholamines are mediated by two distinct pharmacological receptors. Experiments designed to detect an effect of noradrenaline released within the ganglion by pre-synaptic volleys gave negative results. There is no evidence for a modulation of synaptic transmission by adrenergic mechanisms in this particular ganglion.

ACKNOWLEDGEMENT

The skillful technical assistance of Miss Ursula Hotz and Mr. Max Fischer is gratefully acknowledged.

REFERENCES

Andén, N.-E., Dahlström, A., Fuxe, K., Larsson, K., Olson, L., and Ungerstedt, U., (1966); Ascending monoamine neurons to the telencephalon and diencephalon. *Acta physiol. scand.*, **67**, 316–326.

Birks, R., and MacIntosh, F. C., (1961); Acetylcholine metabolism of a sympathetic ganglion. *Canad. J. Biochem.*, **39**, 787–827.

Costa, E., Revzin, A. M., Kuntzman, R., Spector, S., and Brodie, B. B., (1961); Role for ganglionic norepinephrine in sympathetic synaptic transmission. *Science*, **133**, 1822–1823.

DE GROAT, W. C., AND VOLLE, R. L., (1966a); The actions of the catecholamines on transmission in the superior cervical ganglion of the cat, *J. Pharmacol. exp. Ther.*, **154**, 1–13.

DE GROAT, W. C., AND VOLLE, R. L.,(1966b); Interactions between the catecholamines and ganglionic stimulating agents in sympathetic ganglia. *J. Pharmacol. exp. Ther.*, **154**, 200–215.

DE RIBAUPIERRE, F., SIEGRIST, G., DUNANT, Y., AND DOLIVO, M., (1966); Étude de la morphologie et de la fonction probable des cellules chromaffines du ganglion sympathique cervical supérieur du rat. *J. Physiol. (Paris)*, **58**, 601.

ECCLES, J. C., (1935a); The action potential of the superior cervical ganglion. *J. Physiol. (Lond.)*, **85**, 179–206.

ECCLES, J. C., (1935b); Facilitation and inhibition in the superior cervical ganglion. *J. Physiol. (Lond.)*, **85**, 207–238.

ECCLES, R. M., AND LIBET, B., (1961); Origin and blockade of the synaptic responses of curarized sympathetic ganglia. *J. Physiol. (Lond.)*, **157**, 484–503.

GOFFART, M., AND HOLMES, O., (1962); The effect of adrenaline on mammalian C and A nerve fibres. *J. Physiol. (Lond.)*, **162**, 18P–19P.

HAEFELY, W., HÜRLIMANN, A., AND THOENEN, H., (1964); Interferenz von Gefässeffekten eines Pharmakons mit seinen anderen nichtvasculären pharmakologischen Wirkungen. *Naunyn-Schmiedeberg's Arch. exp. Path. Pharmak.*, **249**, 267–278.

HAEFELY, W., HÜRLIMANN, A., AND THOENEN, H., (1967); Wirkungen von Nikotin, DMPP, TMA, Amphetamin und KCl auf das Demarkationspotential des Ganglion cervicale superius und die ganglionäre Transmission. *Helv. physiol. pharmacol. Acta*, **25**, CR 418–CR 419.

KONZETT, H., (1950); Sympathomimetica und Sympathicolytica am isoliert durchströmten Ganglion cervicale superius der Katze. *Helv. physiol. pharmacol. Acta.*, **8**, 245–258.

LISSÁK, K., (1939); Liberation of acetylcholine and adrenaline by stimulating isolated nerves. *Amer. J. Physiol.*, **127**, 263–271.

LUNDBERG, A., (1952); Adrenaline and transmission in the sympathetic ganglion of the cat. *Acta physiol. scand.*, **26**, 252–263.

MARRAZZI, A. S., (1939a); Adrenergic inhibition at sympathetic synapses. *Amer. J. Physiol.*, **127**, 738–744.

MARRAZZI, A. S., (1939b); Electrical studies on the pharmacology of autonomic synapses. II. The action of a sympathomimetic drug (epinephrine) on sympathetic ganglia. *J. Pharmacol. exp. Ther.*, **65**, 395–404.

MATTHEWS, R. J., (1956); The effect of epinephrine, levarterenol, and DL-isoproterenol on transmission on the superior cervical ganglion of the cat. *J. Pharmacol. exp. Ther.*, **116**, 433–443.

MCISAAK, R. J., (1966); Ganglionic blocking properties of epinephrine and related amines. *Int. J. Neuropharmacol.*, **5**, 15–26.

MUSCHOLL, E., AND VOGT, M., (1958); The action of reserpine on the peripheral sympathetic system. *J. Physiol. (Lond.)*, **141**, 132–155.

NORBERG, K.-A., (1967); Transmitter histochemistry of the sympathetic adrenergic nervous system. *Brain Res.*, **5**, 125–170.

PARDO, E. G., CATO, J., GIGÓN, E., AND ALONSO-DE-FLORIDA, F., (1963); Influence of several adrenergic drugs on synaptic transmission through the superior cervical and the ciliary ganglia of the cat. *J. Pharmacol. exp. Ther.*, **139**, 296–303.

PATON, W. D. M., AND THOMPSON, J. W., (1953); The mechanism of action of adrenaline on the superior cervical ganglion of the cat. *Abstr. XIX Int. Physiol. Congress*, pp. 664–665.

REINERT, H., (1962); Role and origin of noradrenaline in the superior cervical ganglion. *J. Physiol. (Lond.)*, **167**, 18–29.

SANAN, S., AND VOGT, M., (1962); Effect of drugs on the noradrenaline content of brain and peripheral tissues and its significance. *Brit. J. Pharmacol.*, **18**, 109–127.

TOSAKA, T., CHICHIBU, S., AND LIBET, B., (1968); Intracellular analysis of slow inhibitory and excitatory postsynaptic potentials in sympathetic ganglia of the frog. *J. Neurophysiol.*, **31**, 396–409.

VIZI, E. S., (1967); The inhibitory action of noradrenaline on release of acetylcholine from guinea-pig ileum longitudinal strips. *Arch. Pharmakol. exp. Path.*, **259**, 199–200.

VOLLE, R. L., (1967); Hyperpolarization and blockade of ganglionic transmission. *Arch. int. Pharmacodyn.*, **169**, 35–43.

WEIR, M. C. L., AND MCLENNAN, H., (1963); The action of catecholamines in sympathetic ganglia. *Canad. J. Biochem.*, **41**, 2627–2636.

The Pharmacological Importance of the Uptake Mechanism for Sympathomimetic Amines

U. TRENDELENBURG*

Department of Pharmacology, Harvard Medical School, Boston, Mass. (U.S.A.)

Until about 10 years ago the mechanisms responsible for the termination of the action of norepinephrine at the receptors of effector organs were not known. Although both monoamine oxidase and catechol-*O*-methyl transferase (COMT) were found to be very important in the degradation of norepinephrine, the use of specific inhibitors of these enzymes revealed that the two enzymes do not play the same role in the fate of norepinephrine which acetylcholinesterase plays in the fate of acetylcholine. It was the discovery of the uptake of sympathomimetic amines by adrenergic nerve endings (Axelrod *et al.*, 1959) which seemed to offer the solution of the problem.

Most workers now believe that the intraneuronal uptake of norepinephrine is the most important factor involved in determining the concentration of norepinephrine at the receptors. If one considers steady-state conditions after an administration of exogenous norepinephrine *in vivo* or *in vitro* a certain concentration of norepinephrine is reached in the circulating plasma or in the bath medium, respectively. According to the concept outlined above, intraneuronal uptake of norepinephrine results in a concentration gradient from the plasma (or the medium) to the neighborhood of the nerve endings. If the receptors are located in the close vicinity of the adrenergic nerve endings, the concentration of norepinephrine there is only a fraction of the concentration in the plasma (or in the medium). Since sympathetic denervation leads to the degeneration of the adrenergic nerve endings, the resulting lack of uptake greatly reduces or abolishes the concentration gradient; this leads to supersensitivity. Since cocaine impairs the intraneuronal uptake of norepinephrine, a similar supersensitivity ensues. In both cases the supersensitivity is the result of a change in the concentration of the amine at the receptors and not of a change in the response of the effector cell to a given concentration at the receptors. This type of supersensitivity differs qualitatively from that observed after chronic decentralization which seems to be due to an increase in the response of the effector organ to a given concentration of the amine at the receptors. For this reason the supersensitivity produced by denervation or cocaine may be called presynaptic, while decentralization supersensitivity may be regarded as postsynaptic (Trendelenburg, 1966).

While a very large body of evidence is compatible with these views, there is no

* Present address: Department of Pharmacology, University of Würzburg (Germany).

direct evidence to prove a causal relationship between uptake and its influence on the concentration of norepinephrine at the receptors. The proposed explanation for denervation and cocaine supersensitivity still rests on circumstantial evidence. There are three lines of evidence which provide the main arguments in favor of the hypothesis:

(1) If the hypothesis is true, the degree of denervation or cocaine supersensitivity should be proportional to the rates of uptake of different amines. Although ample information is available on the degree of presynaptic supersensitivity to many different sympathomimetic amines after denervation of the cat's nictitating membrane, relative rates of uptake have been determined for only a few amines. However, where evidence is available, it agrees with the hypothesis. For instance, as in the rat heart (Hertting, 1964; Iversen, 1965) relative rates for the intraneuronal uptake in the isolated nictitating membrane are: norepinephrine > epinephrine >> isoproterenol (Draskóczy and Trendelenburg, 1969). Degrees of denervation supersensitivity for isolated nictitating membranes have to be ranked in the same order. Since the effects of norepinephrine and epinephrine on the nictitating membrane are mediated by alpha-receptors, isoproterenol was tested in the presence of a beta-receptor antagonist, propranolol, so as to determine its alpha-effects. Although isoproterenol has a low potency as an alpha-agonist, it is possible to determine dose–response curves under such conditions. It is of interest that there is no denervation supersensitivity to isoproterenol (Pluchino and Trendelenburg, 1968) for which no intraneuronal uptake was demonstrable (Draskóczy and Trendelenburg, 1968).

(2) A detailed study of the time course of the development of denervation supersensitivity to norepinephrine (Langer and Trendelenburg, 1966; Langer et al., 1967), of the time course of the decline of the ability of denervated nerve endings to accumulate [^{3}H]norepinephrine (Smith et al., 1966) and of the time course of the morphological degeneration of the adrenergic nerve endings of the nictitating membrane (Van Orden et al., 1967) showed convincingly that there is good temporal agreement between the development of supersensitivity, the decline in intraneuronal uptake and the progression of degeneration. Hence, the observations are in agreement with the hypothesis.

(3) All agents which block intraneuronal uptake should cause supersensitivity, while the presynaptic type of supersensitivity should not be observed after agents which fail to impair uptake. Evidence for this view has been presented earlier (Trendelenburg, 1966), and the author is unaware of any recent reports to the contrary.

While the available evidence is in agreement with the proposed hypothesis, there is a number of observations indicating that, if the hypothesis is true, there must be factors able to modify the postulated concentration gradient from the medium to the receptors. For instance, the degree of denervation or cocaine supersensitivity to *l*-norepinephrine differs markedly between organs or species; cocaine is known to fail to potentiate the effects of at least one sympathomimetic amine in spite of the fact that the amine is taken up at a rate similar to that of *l*-norepinephrine; on the normal nictitating membrane dose–response curves for different sympathomimetic amines are not parallel; in the same tissue a competitive blocker of alpha-receptors causes shifts of dose–response curves for norepinephrine which are much smaller than expected from the kinetics of competition for receptors. In the following discussion, an attempt is made to delineate some of the factors that appear to influence the postulated concentration gradient.

SATURABILITY OF UPTAKE AS AN EXPLANATION FOR THE STEREOSELECTIVITY OF THE SENSITIZING ACTION OF COCAINE

On the nictitating membrane of the spinal cat cocaine potentiates the *l*-isomer of norepinephrine much more than the *d*-isomer (Trendelenburg, 1965; Seidehamel *et al.*, 1966). It was tempting to ascribe the stereoselectivity of the sensitizing effect of cocaine to the stereoselectivity of the uptake mechanism since some reports seemed to indicate that *l*-norepinephrine is much more easily taken up than its *d*-isomer (Iversen, 1963; Maickel *et al.*, 1963). However, there is no agreement on this point (Kopin and Bridgers, 1963). Hence, we studied the uptake of both isomers by the rabbit heart as well as the sensitizing effect of cocaine (Draskóczy and Trendelenburg, 1968). According to Lindmar and Muscholl (1964) a reliable measure of uptake is obtained by the determination of the arteriovenous difference in the norepinephrine concentration of a norepinephrine solution perfused through isolated hearts. With this method we found equal rates of uptake of both isomers; hence the stereoselectivity of the sensitizing effect of cocaine observed in this organ cannot be related to differences in the rates of uptake of the two isomers. Moreover, the impairment by cocaine of the uptake of both isomers was equal. An explanation for the stereoselectivity of the sensitizing effect of cocaine was found in the following observations: in agreement with Iversen (1963) uptake of *l*-norepinephrine by the perfused rabbit heart is saturable when the concentration in the perfusate approaches 1 μg/ml; similar saturation was observed with *d*-norepinephrine. Because there is a marked difference in the potency of the two isomers, the following situation arises. *l*-Norepinephrine is pharmacologically effective in very low concentrations which do not yet saturate the uptake mechanism; hence, an impairment of the uptake by cocaine causes pronounced supersensitivity. However, equieffective concentrations of the much less potent *d*-isomer are so high that they saturate the uptake mechanism. Although more *d*-norepinephrine is taken up by adrenergic nerve endings than at lower concentrations of the amine, uptake can remove from the receptors only a very small fraction of the amine. Hence, uptake becomes ineffective in reducing the concentration of *d*-norepinephrine at the receptors, and an impairment of the uptake mechanism by cocaine fails to cause supersensitivity to the *d*-isomer.

This observation should not be interpreted as ruling out the possibility that uptake is stereoselective in other organs or other species. In fact, Iversen (1963 and personal communication) has obtained evidence for stereoselectivity of uptake of norepinephrine in rat but not in guinea-pig hearts.

Apparently saturability is a pharmacologically important characteristic of the uptake mechanism which moves sympathomimetic amines across the nerve membrane. For a proper assessment of the importance of uptake for the concentration of sympathomimetic amines at the receptors, it is not enough to know the relative rates of uptake of various amines; the relation between pharmacologically effective concentrations (*i.e.*, potency) and the point at which uptake of any given amine becomes saturated is equally important. The possible importance of this second factor is emphasized by the fact that most sympathomimetic amines are less potent than *l*-norepinephrine. If they are taken up at rates roughly similar to that of *l*-norepinephrine, and if their uptake is saturable at concentrations similar to those of *l*-norepinephrine, their pharmacological behavior should fall between that of *l*- and *d*-norepinephrine. That is, amines with a low potency have to be administered in concentrations which may saturate uptake; consequently, uptake would be relatively ineffective on the concentration of the amine at the receptors in spite of the fact that the amine may be taken up at a rate quite similar to that of *l*-norepinephrine. In that case, neither denervation nor cocaine should cause pronounced supersensitivity. One has to conclude that the lack of sensitization by either denervation or cocaine cannot be taken as evidence that the amine under study is not taken up. However, the reverse argument still remains true, namely that an amine which is not taken up should not be potentiated by either denervation or cocaine.

SATURABILITY OF UPTAKE AS A DETERMINANT OF THE SLOPES OF DOSE–RESPONSE CURVES FOR SYMPATHOMIMETIC AMINES

On the normal nictitating membrane of the pithed cat dose–response curves for different sympathomimetic amines are not parallel. For 10 directly acting amines there was a highly significant negative correlation between the slope of dose–response curves and the potency of the amines; the lower the potency of any given amine the steeper was its dose–response curve (Langer and Trendelenburg, 1969). Again, saturability of the uptake mechanism seems to account for the phenomenon. Two assumptions may be made: (*a*) that a hypothetical amine is taken up by adrenergic nerve endings, and (*b*) that its dose–response curve falls into that range of concentrations where a gradual increase in the concentration in the plasma (or in the bath solution) causes a gradual saturation of the uptake mechanism. In that case only a small fraction of the ED10 should reach the receptors (because of the effectiveness of uptake), while a large fraction of the ED90 should contribute to the concentration at the receptors (because of saturation of uptake). Thus, a given increase in the concentration of the amine in the plasma (or in the bath) should lead to disproportionately greater increases in the concentration at the receptors. As a result, the dose–response curve of such an amine should be steeper than that of an amine whose dose–response curve falls within the region of linear relation between plasma (or bath) concentration and uptake.

Experimental evidence supporting this working hypothesis is provided by the following observations:

(*1*) A negative correlation between the slope of dose–response curves and the potency of the amine was observed not only *in vivo* but also *in vitro* experiments with isolated nictitating membranes; thus, all factors outside of the nictitating membrane can be excluded.

(*2*) The same correlation was observed *in vivo* when the potency of a given amine (*l*-phenylephrine) was modified experimentally by decentralization (to increase potency without affecting the uptake mechanism) or by the administration of a competitive alpha-receptor antagonist (to decrease potency without affecting uptake).

(*3*) Slopes of dose–response curves of different amines were not related to potency whenever the uptake mechanism was impaired by either denervation or cocaine; this was found both *in vivo* and *in vitro*.

(*4*) In the presence of increasing concentrations of a competitive blocker of alpha-receptors (phentolamine) slopes of dose–response curves for *l*-norepinephrine increased on the normal but not on the denervated isolated nictitating membrane.

(*5*) In the presence of increasing concentrations of a competitive blocker of muscarinic receptors (atropine) slopes of dose–response curves for acetylcholine were parallel irrespective of whether the isolated nictitating membrane was normal or denervated.

These observations indicate clearly that the characteristic relationship between the slope of dose–response curves and the potency of an amine was observed only when the uptake mechanism was intact (*i.e.*, in normal or decentralized muscles). It was not observed when uptake was impaired (after denervation or cocaine) or when the agonist was not taken up (acetylcholine).

If saturability of the uptake mechanism is responsible for the observed phenomena, one can make an additional postulate. Dose–response curves for a given amine should become flat again when they are determined in a region of concentrations high enough to cause nearly complete saturation of the uptake mechanism. This should be so because the ineffectiveness of the saturated uptake mechanism in reducing the concentration of the amine at the receptors must result in a marked reduction or abolition of the postulated concentration gradient from the medium to the receptors. In that case, any given increase in the concentration of the medium should lead to a nearly equal increase in the concentration of the amine at the receptors. Thus, dose–response curves should have slopes identical with those for amines whose dose–response curves fall into the region of unsaturated uptake. Experimental observations agree with the postulate, since dose–response curves for *l*-norepinephrine (determined on the normal isolated nictitating membrane) become flat again in the presence of very high concentrations of phentolamine.

The evidence indicates that differences in the slopes of dose–response curves for different amines (as well as differences in the slopes of dose–response curves for *one* amine determined in the presence of various concentrations of phentolamine) can be attributed to the fact that the saturability of the uptake mechanism results in a non-linear relationship between the bath concentration and the concentration of the amine at the receptors.

Since the ED50 for *l*-norepinephrine on the normal isolated nictitating membrane is about 1 μg/ml, it is very close to that concentration which, according to Iversen (1963), causes partial saturation of the uptake mechanism. Moreover, our own determinations of the uptake of [^{3}H]norepinephrine (Draskóczy and Trendelenburg, 1969; see below) indicate that partial saturation of the uptake into the adrenergic nerve endings of the nictitating membrane occurs with a bath concentration of 1 μg/ml of *dl*-norepinephrine. Apparently, there is good agreement between studies of uptake and the observations discussed above. It should be noted that if an organ is much more sensitive to *l*-norepinephrine than the isolated nictitating membrane, the ED50 of this amine may fall into a range of concentrations which do not yet saturate uptake. In that case experimental results should differ from those reported here for the nictitating membrane. Or in other words, there is good reason to believe that organ differences must exist.

A further reason for differences between organs lies in the morphology of the synapse. The nictitating membrane has a dense adrenergic innervation (as indicated by its high norepinephrine content of about 9 μg/g; Trendelenburg *et al.*, 1969) and the gap between the nerve endings and the effector cells is narrow (Van Orden *et al.*, 1967); hence, the morphology of the synapse favors uptake. Uptake may play only a minor role in determining the concentration of an amine at the receptors if the organ is sparsely innervated by adrenergic fibers or if the distance between nerve endings and receptors is substantially greater than in the nictitating membrane. In that case, saturation of the uptake mechanism should be of minor pharmacological importance, and the relation between potency of amines and slopes of their dose–response curves described for the nictitating membrane may well be absent. The rabbit aorta seems to be a tissue in which there is a wide gap between the adrenergic innervation and the smooth muscle (Bevan and Verity, 1967); changes in the potency of *l*-norepinephrine by various concentrations of phentolamine fail to cause changes in the slopes of dose–response curves in this organ (Trendelenburg, unpublished observations).

It is concluded that under appropriate conditions (*i.e.*, when the adrenergic innervation is dense, when the synaptic gap is narrow, when the amine is taken up, and when its ED50 does not yet cause pronounced saturation of uptake) the saturability of the uptake mechanism has a pronounced influence on the slopes of dose–response curves of sympathomimetic amines.

SATURABILITY OF UPTAKE AS A DETERMINANT OF THE ANTAGONISTIC POTENCY OF A COMPETITIVE BLOCKER OF ADRENERGIC RECEPTORS

If the concentration of an agonist at the receptors is linearly related to the bath concentration, the plot of log (dose-ratio —1) of the agonist against the log molar concentration of a competitive antagonist should yield a straight line with a slope of unity (Arunlakshana and Schild, 1959). If it is true that saturability of the uptake mechanism results in a non-linear relationship between the concentration in the bath and the concentration at the receptors, this plot cannot be expected to yield a straight line with a slope of unity. In fact, shifts of dose–response curves for *l*-norepinephrine in the presence of various concentrations of phentolamine should be smaller on the normal nictitating membrane (in which the saturable uptake mechanism is functioning) than on the denervated membrane (which lacks the intraneuronal uptake mechanism). The postulate is borne out by experimental results. The antagonism of phentolamine to *l*-norepinephrine complies with the postulate of Arunlakshana and Schild (1959) only on the denervated but not on the normal nictitating membrane. The antagonism of atropine to acetylcholine, on the other hand, is typical for that of a competitive antagonist on both the normal and the denervated nictitating membrane (Langer and Trendelenburg, 1969).

It is concluded that the saturability of the uptake mechanism for sympatho-mimetic amines has a pronounced influence on the magnitude of shifts of dose–response curves by a competitive antagonist, phentolamine. Again, it has to be emphasized that such findings cannot be expected with organs in which uptake is less important than in the nictitating membrane in influencing the concentration of sympathomimetic amines at the receptors.

THE INTRANEURONAL AND EXTRANEURONAL ACCUMULATION OF [³H]NOREPINEPHRINE IN THE ISOLATED NICTITATING MEMBRANE

When isolated normal nictitating membranes were incubated with concentrations of dl-[³H]norepinephrine ranging from 0.6 ng/ml to 100 μg/ml (*i.e.*, over a range of more than 5 log units) the [³H]norepinephrine content was found to be linearly related to the bath concentration (Draskóczy and Trendelenburg, 1969). These findings are in agreement with those of Cervoni and McCullough (1967). They were surprising in that uptake in other organs is known to be saturable and also because our pharma-cological evidence indicated that uptake in the nictitating membrane is saturable (see above). The reason for this unexpected linearity between bath concentration and rate of uptake in the normal nictitating membrane became evident when it was found that substantial extraneuronal binding of [³H]norepinephrine takes place in denervated muscles exposed to concentrations of dl-[³H]norepinephrine greater than 0.1 μg/ml. If it is assumed that extraneuronal uptake in the normal muscle is as great as in the denervated muscle, the difference in [³H]norepinephrine content between the normal and the denervated muscle may be regarded as a measure of the intra-neuronal accumulation of the amine. Since the relation between the accumulation of [³H]norepinephrine and the concentration in the medium yields a regression line which is considerably steeper for the denervated than for the normal membrane, the dif-ference in [³H]norepinephrine content between the two membranes (studied under identical conditions) shows a non-linear relation when plotted against the bath concentration. Or in other words, a curve results which is typical for saturation of the intraneuronal uptake mechanism. Moreover, fluorimetric determinations of the sum of endogenous and exogenous norepinephrine recovered from normal muscles indicated that the intraneuronal accumulation of the [³H]norepinephrine in this preparation is only partially due to a net accumulation of exogenous norepineph-rine. A considerable proportion of the intraneuronal [³H]norepinephrine must be due to exchange of exogenous [³H]norepinephrine with endogenous transmitter, since the content in endogenous (non-labeled) norepinephrine fell significantly when muscles were exposed to concentrations of more than 1 μg/ml of dl-[³H]norepineph-rine. The concentration of norepinephrine at the receptors should be decreased only by the net movement of norepinephrine across the nerve membrane and not by an exchange of exogenous with endogenous amine. Hence, the non-linearity of the relation between the concentration in the bath and that at the receptors must have been greater than indicated by the "saturation curve" obtained by plotting the intraneuronal accumulation of [³H]norepinephrine in the way described above. It is concluded that saturation of the uptake mechanism of the nictitating membrane seems to take place at concentrations of norepinephrine which are virtually identical with the ED50. Or in other words, saturation of uptake is observed for concentrations of norepinephrine which had been used in our determinations of slopes and shifts of dose–response curves (see above).

The intraneuronal binding of [³H]norepinephrine in the nictitating membrane is characterized by the following observations: the accumulated [³H]norepinephrine is retained for a long time; intraneuronal binding is antagonized by pretreatment with reserpine, by cocaine and by phenoxybenzamine; it is not affected by meta-nephrine or by block of COMT; it is increased by block of monoamine oxidase. Thus, the intraneuronal accumulation of norepinephrine in the normal nictitating membrane does not differ from that in other organs; the uptake mechanism seems to be pharmaco-logically identical with uptake₁ of Iversen (1967).

Extraneuronal binding of [³H]norepinephrine in the nictitating membrane seems to have quite different pharmacological properties: extraneuronally bound [³H]-norepinephrine has a half life of only about 10 min; extraneuronal binding is antagonized by metanephrine and by phenoxybenzamine; it is not affected by pre-treatment with reserpine or by cocaine; block of COMT increases extraneuronal binding if the concentration of [³H]norepinephrine is low (*i.e.*, does not exceed 1 μg/ml). It is of interest to note that the extraneuronal binding of norepinephrine in the nictitating membrane is similar to or identical with certain uptake mechanisms described very recently. For instance, uptake₂ of Iversen (1967) is cocaine-resistant and metanephrine-sensitive; Gillespie and Hamilton (1967) observed a phenoxy-benzamine-sensitive accumulation of norepinephrine in vascular smooth muscle of the cat's spleen which had a half life of about 10 min; Eisenfeld *et al.* (1967a, b) described a cocaine-resistant and phenoxybenzamine-sensitive extraneuronal uptake of norepinephrine in rat hearts; and Simmonds and Gillis (1968) also obtained evidence for both intra- and extra-neuronal uptake of norepinephrine in the rat heart.

Further differences in the properties of intra- and extra-neuronal binding became apparent when the accumulation of three amines was studied in the nictitating mem-brane. For intraneuronal binding, the accumulation was found to be: [³H]norepi-nephrine $>$ [³H]epinephrine $>>$ [³H]isoproterenol (for which no intraneuronal accumulation was demonstrable). However, for extraneuronal accumulation the ranking order was isoproterenol $>>$ epinephrine $\geqq$ norepinephrine. Thus, it is evident that the importance of intraneuronal binding relative to the extraneuronal binding differs greatly for different amines. Apparently, the structural requirements for intra- and extra-neuronal accumulation are quite different.

It is not yet clear whether extraneuronal binding of sympathomimetic amines has an influence on the concentration gradient from the medium to the receptors. How-ever, this is quite a possibility in the nictitating membrane, since substantial extraneuronal binding is observed with concentrations which are equal to or greater than the ED50 of *l*-norepinephrine. Thus, extraneuronal uptake is observed with concentrations of norepinephrine (and epinephrine) which fall within the range of the dose–response curve for the normal nictitating membrane. Again, it should be emphasized that there are organs which are much more sensitive to norepinephrine; in that case, extraneuronal binding may occur only with concentrations of norepinephrine which are in excess of the ED100.

There is one indication that extraneuronally bound norepinephrine influences the concentration of this amine at the receptors. After termination of an exposure of the denervated isolated nictitating membrane to various concentrations of norepinephrine the time course of the relaxation of the muscle was followed. It is striking that relaxation is very fast when muscles had been exposed to not more than 1 μg/ml of norepinephrine. After an exposure to higher concentrations (10 or 100 μg/ml of norepinephrine), on the other hand, relaxation was much slower than one would have to expect from simple diffusion. Since extraneuronally bound norepinephrine leaves the stores with a half-life time of about 10 min (see above), it is likely that at least some of this norepinephrine leaves the stores unchanged and contributes to the concentration at the receptors.

From these observations two conclusions may be drawn: (*1*) the intraneuronal uptake mechanism of the adrenergic nerve endings of the nictitating membrane is saturable; and (*2*) concentrations of norepinephrine which begin to saturate the intraneuronal uptake mechanism lead to the extraneuronal accumulation of norepinephrine. Moreover, it is important to realize that all these observations were made with concentrations of norepinephrine which are below the ED100, *i.e.*, which fall within the range of a normal dose–response curve.

THE INFLUENCE OF COMT ON THE CONCENTRATION OF SYMPATHO-MIMETIC AMINES AT THE RECEPTORS

Block of COMT fails to alter the sensitivity of the isolated normal nictitating membrane to *l*-norepinephrine but causes a 4-fold increase in the sensitivity of the denervated muscle (Trendelenburg, unpublished observations). It is tempting to suggest that the influence of COMT on the concentration of norepinephrine at the receptors is much smaller than that of the intraneuronal uptake mechanism; hence, this weak influence is demonstrable only in the absence of intraneuronal uptake. However, as already pointed out by Eisenfeld *et al.* (1967a, b) access to COMT seems to be a saturable process. This view is supported by the fact that the contribution of *O*-methylated metabolites to the total radioactivity of the denervated muscle after an incubation with *dl*-[³H]norepinephrine, *dl*-[³H]epinephrine or *dl*-[³H]isoproterenol is inversely proportional to the concentration of the amines in the bath (Draskóczy and Trendelenburg, 1969). Thus, denervation not only removes the intraneuronal uptake mechanism and thereby enables COMT to exert its modest influence on the concentration of norepinephrine at the receptors, the increase in sensitivity shifts the whole dose–response curve for norepinephrine so far to the left that pharmacologically

References p. 84–85

effective concentrations are then below the range in which saturation of the access to COMT is observed.

This problem of saturability of access to COMT is also illustrated by the following observations. Isoproterenol has a very high potency as a beta-agonist (causing relaxation of the nictitating membrane; Thompson, 1958; Smith, 1963), and its beta-effects are potentiated by block of COMT. On the other hand, this amine has a low potency as an alpha-agonist (causing contraction of the nictitating membrane in the presence of a beta-receptor antagonist, propranolol), and its alpha-effects are not potentiated by block of COMT (Pluchino and Trendelenburg, unpublished observations). Determinations of the O-methylated metabolites of [^{3}H]isoproterenol indicate that saturation of the access to the enzyme is pronounced for concentrations required to elicit alpha-effects, while it is minimal for concentrations effective on beta-receptors.

Apparently, two factors determine the importance of COMT for the concentration of a given amine at the receptors. (*1*) the relative importance of COMT with regard to that of the intraneuronal uptake mechanism; if an amine is taken up at a high rate, if the innervation is dense, if the synaptic gap is narrow, and if intraneuronal uptake is not saturated, COMT probably plays a very minor role in influencing the concentration of the amine at the receptors; if, on the other hand, the various factors governing the importance of the uptake mechanism are less favorable, COMT may well gain in importance; (*2*) the access to COMT seems to be a saturable process; hence, the importance of COMT is also dependent on the concentration of the amine under study.

THE DENSITY OF ADRENERGIC INNERVATION AS A DETERMINANT OF THE SENSITIVITY OF AN ORGAN TO SYMPATHOMIMETIC AMINES

The nictitating membrane is inserted by the medial and inferior smooth muscles (Acheson, 1938). The norepinephrine content of the medial muscle is consistently higher than that of the inferior muscle (Trendelenburg et al., 1969). This difference is not due to differences in the amount of connective tissue in the isolated muscle preparations; the norepinephrine content per gram of muscle protein of the inferior muscle is only 53% of that for the medial muscle. Apparently, the difference in endogenous norepinephrine content reflects a difference in density of adrenergic innervation; two additional observations are consistent with this view. (*1*) When the accumulation of [^{3}H]norepinephrine (after an incubation of the muscles with the amine) is expressed as μg of amine per gram of tissue, the medial muscle contains nearly twice as much [^{3}H]norepinephrine as the inferior muscle; however, there is no difference when the [^{3}H]norepinephrine content is related to the amount of endogenous norepinephrine (determined fluorimetrically). (*2*) The sensitivity of the more densely innervated medial muscle to l-norepinephrine and l-epinephrine is slightly but significantly lower than that of the less densely innervated inferior muscle. This difference in sensitivity is observed only for normal muscles; it is absent after denervation. Moreover, there is no difference in the sensitivity of normal muscles if the agonist is not taken up by the nerve endings (*e.g.*, isoproterenol and acetylcholine).

It is concluded that a more densely innervated smooth muscle takes up more norepinephrine per unit of weight of the tissue, and has a lower sensitivity to norepinephrine (or epinephrine) than the less densely innervated muscle. The importance of the intraneuronal uptake for the concentration of amines at the receptors seems to be proportional to the density of adrenergic innervation.

THE MORPHOLOGICAL RELATION BETWEEN ADRENERGIC NERVE ENDINGS AND EFFECTOR CELLS

There is increasing evidence that the morphological relation between nerve endings and receptors differs markedly from organ to organ. For instance, adrenergic nerve endings are found in close vicinity of the smooth muscle cells of the nictitating membrane (Van Orden *et al.*, 1967). In many types of blood vessels, on the other hand, the smooth muscle cells (of the media) seem to be at quite a distance from the adrenergic nerve endings which terminate in the adventitia or, at best, in the outer layers of the media. For the rabbit aorta there is both morphological and pharmacological evidence indicating that the distance between nerve endings and smooth muscle cells is very considerable (Bevan and Verity, 1967).

The effectiveness with which the intraneuronal uptake mechanism removes norepinephrine from the neighborhood of the receptors should be dependent on the width of the synaptic gap. If the gap is wide, impairment of uptake by either denervation or cocaine should cause only a small degree of supersensitivity to norepinephrine in spite of the fact that norepinephrine is easily taken up into the adrenergic neurons. For the isolated rabbit aorta results agree with the postulate: the degree of supersensitivity after denervation or after cocaine is much smaller than that observed for the nictitating membrane (Bevan and Verity, 1967; Trendelenburg *et al.*, 1969).

A very elegant illustration of the importance of the morphological relation between the sites of uptake (*i.e.*, the nerve endings) and the sites of action (*i.e.*, the receptors) is provided by the experiments of De la Lande and Waterson (1967). The authors administered norepinephrine either intraluminally or extraluminally to the perfused ear artery of the rabbit. Intraluminal norepinephrine reaches the smooth muscle of the media before it diffuses to the adrenergic nerve endings which are located at the border of the media and the adventitia. As a consequence, intraneuronal uptake is relatively unimportant for the concentration of norepinephrine at the receptors, the sensitivity of the perfused artery is high, and cocaine causes only a small degree of supersensitivity. Extraluminally administered norepinephrine, on the other hand, reaches the sites of action only after having passed by the sites of uptake. Consequently, intraneuronal uptake has a pronounced influence on the concentration of norepinephrine at the receptors, the sensitivity of the tissue to the amine is low, and cocaine causes marked supersensitivity.

Although there is a lack of systematic comparative studies of the pharmacology and morphology of different organs, the available evidence is in favor of the view that the morphological organization of adrenergic synapses is an important determinant of their pharmacology.

CONCLUSIONS

A few years ago it became evident that the intraneuronal uptake of sympathomimetic amines was the most important mechanism involved in influencing the concentration of the amines at the receptors. Evidence obtained in recent years (and reviewed in this article) is in agreement with this view. Moreover, it has become evident that there are various factors which can modify the importance of the uptake mechanism.

For an assessment of the importance of the intraneuronal uptake mechanism in influencing the concentration of sympathomimetic amines at the receptors, the following factors should be known: (1) The rate of intraneuronal uptake (determined at concentrations which do not saturate the uptake mechanism). (2) The relation between potency of the amine and the concentration which causes partial saturation of uptake. (3) The degree of extraneuronal binding observed with pharmacologically effective concentrations of the amine under study. (4) The effect of enzymes (i.e., of COMT and monoamine oxidase) on the concentration of sympathomimetic amines at the receptors with particular attention to the possibility of saturation of the enzymes or of access to the enzymes. (5) The density of adrenergic innervation. (6) The morphological relationship between effector cells and adrenergic nerve endings.

Although our knowledge of these factors is still incomplete, it seems to be safe to state that most (and perhaps all) are able to modify the pharmacological importance of the intraneuronal uptake mechanism.

REFERENCES

ACHESON, G. H., (1938); The topographical anatomy of the smooth muscle of the cat's nictitating membrane. *Anat. Rec.*, **71**, 297–311.

ARUNLAKSHANA, O., AND SCHILD, H. O., (1959); Some quantitative uses of drug antagonists. *Brit. J. Pharmacol.*, **14**, 48–58.

AXELROD, J., WEIL-MALHERBE, H., AND TOMCHICK, R., (1959); The physiological disposition of H^3-epinephrine and its metabolite metanephrine. *J. Pharmacol. exp. Ther.*, **127**, 251–256.

BEVAN, J. A., AND VERITY, M. A., (1967); Sympathetic nerve-free vascular muscle. *J. Pharmacol. exp. Ther.*, **157**, 117–124.

CERVONI, P., AND MCCULLOUGH, J., (1967); Uptake of catecholamines in normal, decentralized and denervated cat nictitating membrane *in vivo* and *in vitro. Fed. Proc.*, **26**, 509.

DE LA LANDE, I. S., AND WATERSON, J. G., (1967); Site of action of cocaine on the perfused artery. *Nature (Lond.)*, **214**, 313–314.

DRASKÓCZY, P. R., AND TRENDELENBURG, U., (1968); The uptake of *l*- and *d*-norepinephrine by the isolated perfused rabbit heart in relation to the stereospecificity of the sensitizing action of cocaine. *J. Pharmacol. exp. Ther.*, **159**, 66–73.

DRASKÓCZY, P. R., AND TRENDELENBURG, U., (1969); Intra- and extraneuronal uptake of various sympathomimetic amines in the isolated cat's nictitating membrane. In preparation.

EISENFELD, A. J., AXELROD, J., AND KRAKOFF, L., (1967a); Inhibition of the extraneuronal accumulation and metabolism of norepinephrine by adrenergic blocking agents. *J. Pharmacol. exp. Ther.*, **156**, 107–113.

EISENFELD, A. J., LANDSBERG, L., AND AXELROD, J., (1967b); Effect of drugs on the accumulation and metabolism of extraneuronal norepinephrine in the rat heart. *J. Pharmacol. exp. Ther.*, **158**, 378–385.

GILLESPIE, J. S., AND HAMILTON, D. N. H., (1967); A possible active transport of noradrenaline into arterial smooth muscle cells. *J. Physiol. (Lond.)*, **192**, 30P.

HERTTING, G., (1964); The fate of ^{3}H-isoproterenol in the rat. *Biochem. Pharmacol.*, **13**, 1119–1128.

IVERSEN, L. L., (1963); The uptake of noradrenaline by the isolated perfused rat heart. *Brit. J. Pharmacol.*, **21**, 523–537.

IVERSEN, L. L., (1965); The uptake of adrenaline by the rat isolated heart. *Brit. J. Pharmacol.*, **24**, 387–394.

IVERSEN, L. L., (1967); *The Uptake and Storage of Noradrenaline in Sympathetic Nerves*, Cambridge University Press, Cambridge, England.

KOPIN, I. J., AND BRIDGERS, W., (1963); Differences in *d*- and *l*-norepinephrine-H^3. *Life Sci.*, **2**, 356–362.

LANGER, S. Z., DRASKÓCZY, P. R., AND TRENDELENBURG, U., (1967); Time course of the development of supersensitivity to various amines in the nictitating membrane of the pithed cat after denervation or decentralization. *J. Pharmacol. exp. Ther.*, **157**, 255–273.

LANGER, S. Z., AND TRENDELENBURG, U., (1966); The onset of denervation supersensitivity. *J. Pharmacol. exp. Ther.*, **151**, 73–86.

LANGER, S. Z., AND TRENDELENBURG, U., (1969); The effect of a saturable uptake mechanism on the slopes of dose–response curves for sympathomimetic amines and on the shifts of dose–response curves by a competitive antagonist. *J. Pharmacol. exp. Ther.*, in the press.

LINDMAR, R., AND MUSCHOLL, E., (1964); Die Wirkung von Pharmaka auf die Elimination von Noradrenalin aus der Perfusionsflüssigkeit und die Noradrenalinaufnahme in das isolierte Herz. *Naunyn-Schmiedeberg's Arch. exp. Path. Pharmak.*, **247**, 469–492.

MAICKEL, R. P., BEAVEN, M. A., AND BRODIE, B. B., (1963); Implications of uptake and storage of norepinephrine by sympathetic nerve endings. *Life Sci.*, **2**, 953–958.

PLUCHINO, S., AND TRENDELENBURG, U., (1968); The influence of denervation and of decentralization on the α- and β-effects of isoproterenol on the nictitating membrane of the pithed cat. *J. Pharmacol. exp. Ther.*, **163**, 257–265.

SEIDEHAMEL, R. J., PATIL, P. N., TYE, A., AND LAPIDUS, J. B., (1966); The effects of norepinephrine isomers on various supersensitivities of the cat nictitating membrane. *J. Pharmacol. exp. Ther.*, **153**, 81–89.

SIMMONDS, M. A., AND GILLIS, C. N., (1968); Uptake of normetanephrine and norepinephrine by cocaine-treated rat heart. *J. Pharmacol. exp. Ther.*, **159**, 283–289.

SMITH, C. B., (1963); Relaxation of the nictitating membrane of the spinal cat by sympathomimetic amines. *J. Pharmacol. exp. Ther.*, **142**, 163–170.

SMITH, C. B., TRENDELENBURG, U., LANGER, S. Z., AND TSAI, T. H., (1966); The relation of retention of norepinephrine-H^3 to the norepinephrine content of the nictitating membrane of the spinal cat during development of denervation supersensitivity. *J. Pharmacol. exp. Ther.*, **151**, 87–94.

THOMPSON, J. W., (1958); Studies on the response of the isolated nictitating membrane of the cat. *J. Physiol. (Lond.)*, **141**, 46–72.

TRENDELENBURG, U., (1965); Supersensitivity by cocaine to dextrorotatory isomers of norepinephrine and epinephrine. *J. Pharmacol. exp. Ther.*, **148**, 329–338.

TRENDELENBURG, U., (1966); Mechanisms of supersensitivity and subsensitivity to sympathomimetic amines. *Pharmacol. Rev.*, **18**, 629–640.

TRENDELENBURG, U., DRASKÓCZY, P. R., AND PLUCHINO, S., (1969); The density of adrenergic innervation of the cat's nictitating membrane as a factor influencing the sensitivity of the isolated preparation to *l*-norepinephrine. *J. Pharmacol. exp. Ther.*, in the press.

VAN ORDEN III, L. S., BENSCH, K. G., LANGER, S. Z., AND TRENDELENBURG, U., (1967); Histochemical and fine structural aspects of the onset of denervation supersensitivity in the nictitating membrane of the spinal cat. *J. Pharmacol. exp. Ther.*, **157**, 274–283.

Microfluorimetric Investigations of Catecholamine-Containing Neurons*

W. LICHTENSTEIGER AND H. LANGEMANN

Department of Pharmacology, University of Zürich (Switzerland)

A topographical differentiation of findings related to monoamine-containing neurons has become feasible with the development of the histochemical fluorescence method of Falck *et al.* (1962). However, if one intends to use this method for the detection of minor variations in the monoamine concentration that might possibly accompany functional changes, a microfluorimetric analysis of the monoamine fluorescence is necessary. Within certain limits, the fluorescence method of Falck *et al.* is suited for such an adaptation (Ritzén, 1966). We decided to start with measurements of the fluorescence intensity of catecholamine-containing nerve cell bodies. Although this site is somewhat remote from the adrenergic synapse, we think it appropriate to discuss our results in this Symposium, because they illustrate an approach at the topographical differentiation of quantitative analysis.

The catecholamine-containing nerve cells we have studied are situated in the arcuate and periventricular nuclei of the hypothalamus and in the substantia nigra. Those of the *tuberal group* have been shown — by pharmacological experiments (Lichtensteiger and Langemann, 1965, 1966) and by degeneration studies (Fuxe and Hökfelt, 1966) — to send their axons down to the external layer of the median eminence. They terminate in the region of the primary plexus of the hypophysial portal system (Fuxe, 1964; Lichtensteiger and Langemann, 1966; and unpublished observations). In the same location, small dense-core vesicles that could contain catecholamines have been observed in some nerve endings in the neighborhood of capillaries (Hökfelt, 1967; Pellegrino de Iraldi and Etcheverry, 1967). These topographical relationships strongly suggest that the catecholamine-containing tubero-infundibular neurons might be involved in the control of anterior pituitary function. Therefore, we investigated the intensity of the catecholamine fluorescence in the nerve cell bodies of this neuron group first during the estrous cycle.

Female albino rats were kept under controlled lighting and temperature conditions (light period from 05.00 to 19.00 h; 22°). Only rats that showed a regular 4-day estrous cycle in their vaginal smears were studied. They were killed by decapitation between 14.00 and 14.15 h in order to avoid possible diurnal variations, and their brains were worked up according to the method of Falck *et al.* in a strictly standardized

* Supported by the Swiss National Foundation for Scientific Research (Grants Nos. 4309 and 4563).

References p. 92–93

manner. A detailed description of the method is given elsewhere (Lichtensteiger, 1969); therefore, we shall content ourselves with a brief survey of the essential points of the microfluorimetric analysis. The measurements were performed in epi-illumination at a magnification of 700 ×. The exciting light from a stabilized xenon lamp was conducted through a Schott BG 3 filter, and the emitted light passed through a Leitz K470 filter. A rectangular diaphragm was inserted in the course of the emitted light and adjusted to give a measuring field of 2.8 × 2.8 μ in the section. It was centered on a portion of the fluorescent cell body. In order to avoid scattering of light, the illuminated area was reduced to a diameter of 19 μ before every measurement by closing an illumination field diaphragm. The emitted light was detected by a photomultiplier and recorded. The absolute intensity readings of the nerve cells were referred to the fluorescence intensity of a gelatin standard containing norepinephrine (NE) and ascorbic acid as a reducing agent. Small blocks of this and of a NE-free standard were processed, embedded and cut together with the brain tissue. The relative fluorescence intensity of a nerve cell was then obtained from the equation

$$I_r = \frac{c-t}{g_{NE}-g_f}$$

where c is the absolute fluorescence intensity of the cell, t the mean intensity (3 measurements) of the background fluorescence of that section serving as an approximation of the non-specific fluorescence of the cell, and where g_{NE} and g_f are the mean intensities of the NE-containing (4–6 measurements) and of the NE-free (3 measurements) standards of the same section. In this way the fluorescence readings were corrected with respect to the reaction conditions and to the thickness of the section. In a series of about 30 sections of 7 μ taken at regular intervals through the tuberal region, every nerve cell that exhibited a visible catecholamine fluorescence in the monocular tube was measured, whereas in the substantia nigra the measurements were started at the lateral border of the region and continued until a fixed number (17) of neighboring cells per section had been investigated. The cells were grouped according to their relative fluorescense intensity I_r into 22 classes, each class representing a 10% change in I_r.

The frequency distributions of relative fluorescence intensity that were derived from these data showed characteristic changes during the *estrous cycle*. Preliminary results (Lichtensteiger, 1967) have subsequently been confirmed in a different strain of albino rats (Lichtensteiger, 1969), where 5 females (2000–2500 nerve cells in the tuberal region and about 400 nerve cells in the substantia nigra) were studied for each of the four days of the estrous cycle.

In the *tuberal region* maximal frequencies are observed at 14.00 h on diestrous day 1 in classes of low relative fluorescence intensity, but a few cells with high fluorescence intensity also occur. Accordingly, the frequency distribution is distinctly unsymmetrical. Between diestrous days 1 and 2 a considerable shift to classes of higher fluorescence intensity takes place. It continues until the estrous day. At the same time, the symmetry of the frequency distributions increases. The transition to diestrous day 1 is then characterized by a marked decrease in the frequency of cells with high and medium fluorescence intensity as well as by a loss of symmetry of the frequency distribution. These changes are reflected by the mean relative fluorescence intensities of the four groups which are: 41.2% of NE standard on diestrous day 1, 57.5% on diestrous day 2, 63.4% on proestrous day and 67.2% on estrous day (Fig. 1). The changes in symmetry can be expressed in terms of the coefficient $\beta_1 = \mu_3{}^2/\mu_2{}^3$ of the skewness, where μ_2 and μ_3 are the 2nd and 3rd central moments, respectively. This coefficient is equal to zero in a completely symmetrical distribution ($\mu_3 = 0$) and increases with decreasing symmetry. The estimates b_1 of β_1 that were calculated on the basis of the actual frequency distributions show a continuous decrease from diestrous day 1 to estrous day which confirms the increase in symmetry of the frequency distributions during this period (Fig. 1). Significant differences ($p \leqslant 0.001$) are found between the distributions of the four groups, between the means and between the coefficients b_1 of diestrous day 1 against diestrous day 2, of diestrous day 2 against proestrous day and of estrous day against diestrous day 1. [For details of the statistical analysis, the reader is referred to Lichtensteiger (1969).] The frequency distributions of the four days of the cycle are thus well characterized, those of proestrous and estrous days being rather similar.

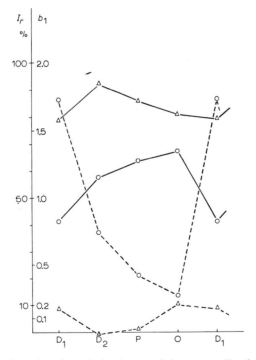

Fig. 1. The fluorescence intensity of catecholamine-containing nerve cells of the tuberal region (○) and of the substantia nigra (△) of the rat during the 4-day estrous cycle. Solid lines: mean relative intensity I_r of catecholamine fluorescence in percent of the fluorescence intensity of the NE standard. Broken lines: coefficients b_1 of skewness of the frequency distributions. D_1 = diestrous day 1; D_2 = diestrous day 2; P = proestrous day; O = estrous day. The values are calculated from the total cell counts of 5 rats for each of the four days of the cycle. For further explanations, the reader is referred to the text.

The catecholamine-containing nerve cells of the *substantia nigra* were chosen for comparison, because they are not connected directly to the median eminence. Their frequency distributions present an entirely different picture. There occur rather slight changes in the mean relative fluorescence intensity, but their sequence differs from that found in the tuberal region (Fig. 1). Maximal values are reached on diestrous day 2 with 92.0% of NE standard intensity. The means of the other days are 78.8% for diestrous day 1, 85.7% for proestrous day and 80.7% for estrous day. Values of the coefficients b_1 of the skewness that are lower than those observed in the tuberal region indicate a higher degree of symmetry in the frequency distributions. It does not vary significantly during the cycle (Fig. 1). In marked contrast to the tuberal region, the distribution of diestrous day 1 and estrous day are here very similar.

If we restrict our discussion to the possible occurrence of primary catecholamines, then a change in the intensity of the catecholamine fluorescence can be explained by a change in the concentration of the amine. Since increased neuronal activity is reported to provoke an increase in catecholamine concentration in central nerve cell bodies (Andén *et al.*, 1966; Corrodi *et al.*, 1967) and also to enhance transmitter synthesis in peripheral adrenergic neurons (Austin *et al.*, 1967; Roth *et al.*, 1966; Sedvall and Kopin, 1967), the increase in fluorescence intensity that was observed in a majority of tuberal catecholamine-containing nerve cells between diestrous day 1 and estrous day may also be due to a stimulation of these neurons. The considerable variations in the symmetry of the frequency distributions appear to indicate that not all of these nerve cells were in the same reactive state at the same time. This is especially evident on diestrous day 1, when a few strongly fluorescent nerve cells are still present, although the majority of them develop a comparatively weak fluorescence.

With only slight changes in the mean fluorescence intensity and no change in the symmetry of the frequency distributions, the catecholamine-containing nerve cells of the substantia nigra show an entirely different reactive pattern. These findings strongly suggest that the variations observed in the tuberal region are caused by a special functional involvement of the tubero-infundibular catecholamine-containing neurons during the estrous cycle. Accordingly, we have tried to answer the question whether disturbances of the pituitary-gonadal axis could exert some influence on the catecholamine content of the tuberal nerve cells (Lichtensteiger *et al.*, 1968a, b).

In one series of experiments, three groups of 5 female rats that had previously shown a regular 4-day estrous cycle were ovariectomized on diestrous day 1 and investigated 4, 7 and 8 days later. If the cyclic changes of fluorescence intensity in the tuberal catecholamine-containing nerve cells had not been influenced, days 4 and 8 should exhibit frequency distributions of the diestrous day 1 type and day 7 one of estrous day type. However, the frequency distribution of day 7 resembles that of diestrous day 1 as shown by the mean relative fluorescence intensity of 40.9%, whereas the values of days 4 and 8 (49.4 and 48.3% respectively) are intermediary between diestrous days 1 and 2. The distributions are rather unsymmetrical. At present we cannot give a complete description of the sequence of changes in fluorescence intensity that is induced by ovariectomy, but it is evident from our results that the original cycle is interrupted.

Six rats have so far been studied three or more weeks (3–7 weeks) after ovariectomy. At this time, the frequency distribution strongly resembles that of diestrous day 2. The mean relative fluorescence intensity (54.9%) corresponds to that of diestrous day 2, and the symmetry is also similar. When we treated the ovariectomized animals with 10 μg of estradiol dipropionate (s.c. in oily solution) at this stage, we induced a marked dislocation of the frequency distribution towards classes of lower fluorescence intensity (Fig. 2). The fluorescence intensity of the tuberal catecholamine-containing nerve cells was determined 24 and 48 h after the injection. In the latter group of 5 rats that has already been completed, the frequency distribution is similar to that of diestrous day 1, with a mean fluorescence intensity of 37.7%. This value is significantly different ($p \leqslant 0.01$) from that of the ovariectomized control animals. The symmetry of the frequency distribution appears to be even lower than on diestrous day 1 and differs considerably from that of the ovariectomized controls. Whether this change is related to a direct or indirect feedback action of the steroid itself or to its influence on the level of gonadotropins, remains to be established.

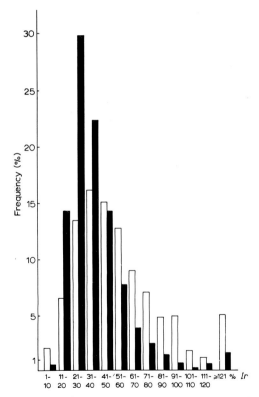

Fig. 2. Tuberal region. Frequency distributions of catecholamine-containing nerve cells classified according to their relative fluorescence intensities at 14.00 h. Abscissae: relative intensities of catecholamine fluorescence in percent of the fluorescence intensity of the NE standard. Ordinate: cell frequencies in percent of the total cell number of each group. The rats had been ovariectomized for 3 weeks or more. After treatment with 10 μg of estradiol dipropionate, a marked shift of the frequency distribution to classes of lower fluorescence intensity was observed. □, ovariectomized controls; ■, oestradiol dipropionate 1 × 10 μg, 48 h.

References p. 92–93

On the other hand, a 2-days' treatment of 5 ovariectomized rats with 2×2 mg progesterone s.c. did not significantly change the mean relative fluorescence intensity which has been calculated as 52.9%. A certain loss of symmetry of the frequency distribution is indicated by the increase in the coefficient b_1. Its interpretation is uncertain.

The results of this second series of experiments clearly demonstrate that the catecholamine content of the tuberal nerve cells is influenced by ovariectomy and by estrogen. They further support the hypothesis of a role of these tubero-infundibular neurons in the control of anterior pituitary function. It is interesting to note that some time after ovariectomy the frequency distribution assumes an intermediary position similar to that of diestrous day 2, which can be displaced towards lower values of fluorescence intensity by the administration of estrogen. On the other hand, frequency distributions similar to those of proestrous or estrous day with a considerable proportion of intensely fluorescent nerve cells and high degrees of symmetry, have not so far been observed in the experimental animals. In other words, we have not yet created conditions that could provoke this additional increase in fluorescence intensity. It might be related to ovulation.

While these and other studies (Fuxe *et al.*, 1967) indicate that the catecholamine-containing tubero-infundibular neurons probably take part in the control of anterior pituitary function, we do not know the mechanism by which this control is exerted. This question has recently been discussed in some detail (Lichtensteiger, 1969).

In the context of the present Symposium, our results are meant to serve as an example of a functional analysis of the catecholamine content of single neurons.

SUMMARY

The intensity of the catecholamine fluorescence was measured in nerve cells of the tuberal region and of the substantia nigra of female rats by means of an adaptation for microfluorimetry of the fluorescence method of Falck *et al.* Frequency distributions of these nerve cells were established on the basis of their relative fluorescence intensities (referred to a norepinephrine standard). During the 4-day estrous cycle, marked changes of the frequency distributions were observed in the tuberal region, whereas the substantia nigra showed only slight changes of a different rhythm. The catecholamine fluorescence of the tuberal nerve cells has further been found to be influenced by ovariectomy and by subsequent estrogen treatment. The findings are interpreted as reflecting activity changes of these neurons. They illustrate a possible approach to a quantitative functional analysis of the catecholamine content of single neurons.

REFERENCES

ANDÉN, N.-E., DAHLSTRÖM, A., FUXE, K., LARSSON, K., OLSON, L., AND UNGERSTEDT, U., (1966); Ascending monoamine neurons to the telencephalon and diencephalon. *Acta physiol. scand.*, **67**. 313–326,

AUSTIN, L., LIVETT, B. G., AND CHUBB, I. W., (1967); Increased synthesis and release of noradrenaline and dopamine during nerve stimulation. *Life Sci.*, **6**, 97–104.

CORRODI, H., FUXE, K., AND HÖKFELT, T., (1967); The effect of neuroleptics on the activity of central catecholamine neurons. *Life Sci.*, **6**, 767–774.

FALCK, B., HILLARP, N.-Å., THIEME, G., AND TORP, A., (1962); Fluorescence of catecholamines and related compounds condensed with formaldehyde. *J. Histochem. Cytochem.*, **10**, 348–354.

FUXE, K., (1964); Cellular localization of monoamines in the median eminence and the infundibular stem of some mammals. *Z. Zellforsch.*, **61**, 710–724.

FUXE, K., AND HÖKFELT, T., (1966); Further evidence for the existence of tubero-infundibular dopamine neurons. *Acta physiol. scand.*, **66**, 245–246.

FUXE, K., HÖKFELT, T., AND NILSSON, O., (1967); Activity changes in the tubero-infundibular dopamine neurons of the rat during various states of the reproductive cycle. *Life Sci.*, **6**, 2057–2061.

HÖKFELT, T., (1967); The possible ultrastructural identification of tubero-infundibular dopamine-containing nerve endings in the median eminence of the rat. *Brain Res.*, **5**, 121–123.

LICHTENSTEIGER, W., (1967); Mikrofluorimetrische Studien an katecholaminhaltigen hypothalamischen Nervenzellen der Ratte in den verschiedenen Phasen des viertägigen Oestruszyklus. *Helv. physiol. pharmacol. Acta*, **25**, CR 423–CR 425.

LICHTENSTEIGER, W., (1969); Cyclic variations of catecholamine content in hypothalamic nerve cells during the estrous cycle of the rat, with a concomitant study of the substantia nigra. *J. Pharmacol. exp. Ther.*, in the press.

LICHTENSTEIGER, W., AND LANGEMANN, H., (1965); Aufnahme exogener Katecholamine in monoaminhaltige Neurone des ZNS. *Helv. physiol. pharmacol. Acta*, **23**, C 31–C 33.

LICHTENSTEIGER, W., AND LANGEMANN, H., (1966); Uptake of exogenous catecholamines by monoamine-containing neurons of the central nervous system: Uptake of catecholamines by arcuato-infundibular neurons. *J. Pharmacol. exp. Ther.*, **151**, 400–408.

LICHTENSTEIGER, W., KORPELA, K., AND LANGEMANN, H., (1968a); Mikrofluorimetrische Studien an katecholaminhaltigen hypothalamischen Nervenzellen der Ratte. Der Einfluss von Ovariektomie und gonadalen Steroiden. *Helv. physiol. pharmacol. Acta*, in the press.

LICHTENSTEIGER, W., KORPELA, K., LANGEMANN, H., AND KELLER, P. J., (1968b); The influence of ovariectomy, estrogen, and progesterone on the catecholamine content of hypothalamic nerve cells in the rat. To be published.

PELLEGRINO DE IRALDI, A., AND ETCHEVERRY, G. J., (1967); Ultrastructural changes in the nerve endings of the median eminence after nialamide–DOPA administration. *Brain Res.*, **6**, 614–618.

RITZÉN, M., (1966); Quantitative fluorescence microspectrophotometry of catecholamine–formaldehyde products. *Exp. Cell Res.*, **44**, 505–520.

ROTH, R. H., STJÄRNE, L., AND EULER, U. S. VON, (1966); Acceleration of noradrenaline biosynthesis by nerve stimulation. *Life Sci.*, **5**, 1071–1075.

SEDVALL, G. C., AND KOPIN, I. J., (1967); Acceleration of norepinephrine synthesis in the rat submaxillary gland *in vivo* during sympathetic nerve stimulation. *Life Sci.*, **6**, 45–51.

Metabolic Effects of Nerve Impulses and Nerve-Growth Factor in Sympathetic Ganglia

M. G. LARRABEE

Thomas C. Jenkins Department of Biophysics, The Johns Hopkins University, Baltimore, Md. (U.S.A.)

Sympathetic ganglia are portions of the nervous system which are relatively accessible and relatively easy to bring under experimental control. Therefore numerous studies have been made of their synaptic mechanisms, of their cellular metabolism, and of the modification of their properties by various environmental changes. Not only are they significant in the economy of the total organism and therefore worthy of investigation in their own right, but the study of such experimentally advantageous and relatively simple systems is a useful prelude to the investigation of more complex arrangements, such as those in the brain.

The experiments I shall be discussing were mostly conducted on ganglia after excision from the animal, in order to obtain better controlled conditions. In choosing the species for such purposes one must make a balanced selection between very small ganglia, which may be best supported by diffusion exchange, and larger ganglia, on which quantitative measurements are easier. For the readily accessible superior cervical ganglia of mammals, the available range of sizes is indicated in Fig. 1. Over the extraordinary weight range from a young mouse of 2 g to an adult man of 70 kg, these ganglia vary approximately with the 2/3 power of the body weight. We have found that 50 μg ganglia excised from mice as young as two days of age can be used for electrical studies of synaptic transmission. For a biochemist who might like as much as 1 g of tissue, I recommend an elephant — rather a small one should suffice, according to extrapolation of the data in Fig. 1. For our own purposes we have usually been satisfied with 1 mg ganglia from rats, which are somewhat easier than elephants to obtain in large numbers.

In this paper, I will discuss certain metabolic adjustments accompanying two different kinds of nerve-cell activity. The first is the kind which is usually considered, namely the discharge and conduction of nerve impulses. This was studied in rat ganglia. The second kind of activity is the outgrowth of nerve fibers, whose study

Investigations reported in this paper were supported by Research Grant No. NB-00702 from the National Institute of Neurological Diseases and Blindness, National Institutes of Health, U.S. Public Health Service. We are indebted to Dr. Rita Levi-Montalcini for a gift of nerve-growth factor and to Dr. D. Caird Edwards of the Wellcome Research Laboratories, Beckenham, Kent, England, for a gift of antiserum to nerve-growth factor.

References p. 109–110

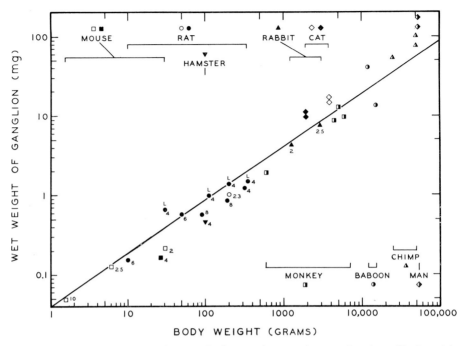

Fig. 1. Wet weight of superior cervical ganglia from various species, as a function of body weight. For the filled symbols the wet weights were determined directly. For the unfilled symbols, dry weights were multiplied by 5. For the half-filled symbols the wet weights were assumed equal to the volumes estimated from serial sections by Ebbeson (1968), although the volumes in this case may have been considerably reduced by fixation. Points marked L (for Lausanne) are from Roch-Ramel and Dolivo (1967). The solid line represents: Wet weight of ganglion in mg $= 4 \times$ (Body weight of animal in kg)$^{2/3}$. Numbers of ganglia averaged are indicated beside some points. Other points represent single ganglia.

has become possible through the discovery of a growth-controlling protein by Rita Levi-Montalcini and her colleagues. These investigations are now in progress, using ganglia from chicken embryos.

I. IMPULSE ACTIVITY

First let us consider two examples of the way in which impulse activity affects metabolism. Interest in this subject has been stimulated by advances in the understanding of related physiological mechanisms, such as active transport, rapid changes in membrane permeability during nerve action, and synthesis and release of transmitters. Each of these mechanisms places demands on the cellular metabolism which are unique to neurons and are initiated or intensified on activation of the nerve cell. Moreover, recent speculations on learning and memory have suggested that certain chemical changes produced by neuronal activity may possibly play an important role, but do not fully specify how these changes are initiated, maintained or expressed. Further illumination of many problems thus depends on a fuller understanding of the metabolic differences between resting and active neurons.

For the study of activity metabolism, sympathetic ganglia offer a combination of advantages which is unique among mammalian neuronal preparations. They contain synapses and nerve-cell bodies as well as axons. The neurons are normally at rest unless stimulated. Impulse conduction and discharge can readily be evoked and measured by conventional electrophysiological techniques. Moreover the activation can be achieved by stimulating the preganglionic nerve at a point relatively remote from the ganglion, so that the observed effects are those of conducted impulses and cannot be direct effects of the electric shocks used for stimulation.

The rat's superior cervical sympathetic ganglion survives at 37° in a modified Krebs' solution for about one day: after this time the postganglionic action potential evoked by preganglionic nerve stimulation declines to about half its initial value, both in Baltimore and in Lausanne (Larrabee and Klingmann, 1962; Roch-Ramel, 1962). Most experiments can be completed within 5 or 10 h after excision, at which time the response is usually greater than at the beginning. The ability of these excised preparations to maintain various aspects of metabolism as well as their normal internal potassium and sodium concentrations has been discussed elsewhere (Larrabee and Klingman, 1962; Larrabee *et al.*, 1963; Garlid and Larrabee, 1965; Garlid, 1968; Brinley, 1967). It has recently been observed at Lausanne that ganglia kept in a typical culture medium can discharge impulses in response to acetylcholine as long as 15 days after excision (A.-C. Gaide-Huguenin, personal communication, 1968).

Carbohydrate metabolism

It has long been known that impulse conduction causes a prompt increase in the rate of oxygen consumption by nervous tissue. It is obvious that this extra oxygen is required to supply energy for restorative processes, including ion transport and possibly membrane rebuilding. It is less certain what material is used as substrate for the extra oxidations. Some clarification of the controversial literature on activity substrates is possible in the light of experiments on sympathetic ganglia. The uncertainties seem to have arisen from the use of radioactively labelled glucose in experiments of relatively short duration.

In our experiments the output of labelled CO_2 from an excised ganglion, which was consuming glucose labelled with C-14, was measured continuously for many hours (Horowicz and Larrabee, 1962a). In the experiment of Fig. 2, the bathing medium was exchanged at zero time for one containing uniformly labelled glucose. The rate of output of labelled CO_2 rose progressively, not reaching a final steady state until after 3 or 4 h. This delay was not due to instrumental lags or to the time for diffusion of labelled glucose into the extracellular spaces; these were both much shorter. The delay in reaching a steady output was due to the time required for the specific activity of carbon in the metabolic intermediates to become equal to that in the glucose of the bathing fluid. This equilibration process is governed by a time constant of 3/4 h, according to which the smooth curve in Fig. 2 has been drawn. The intermediates involved must include those of glycolysis and the tricarboxylic acid cycle, and possibly some closely related products, such as certain amino acids. Although their equilibration may seem relatively slow from some points of view,

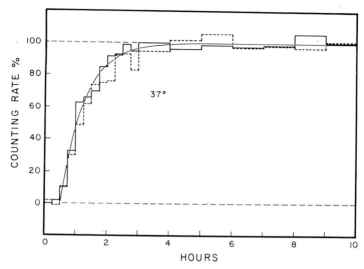

Fig. 2. Production of labelled CO_2 by a superior cervical ganglion excised from a rat. Glucose uniformly labelled with C-14 was added at 0 h. The counting rate was directly proportional to the rate of release of labelled CO_2. Two different experiments are represented by the solid and dashed lines. The smooth curve has been drawn with an exponential time constant of 3/4 h. (Horowicz and Larrabee, 1962a.)

we will be referring to them as rapidly equilibrating intermediates, for reasons which will become apparent.

There are other substances through which carbon finds its way to CO_2 and which equilibrate much more slowly than those just discussed. These include lipids, proteins, and nucleic acids. The labelling of such substances was studied by measuring the rate of change of total C-14 content of ganglia after the rapidly equilibrating intermediates had been fully equilibrated (Horowicz and Larrabee, 1962b). Later experiments allowed the incorporation of C-14 into phospholipids to be distinguished from that into the other substances (Larrabee et al., 1963; Larrabee and Leicht, 1965). All of these materials equilibrate with carbon from labelled glucose according to a time constant which considerably exceeds 10 h. The result is that no detectable labelled carbon reaches CO_2 through them in relatively short experiments. We will refer to them as slowly equilibrating intermediates.

The flux rates for carbon through various intermediates in resting ganglia are compared in Fig. 3. One pathway, that to lactate, is indicated in addition to those leading to CO_2. The fluxes were all measured independently and it is a matter of chance that they happened to add up to exactly 100% of the rate at which glucose was utilized, as shown on the left of the figure. Most of the glucose carbon went directly to CO_2 through the rapidly equilibrating intermediates. About 12% went into the slowly equilibrating intermediates. If we assume that these latter intermediates were in a steady state, this carbon influx would have to be balanced by an equal rate of release of CO_2, indicated by dashed lines. The CO_2 from this source is essentially unlabelled during short experiments. If we add this assumed rate for unlabelled CO_2 to the rate which we have measured for labelled CO_2 in the rapid pathways, the total

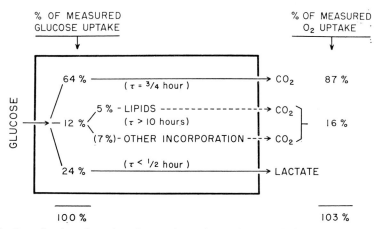

Fig. 3. The flow of carbon through various pathways in a rat's sympathetic ganglion. (From the data of Horowicz and Larrabee, 1962b; and Larrabee et al., 1963.)

measured oxygen consumption is well accounted for, as shown on the right of the figure. This supports our assumptions.

Such results suggest a possible explanation for reports that the specific activity of the CO_2 by nervous tissue is less than that of the glucose being consumed (e.g. Geiger et al., 1960; for summary, see Larrabee, 1967). The slowly equilibrating substances, such as lipids and proteins, which are here somewhat unconventionally regarded as intermediates of carbohydrate metabolism, presumably have not had enough time to begin delivering labelled carbon to CO_2 during the relatively short experiments which have so far been performed.

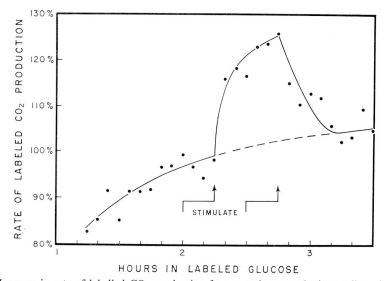

Fig. 4. Increase in rate of labelled CO_2 production from a rat's sympathetic ganglion, during repetitive stimulation of the preganglionic nerve. Each point is the average of 10 ganglia, bathed with glucose uniformly labelled with C-14. (Horowicz and Larrabee, 1962a.) Offsets in arrows represent instrumental delays.

How does the presence of the two classes of intermediates affect measurements of activity metabolism? When a sympathetic ganglion consuming labelled glucose is activated by presynaptic impulses, there is a prompt increase in the rate of production of labelled CO_2 (Horowicz and Larrabee, 1962a). This is shown in Fig. 4. Both in time course and in magnitude, the increase in labelled CO_2 suffices to account for the increased rate of oxygen uptake which simultaneously occurs. Thus the increased oxygen uptake in a ganglion results mostly from an increased rate of oxidation of exogenous glucose through rapidly equilibrating intermediates. We have obtained similar results on the frog's sciatic nerve (Larrabee, 1961), despite some puzzling contrary observations, which were made on frog's nerve when isotopes were first becoming available for these purposes (Mullins, 1953).

In sharp contrast with our results on nerve and ganglion are some observations on cat's brain perfused with labelled glucose by Geiger et al. (1960). These workers found that increased neuronal activity, produced by a convulsant drug, failed to cause any measurable change in the output of labelled CO_2. There was however an increased output of unlabelled CO_2. A reasonable explanation is that there was an accelerated oxidation of slowly equilibrating intermediates, which were not significantly labelled under the conditions of the experiments. But oxidation of these intermediates would still be an ultimate oxidation of the glucose from they which arise. In this way, regarding the lipids, proteins and nucleic acids of nervous tissue as intermediates of carbohydrate metabolism brings these experiments on animal brains into line with what is known about human brain, where glucose appears to be the only exogenous oxidative substrate of quantitative significance (Kety, 1957, 1967). Thus the seeming discrepancies may be more apparent than real, resulting from the fact that the same experiments have not been done on the different species (Larrabee, 1967). Accordingly, observations which have been made on the metabolism of perfused animal brains may be of more help in understanding the metabolism of human brain than has sometimes been thought.

My discussion to this point should suffice to demonstrate that glucose is the major or exclusive substrate for oxidation in a sympathetic ganglion, both at rest and in action. It is not surprising that changes in function occur soon after glucose is withdrawn, although the lack of certain expected metabolic effects has been a puzzle (Larrabee and Bronk, 1952; Larrabee, 1961; Larrabee and Klingman, 1962). I will leave the subject of glucose lack for Dolivo and Rouiller (p. 111), who are presenting a paper later in this symposium. They have recently participated in a new and penetrating analysis of the mechanism of functional loss (Nicolescu et al., 1966).

Phospholipid metabolism

The reactions discussed up to this point are commonly associated with energy production. The substances now to be considered — the phospholipids — are usually thought of as structural components of membranes, both at the cell surface and at intracellular organelles. Lowell and Mabel Hokin first discovered in excised nervous tissue that the rate of synthesis of two phospholipids, phosphatidyl inositol and phosphatidic acid, was increased under the application of acetylcholine (*e.g.* Hokin and Hokin, 1955; Hokin *et al.*, 1960). The acetylcholine was used with the intention of increasing nerve-cell activity, but the concentrations employed were unfortunately so high that they were in the range where cellular activity is depressed rather than stimulated. The difficult problems of choosing suitable concentration of chemical stimulants, as well as problems encountered by investigators who have attempted similar studies on brain *in situ*, have been discussed elsewhere (Larrabee, 1967).

We repeated the observations of the Hokins, but activated excised rat ganglia with naturally conducted nerve impulses. We were able to reproduce their effect on phosphatidyl inositol but not on phosphatidic acid (Larrabee *et al.*, 1963; Larrabee and Leicht, 1965). In our experiments the impulses were initiated by electrical stimulation of the preganglionic nerve at a point relatively remote from the ganglion. Two superior cervical ganglia from the same animal were excised and kept together for 4 h at 37° in a modified Krebs' solution, which contained inorganic phosphate labelled with P-32. During the last 3 of these hours, the preganglionic nerve to one ganglion was stimulated repetitively. At the end of stimulation the phospholipids were extracted from both ganglia and separated from one another by paper chromatography. Scans of the radioactivity on typical chromatograms are shown in Fig. 5. The only conspicuous and reproducible difference is an increase in P-32 in phosphatidyl inositol in the stimulated ganglion. There was no consistent effect on phosphatidyl choline, phosphatidyl ethanolamine, or phosphatidic acid.

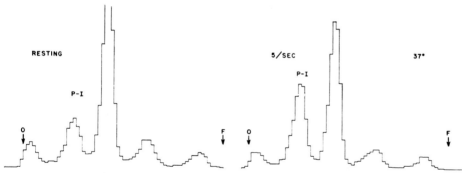

Fig. 5. Distribution of radioactivity on chromatograms of lipids extracted from the two superior cervical ganglia of a rat. After excision the two ganglia were simultaneously exposed for 4 h to inorganic phosphate labelled with P-32. One was kept at rest, while the preganglionic nerve leading to the other was stimulated at a frequency of 5/sec during the last 3 h. The five peaks on each chromatogram represent, from left to right, unidentified material near the origin, phosphatidyl inositol (marked P-I), phosphatidyl choline, phosphatidyl ethanolamine, and phosphatidic acid. (Larrabee *et al.*, 1963.)

Other experiments showed that there was no corresponding increase in the total amount of phosphatidyl inositol, so the effect is best ascribed to accelerated turnover. This inositide effect was also found in the ganglia of other species. Because the effect could be abolished by blocking ganglionic transmission with tubocurarine, it was concluded that the site of the effect must be postsynaptic. Because it could not be

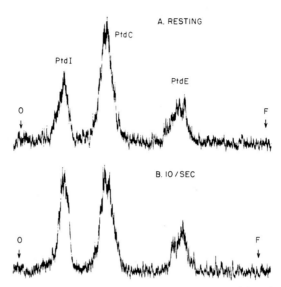

Fig. 6. Increased P-32 labelling of phosphatidyl inositol (PtdI) caused by stimulating the preganglionic nerve to a superior cervical ganglion with natural blood supply. The effect is indicated by the increase in PtdI relative to phosphatidyl choline (PtdC). (Larrabee, 1968.)

reproduced in nerve trunks lacking synapses or by impulses sent antidromically into a sympathetic ganglion, it seemed unrelated to transport of ions, since this is associated with activity in all portions of nerve cells. It was concluded that the inositide effect was probably related to some postsynaptic event caused by the synaptic transmitter, other than impulse conduction. Possible relations to transmitter–receptor reactions or generalized permeability changes might be worthy of consideration.

Since the inositide effect had never to our knowledge been demonstrated on nerve cells *in situ*, we wondered if it could possibly be an artifact of the excised state. Therefore we were recently pleased to find that it could be reproduced in naturally circulated ganglia, by electrical stimulation of the preganglionic nerve (Larrabee, 1968). In the experiment shown in Fig. 6, P-32 was administered to an anesthetized rat by intramuscular injection before the period of stimulation. Both preganglionic nerves were cut at the outset, so that the unstimulated ganglion was at rest. The labelling of phosphatidyl inositol was clearly greater in the stimulated ganglion.

A final question was whether the inositide effect developed at natural levels of activity in the sympathetic nervous system, since electrical stimulation applied to the preganglionic nerve might activate the ganglion cells in greater number and at higher frequencies than ever normally occurs. Therefore the effects of natural activity were investigated. This was readily possible because sympathetic ganglia are paired peripheral structures. First, under temporary ether anesthesia, the preganglionic fibers to one superior cervical ganglion were cut and the P-32 was injected intramuscularly. Thus one ganglion was kept at rest during the labelling period, while the other was stimulated only by impulses which were naturally discharged from the central nervous

TABLE I

EFFECTS OF ACTIVITY ON RELATIVE LABELLING

Mean percent change $\pm$ s.e.m. (P by t-test)
Larrabee, 1968

	N	$PtdI/PtdC$	$PtdE/PtdC$
Breathing air	8	$+ 6 \pm 2$ (0.04)	-2 ± 4
Breathing 10% O_2	6	$+21 \pm 5$ (0.01)	-7 ± 5
Combined	14	$+12 \pm 3$ (0.002)	-4 ± 3

system. The animals quickly recovered from the ether anesthesia and were thus unanesthetized during most of the labelling period. A few hours later the animals were reanesthetized and the two superior cervical ganglia were taken for analysis of their phospholipids.

The effects which were obtained were small and could be seen only in the average of a number of animals (Table I). In order to get the highest reproducibility in studying the inositide, its labelling was measured relative to the labelling of phosphatidyl choline. The latter was thus used as a reference compound, because our earlier studies on excised ganglia had shown that it was unaffected by neuronal activity. On the average of 8 animals, the labelling of the inositide was 6% greater in the active ganglia than in those which had their preganglionic nerves severed. Although this was a difference in the expected direction, it was of dubious statistical significance, with a probability of 0.04 according to Fisher's t-test. Therefore 6 additional animals were made anoxic during the labelling period by letting them breath 10% oxygen. This is known to increase the activity in the sympathetic nervous system. In this series the effect on the inositide was greater, as expected, being 21%, and passed the generally accepted standards for significance, with a probability of 0.01. When the number of observations was increased by combining the two series of experiments, the probability decreased to a very respectable 0.002. Thus the inositide effect clearly occurs under more natural conditions as well as under the artificial situations in which it was originally discovered and could be more rigorously analyzed.

The significance of the inositide effect remains obscure. Apparently this particular phospholipid plays some special role in synaptic transmission. So far the effect has been seen only at a cholinergic junction. Its abolition by tubocurarine implies that the effect which we have seen is related to the action of acetylcholine on nicotinic receptors and not to an action on muscarinic receptors or to some action in the adrenergic system that has recently been found in sympathetic ganglia. Further speculations would be aided if we knew whether the effect is characteristic of all cholinergic junctions and whether it occurs at sites dominated by other transmitters. We have been seeking preparations for such studies, but it is hard to find others as suitable as a sympathetic ganglion.

References p. 109–110

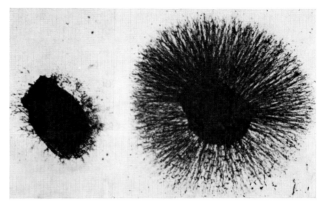

Fig. 7. Halo of fibers growing out from an excised embryonic sensory ganglion in the presence of nerve-growth factor (right), compared to the lack of such outgrowth in the absence of the growth factor (left). (Levi-Montalcini, 1964.) Similar outgrowth occurs around excised embryonic sympathetic ganglia.

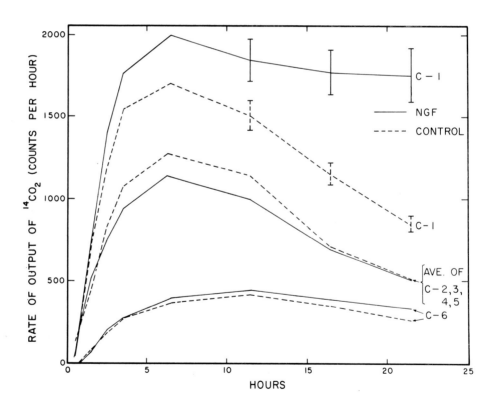

Fig. 8. Release of labelled CO_2 from sympathetic ganglia excised from chicken embryos and supplied with glucose labelled in various positions with C-14, in the presence and absence of nerve-growth factor. The average output for carbons 2, 3, 4, and 5 was calculated by subtracting the output of C-1 and C-6 from the output with uniformly labelled glucose. (Unpublished experiments by W. T. Brown.)

II. GROWTH ACTIVITY

We turn now to the metabolic accompaniments of a second type of nerve-cell activity, that of fiber outgrowth. This was studied with the aid of a protein called nerve-growth factor, which was discovered by Rita Levi-Montalcini and her colleagues, first in tumors, later in snake-venom glands and many other locations. The standard source at present is the salivary gland of the mouse. The extensive investigations that have been performed on it have recently been thoroughly reviewed by Levi-Montalcini and Angeletti (1968). The spectacular effects of the growth factor are well illustrated in a picture, published by Levi-Montalcini (1964), of fiber outgrowth around a sensory ganglion which had been exposed for 24 h to the growth factor in tissue culture (Fig. 7, right). In the absence of the growth factor, there is no outgrowth of fibers, but only the outwandering of a few fibroblasts (Fig. 7, left). The sensory ganglia in this picture were obtained from a chicken embryo. The same profuse halo of fibers grow out around sympathetic ganglia excised from chicken embryos, and it is these which we have recently started to study.

In order to obtain fiber outgrowth, an excised ganglion is embedded in a fibrin clot and bathed with a complex culture medium containing a number of organic and inorganic constituents as well as the nerve-growth factor. The procedure of embedding in a clot, which provides a fibrous matrix to support the outgrowing fibers, was followed in all of our metabolic experiments. This permitted simultaneous observation of the growth, which has turned out to be an important control. The sympathetic ganglia were obtained from chicken embryos about 14 days old, which is the critical age at which the maximum growth response occurs.

The production of labelled CO_2 from ganglia consuming glucose labelled with C-14 was studied in our laboratory by Mr. W. T. Brown, using an adaptation of our earlier procedures for continuous measurements over long periods of time (Horowicz and Larrabee, 1962a). Results with glucose labelled in the C-1 and C-6 positions are shown in Fig. 8. The output from uniformly labelled glucose was also measured: this is not shown here, but the results were used to calculate the average output for carbons 2, 3, 4, and 5, by subtracting the outputs of C-1 and C-6 from that with uniformly labelled glucose. In the absence of growth factor (broken lines), there was first a progressive rise in output from all carbons as the intermediates became equilibrated with the radioactive carbon. This was followed by a progressive decline, ascribable to slow deterioration of the tissue. The growth factor (continuous lines) caused a significant increase in output from only one carbon, that in the C-1 position of glucose. As is well known this particular carbon is released relatively early in carbohydrate metabolism, at the point where the other five carbons of some of the hexose molecules are shunted off to make pentose. Thus the growth factor selectively enhanced synthesis of substances such as nucleotides and nucleic acids, which contain pentoses.

Further examination of Fig. 8 suggests that the growth factor did not cause a significant increase in C-1 release at the earliest times. The impression is that the output was simply sustained at a level from which the control would have started if the earliest measurements had not been obscured by the process of isotopic equilibration. This point was missed in earlier investigations, where observations were limited to 3 h and may have been confounded by the equilibration process (Angeletti *et al.*, 1964). We may possibly be observing the metabolic consequences not of the growth process, but of a second known effect of the growth factor, which is the prevention of cell deterioration (Levi-Montalcini and Angeletti, 1963). Or the effect of the growth factor on C-1 release may result from a combination of both better maintenance and stimulated growth, the relative contribution of these two factors being at present unknown. Obviously the situation is more complicated than was at first thought. We are now seeking ways of obtaining a better baseline on which to study the growth effect.

Another approach is to look at the metabolism of the outgrowing fibers themselves instead of the whole preparation. In experiments on the incorporation of P-32 into lipids, Mr. Lester Partlow of our laboratory succeeded in separating the halo of fibers from the body of the ganglion at the end of the growth period. One of the joys of working with tiny embryonic ganglia was that the usual lipid extraction procedures could be omitted. It sufficed simply to squash the preparations on the origin of the chromatogram and to let the chromatography solvents do all the work. Fig. 9 shows the resulting distribution of radioactivity and demonstrates significant labelling of lipids in the halo as well as the body of the ganglion. The identified labelled materials are all familiar ones. One difference between the chromatogram from the halo and that from the body of the ganglion is a prolongation of the falling phase of the PtdI peak from the halo. This may represent sphingomyelin, which one would not be surprised to find labelled only in freshly growing tissue, since it is known to undergo less subsequent turnover than the other phospholipids. The lipids of the halo are almost certainly extracted from the growing fibres, because there are few if any other kinds of cells located here. This is an advantage over studies of growth in the intact organism, where several kinds of cells are always intermingled. Using variants of this approach we hope to be able to distinguish local synthesis in growing fibers from synthesis in the cell body followed by transport out along the axon.

The next experiment to be described contributes in a negative way to understanding the biochemical mechanism through which nerve-growth factor acts. Because the factor has been found to increase the synthesis of ribonucleic acid, the possibility has arisen that the primary action might be at the chromosomal level, starting the synthesis of some new messenger RNA (Angeletti *et al.*, 1965; Levi-Montalcini and Angeletti, 1968). While our observations generally support the earlier findings, some observations with actinomycin-D suggest caution in interpreting them. Mr. Partlow has confirmed that this inhibitor at suitable concentrations not only stops RNA synthesis in control ganglia, as measured by incorporation of labelled uridine, but also eliminates the stimulant effects of the growth factor on RNA metabolism (Fig. 10). A surprising discovery was that fiber outgrowth was only moderately impaired. As seen in the figure, a concentration of 1 μg/ml, for example, almost entirely stopped uridine incorporation and completely inhibited its stimulation by the growth factor. However, this concentration only reduced the width of the growth halo by about 25%. In subsequent experiments with cycloheximide, an inhibitor

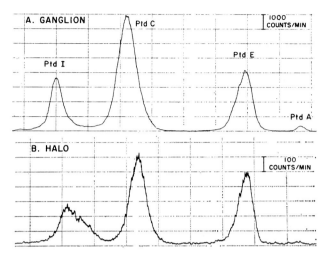

Fig. 9. Radioactivity in chromatograms of lipids extracted from the body of a sympathetic ganglion and from the halo of fibers surrounding it. The preparation had been incubated for 24 h with nerve-growth factor and with inorganic phosphate labelled with P-32. The portions of the chromatograms shown above extend from an R_f of about 0.1 to the front. PtdI = phosphatidyl inositol; PtdC = phosphatidyl choline; PtdE = phosphatidyl ethanolamine; PtdA = phosphatidic acid. (Unpublished experiments by L. M. Partlow.)

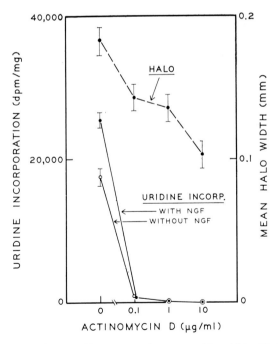

Fig. 10. Effects of actinomycin-D on fiber outgrowth, measured by width of halo in the presence of the nerve-growth factor, and incorporation of labelled uridine into RNA of embryonic sympathetic ganglia with and without the growth factor. Incubation for 15 h. (Unpublished experiment by L. M. Partlow.)

of protein synthesis, it was shown that this small reduction in the fiber outgrowth could be fully accounted for by the small reduction of protein synthesis that is caused by actinomycin-D. The conclusion is that the stimulation of fiber outgrowth is not dependent on modification of RNA synthesis. Therefore it would be well to seek other possible mechanisms for the turning on of fiber growth.

A different aspect of the nerve-growth factor is that it can be used as an antigen to produce an antiserum which causes selective degeneration of the sympathetic nervous system, when injected into a young animal. This is at present a popular pharmacological tool (Levi-Montalcini and Angeletti, 1966). Relatively little is known about its metabolic effects, except for a report of early depression of RNA synthesis (Sabatini *et al.*, 1966) and later changes in catecholamine metabolism which are consequent to the cellular degeneration. Accordingly Mr. David Halstead of our laboratory has started to study the early effects of the antiserum. This is done by administering a single dose of antiserum to a mouse 6–11 days old, removing the superior cervical ganglia a few hours or days later, and measuring their properties

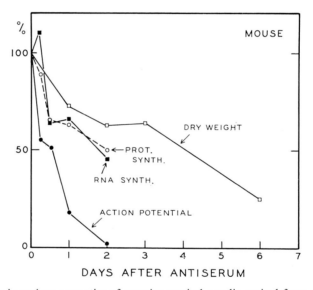

Fig. 11. Decline in various properties of superior cervical ganglia excised from mice which had received a single injection of antiserum to nerve-growth factor. The values are expressed as percent of those for control mice of the same age. The injection was made 6–11 days after birth. (Unpublished experiments by D. C. Halstead.)

in various ways (Fig. 11). Mr. Halstead showed considerable skill in measuring transmission through these extremely small ganglia by standard electrical methods. This is the most rapidly affected variable which he has so far studied. Transmission was markedly depressed as soon as 6 h after the injection, and had completely failed in 2 days. RNA and protein synthesis, as measured by incorporation of labelled precursors were greatly affected within the first day. The tissue rather rapidly wasted away, as quantitatively shown by measurements of dry weight. We are seeking clues concerning the initial events in the antiserum action by these and other metabolic studies.

III. CONCLUSION

In retrospect, this paper has concerned three general topics, which indicate some of the experimental possibilities of excised sympathetic ganglia. The first topic, carbohydrate metabolism, is of possible significance for nerve cells in general and has served to sharpen some questions about brain metabolism. The other two topics, inositide metabolism and nerve-growth factor, are related to properties which at present seem particularly pertinent to sympathetic ganglia. The effect of activity on phosphatidyl inositol needs further analysis in sympathetic ganglia and at other synapses before its significance can be understood. The metabolic actions of the growth factor are relatively complex and at present seem to raise more questions than they answer concerning the mode of action of this fascinating material.

REFERENCES

ANGELETTI, P. U., GANDINI-ATTARDI, D., TOSCHI, G., SALVI, M. I., AND LEVI-MONTALCINI, R., (1965); Metabolic aspects of the effect of nerve growth factor on sympathetic and sensory ganglia: protein and ribonucleic acid synthesis. *Biochim. biophys. Acta (Amst.)*, **95**, 111–120.

ANGELETTI, P. U., LUIZZI, A., LEVI-MONTALCINI, R., AND GANDINI-ATTARDI, D., (1964); Effect of a nerve growth factor on glucose metabolism by sympathetic and sensory nerve cells. *Biochim. biophys. Acta (Amst.)*, **90**, 445–450.

BRINLEY JR., F. J., (1967); Potassium accumulation and transport in the rat sympathetic ganglion. *J. Neurophysiol.* **30**, 1531–1560.

EBBESON, SVEN O. E., (1968); Quantitative studies of superior cervical sympathetic ganglia in a variety of primates including man. II. Neuronal packing density. *J. Morph.*, **124**, 181–186.

GARLID, K. D., (1968); Sodium transport in a mammalian sympathetic ganglion. *Dissertation*, Johns Hopkins University.

GARLID, K. D., AND LARRABEE, M. G., (1965); Sodium and sulphate efflux from the superior cervical ganglion of the rat. *Biophys. Soc., Abstracts of Ninth Annual Meeting*, p. 121.

GEIGER, A., KAWAKITA, Y., AND BARKULSI, S. S., (1960); Major pathways of glucose utilization in the brain in brain perfusion experiments *in vivo* and *in situ*. *J. Neurochem.*, **5**, 323–338.

HOKIN, L. E., AND HOKIN, M. R., (1955); Effects of acetylcholine on phosphate turnover in phospholipids of brain cortex *in vitro*. *Biochim. biophys. Acta (Amst.)*, **16**, 229–237.

HOKIN, M. R., HOKIN, L. E., AND SHELP, W. D., (1960); The effects of acetylcholine on the turnover of phosphatidic acid and phosphoinositide in sympathetic ganglia, and in various parts of the nervous system *in vitro*. *J. gen. Physiol.*, **44**, 217–226.

HOROWICZ, P., AND LARRABEE, M. G., (1962a); Oxidation of glucose in a mammalian sympathetic ganglion at rest and in activity. *J. Neurochem.*, **9**, 1–22.

HOROWICZ, P., AND LARRABEE, M. G., (1962b); Metabolic partitioning of carbon from glucose by a mammalian sympathetic ganglion. *J. Neurochem.*, **9**, 407–420.

KETY, S. S., (1957); The general metabolism of the brain *in vivo*. *The Metabolism of the Nervous System*. D. RICHTER (Ed.), Pergamon, Oxford, pp. 221–237.

KETY, S. S., (1967); Relationships between energy metabolism of the brain and functional activity. *Sleep and Altered States of Consciousness*. SEYMOUR S. KETY (Ed)., Williams and Wilkins, Baltimore, pp. 39–47.

LARRABEE, M. G., (1961); Glucose metabolism in ganglia and nerves. *Biophysics of Physiological and Pharmacological Actions*. A. M. SHANES (Ed.), pp. 199–213.

LARRABEE, M. G., (1967); The influence of neural activity on neural metabolism of glucose and phospholipid. *Sleep and Altered States of Consciousness*. SEYMOUR S. KETY (Ed.), Williams and Wilkins, Baltimore, pp. 64–85.

LARRABEE, M. G., (1968); Transynaptic stimulation of phosphatidylinositol metabolism in sympathetic neurons *in situ*. *J. Neurochem.*, **15**, 803–808.

LARRABEE, M. G., AND BRONK, D. W., (1952); Metabolic requirements of sympathetic neurons. *Cold Spr. Harb. Symp. quant. Biol.*, **17**, 245–266.

LARRABEE, M. G., AND KLINGMAN, J. D., (1962); Metabolism of glucose and oxygen in mammalian sympathetic ganglia at rest and in action. *Neurochemistry*. 2nd ed. K. A. C. ELLIOTT, I. H. PAGE AND J. H. QUASTEL (Eds.), Thomas, Springfield, Ill., pp. 150–176.

LARRABEE, M. G., KLINGMAN, J. D., AND LEICHT, W. S., (1963); Effects of temperature, calcium, and activity on phospholipid metabolism in a sympathetic ganglion. *J. Neurochem.*, **10**, 549–570.

LARRABEE, M. G., AND LEICHT, W. S., (1965); Metabolism of phosphatidyl inositol and other lipids in active neurones of sympathetic ganglia and other peripheral nervous tissues. The site of the inositide effect. *J. Neurochem.*, **12**, 1–13.

LEVI-MONTALCINI, R., (1964); Growth control of nerve cells by a protein and its antiserum. *Science*, **143**, 105–110.

LEVI-MONTALCINI, R., AND ANGELETTI, P. U., (1963); Essential role of the nerve growth factor in the survival and maintenance of dissociated sensory and sympathetic embryonic nerve cells *in vitro*. *Develop. Biol.*, **7**, 653–659.

LEVI-MONTALCINI, R., AND ANGELETTI, P. U., (1966); Immunosympathectomy. *Pharmacol. Rev.*, **18**, 619–628.

LEVI-MONTALCINI, R., AND ANGELETTI, P. U., (1968); Nerve growth factor. *Physiol. Rev.*, **48**, 534–569.

MULLINS, L. J., (1953); Substrate utilization by stimulated nerve. *Amer. J. Physiol.*, **175**, 358–362.

NICOLESCU, P., DOLIVO, M., ROUILLER, C., AND FOROGLOU-KERAMEUS, C., (1966); The effect of deprivation of glucose on the ultrastructure and function of the superior cervical ganglion of the rat *in vivo*. *J. Cell. Biol.*, **29**, 267–285.

ROCH-RAMEL, F., (1962); Métabolisme et "survie fonctionnelle" du ganglion sympathique cervical isolé du rat. *Helv. physiol. pharmacol. Acta*, **Suppl. XIII**, 1-64.

ROCH-RAMEL, F., AND DOLIVO, M., (1967); Activité de quelques enzymes et survie fonctionnelle du ganglion sympathique isolé du rat. *Helv. physiol. pharmacol. Acta*, **25**, 40–61.

SABATINI, M. T., LEVI-MONTALCINI, R., AND ANGELETTI, P. U., (1966); Effetti precoci del siero anti-Nerve Growth Factor sulla cellula nervosa. *Ann. Ist. Super. Sanità*, **2**, 349–355.

Changes in Ultrastructure and Synaptic Transmission in the Sympathetic Ganglion During Various Metabolic Conditions*

M. DOLIVO AND CH. ROUILLER

Department of Physiology, University of Lausanne, and
Department of Histology, University of Geneva (Switzerland)

In trying to establish correlations between metabolism and function in nervous tissue kept *in vitro*, one has to choose a tissue in which the electrophysiological activity may be recorded precisely in terms of conduction and transmission; and one has also to be able, if possible, to control pre- and post-synaptic activities (Larrabee, 1961a; Dunant, 1967; Dunant and Dolivo, 1968a, b). As a second point one has to be able to keep both the electrical activity and the metabolic exchanges under strict control, and both must be measured easily as input *versus* output. Finally — and this is one of the main conditions to make it a valuable enterprise — histology and electron microscopy have to be performed on a tissue that can retain its morphological and ultrastructural characteristics *in vitro*. The superior cervical ganglion, isolated from the rat, is almost the only tissue showing all these qualities (Dolivo, 1966). After having been incubated for 18 h *in vitro* in a bicarbonate buffered Krebs' solution, it still reveals a normal ultrastructure (Fig. 1), transmission being kept for about 36 h and conduction for at least twice as long. Neither cortex slices, homogenates nor perfused tissues offer the possibility of so much control *in vitro* for so long a time without showing major cellular lesions.

Nevertheless nervous tissue *in vitro* cannot be considered as being in a steady state: placed in the best conditions (sterile and enriched medium) it will be submitted to irreversible changes, bound to the degeneration of the preganglionic nerve and the regeneration of the postganglionic one.

TECHNIQUES

Electrophysiological control. The preganglionic fibers were stimulated and the electrophysiological response recorded simultaneously on the preganglionic nerve and the postganglionic axons; thus both the preganglionic and postganglionic activity were tested. The activity of the preganglionic terminals were also recorded sometimes,

---

* This work was supported by the following grants from the Swiss National Fund for Scientific Research 3444, 3893, 4237, 5344, and by a grant from the Fritz Hoffmann-La Roche Foundation.

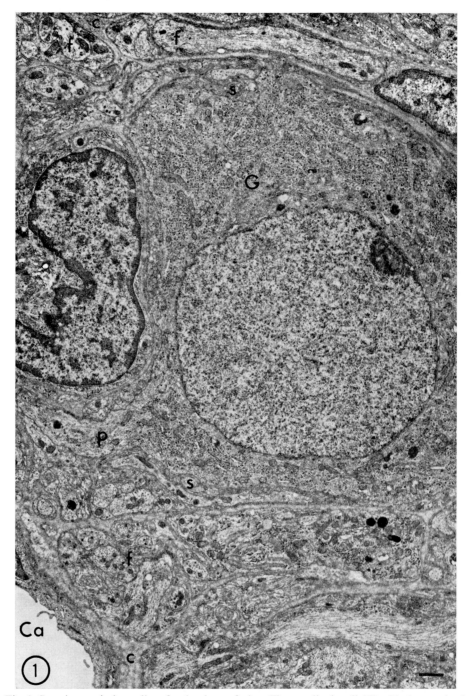

Fig. 1. Superior cervical ganglion, fixation by perfusion. The ganglionic cell (G) with the proximal part of its cell process (p) surrounded by satellite cells (s) and bundles of fibers (f). Ca, capillary. Magnification 6000 ×.

Abbreviations used in all figures: C, connective tissue space; E, endoplasmic reticulum; f, nerve fiber (for the purpose of simplification, the term 'nerve fiber' is used for all sections of cell processes, without distinction between axon and dendrite); G, ganglionic cell; go, Golgi area; S, satellite cell; T, nerve terminal.

using modified electrodes that made it possible to pick up the electrical activity at this level (Dunant and Dolivo, 1968a).

Metabolic conditions. Conditions were so chosen as to be under strict control for the duration of the experiment and to allow measurements of the substrate uptake, enzymatic activities, etc. In almost all these conditions the electrical activity to preganglionic stimulation could be measured.

Histology and histochemistry. The usual techniques, with some modifications, have been used (Winckler, 1959; Pears, 1958; Barka and Anderson, 1963; Mumenthaler and Engels, 1961).

Electron microscopy. After withdrawal from the incubation medium, the ganglions were cut transversely into 2 or 3 fragments, and fixed in a solution of osmium tetroxide–dichromate (Forssmann, 1965) or in a solution of osmium tetroxide buffered with phosphate (Millonig, 1961). After dehydration, the fragments were embedded in Vestopal (Ryter and Kellenberger, 1958) or Epon (Luft, 1961). The sections were cut with lead according to Karnovsky (1961) and studied with the electron microscopes Zeiss EM9, Siemens Elmiskop I and Philips EM 300.

RESULTS

We want to show and discuss here the correlations between the irreversible loss of synaptic transmission, metabolic events and the ultrastructural changes in three well-defined conditions: lack of glucose in the incubation medium, lack of oxygen in presence of glucose, and oxygen under pressure.

1. Glucose lack

In this situation the tissue is oxygenated but gets no substrate from the incubation medium; the oxygen received allows the tissue to use internal substrates.

1.1. Electrophysiological response

(a) Transmission ability is lost irreversibly 2 h after the tissue has been deprived of glucose (Larrabee *et al.*, 1957); (b) the pre- and postganglionic fibers can still be stimulated up to 24–30 h after the loss of the synaptic transmission (Dolivo *et al.*, 1965; Nicolescu *et al.*, 1966); (c) exposing a ganglion to 5 μg/ml of eserine after glucose deprivation makes its neurons respond to acetylcholine added to the incubation medium; (d) on the other hand, in these same conditions (glucose lack and exposure to eserine) these neurons no longer respond to a preganglionic stimulation by the usual long asynchronous discharge shown in normal conditions, in presence of the same dose of eserine; (e) finally one can record an asynchronous spontaneous activity on the postganglionic axons from the 90th minute after glucose has been removed; it lasts for about 60 min (Dolivo *et al.*, 1966).

1.2. Metabolic experiments

(a) The oxygen uptake, as shown by Larrabee (1958), first increases after glucose has been removed and then only slowly decreases, showing that the tissue is able to use some internal substrate; (b) the enzymatic activities, namely those of the* LDH, SDH, GOT and G6PDH, do not decrease significantly for the first hours after glucose deprivation (De Perrot, 1962; Roch-Ramel and Dolivo, 1967); (c) if the tissue has been allowed to synthesize glycogen before glucose is removed, the time between the withdrawal of glucose and the irreversible loss of transmission is longer (De Ribaupierre, 1968); (d) at 6° the tissue may be deprived of glucose for as long as 18 h and still show a normal response to preganglionic stimulation; (e) the loss of K^+ is negligible in absence of glucose (Larrabee, 1961b); (f) the amount of ATP does not seem to change rapidly after glucose withdrawal (Larrabee, 1961b).

All these observations suggest that a loss of function due to a presynaptic lesion must be sought.

1.3. Histology and electron microscopy

Photonic microscopy does not show obvious lesions. Histochemistry, on the other hand, reveals a loss of activity of the cholinesterase (Foroglou-Kerameus and Dolivo, 1968). Electron microscopy has shown an important lesion specifically located at the presynaptic fibers (Nicolescu et al., 1966).

The presynaptic endings are usually swollen and the neurofibrils have disappeared. The mitochondria are rare and their structure modified. Frequently, the swollen cell processes contain vesicles that differ from the presynaptic vesicles as to larger and variable size, wider distribution, and denser contents. Cytolysomes and dense amorphous masses of irregular form and unknown nature are also observed in the swollen endings. The most extensively deteriorated cell processes are practically reduced to their plasma membrane. Synaptic vesicles are extremely rare and synapses cannot be seen.

In this particular condition the ultrastructural findings explain both the irreversible loss of transmission, due to a real destruction of the tissue, and the fact that the neurons still respond to a chemical stimulation because their own structure is preserved, as also is that of their satellite cells.

The histochemical observation on the inactivation of the cholinesterase explains why the neurons show a spontaneous activity at the time when the presynaptic fibers are being destroyed and releasing their content of acetylcholine. This activation of the neurons results in the observed increase in oxygen uptake 1 h after glucose has been removed. Later the oxygen consumption only slowly diminishes because the cells are still able to draw on their internal substrate.

The reason why the presynaptic terminals are more sensitive to the lack of glucose is not yet understood. One possible reason for it might appear to be that the presynaptic terminals are separated from their neurons of origin in an isolated tissue. This hypothesis, however, can be ruled out: ganglia kept in vivo with their preganglionic nerve intact and perfused with a glucose-free solution show exactly the same ultrastructural

---

* Abbreviations: G6PDH, glucose-6-phosphate dehydrogenase; LDH, lactate dehydrogenase; SDH, succinate dehydrogenase; GOT, glutamic–oxaloacetic transaminase.

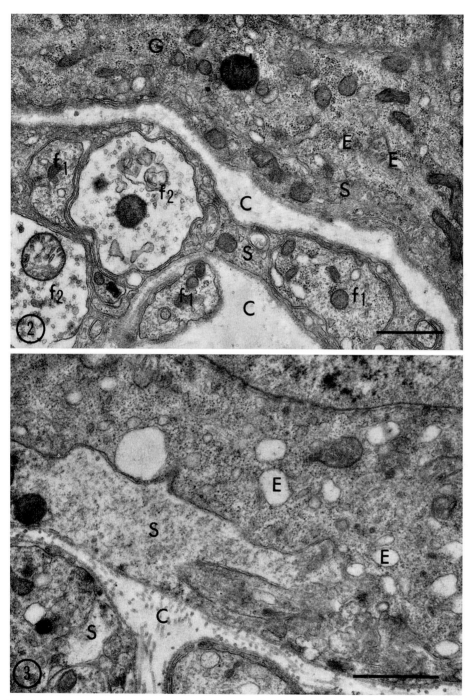

Fig. 2. Superior cervical ganglion deprived of glucose for 5 h (the preganglionic fiber had not been cut). Ganglion (G) and satellite (S) cells are well preserved as the only visible modification is simply a slight swelling of the cisternae of the endoplasmic reticulum (E). Amongst the cell processes, some are preserved (f₁) and others are injured (f₂). L, lysosome. Magnification 18 000 ×.

Fig. 3. Superior cervical ganglion deprived of oxygen for 8 h. Complete degeneration of the satellite cells (S). The ganglion cell shows a swelling of the endoplasmic reticulum (E). Magnification 23 750 ×.

lesion as a ganglion kept *in vitro* without glucose (Fig. 2). Another explanation could be that the presynaptic terminals have much less glycogen to cover their energetic requirements than the cell body itself (De Ribaupierre *et al.*, 1968). It is noteworthy that the glucose is not only necessary to assure the metabolic function of the nervous tissue but is also most important to keep the structural integrity of the cell processes and, after a longer time, the cell integrity itself. The demonstration that the cells themselves eventually suffer from a lack of substrate is indicated by the loss of enzymes occurring after the 10th hour of glucose deprivation.

2. Anoxia

In this metabolic condition the tissue is able to take from the medium as much glucose as it needs, but has to cover all its metabolic requirements with the energy it can draw from anaerobic glycolysis.

2.1. Electrophysiological activity

(*a*) When the standard medium equilibrated with O_2 and CO_2 is suddenly replaced by a solution that has been equilibrated for at least 12 h with 95% N_2 and 5% CO_2 * the ability to transmit through the synapses of the ganglion is lost in a much shorter time than after glucose deprivation: after 15 min the normal postsynaptic response to presynaptic stimulation is lost. (*b*) Some residual response can often be recorded, its amplitude being about 20% of the postganglionic response recorded before the oxygen deprivation. (*c*) The main difference between the consequences of oxygen lack *versus* glucose lack, is that the transmission can be fully restored even after the tissue has been deprived of oxygen during 3 h, namely after the loss of the response to a preganglionic stimulation has lasted for about the same length of time. (*d*) If oxygen deprivation is prolonged for over 3 h, the irreversibility is not complete, about 50% of the initial response reappearing after the tissue has been brought back to an oxygenated solution. (*e*) The time before function is lost can be prolonged by increasing the amount of Ca^{2+} in the solution (Kocsis, to be published).

2.2. Metabolic data

(*a*) Under anaerobic conditions the glucose uptake is greatly increased, reaching the value of 56.7 mg/g dry weight/h, the value in aerobic conditions being 18.7 mg/g dry weight/h. (*b*) Such an uptake of 56.7 mg/g dry weight/h seems the greatest amount of glucose that the tissue can draw from the solution (Berger, to be published; Matthieu, to be published), and in anaerobic conditions it entirely reappears as lactate in the medium. (*c*) The enzymatic mechanisms controling this uptake of glucose are very sensitive to β-irradiation. After the tissue has been exposed to 20 krad the possibility of taking up glucose is decreased by 20%, though no ultrastructural lesion can be seen for such a small dose of β-irradiation and though the electrophysiological

---

* The gas used for equilibrating the solution has always been checked by using a Scholander analyser.

response remains apparently normal (Berger and Dolivo, 1966). (*d*) When the amount of glucose in the solution is increased, the time before transmission is lost after the onset of anoxia is prolonged. Nevertheless over a concentration of 250 mg/100 ml this increase in the glucose content is of no benefit, or even seems to accelerate the loss of function, though in normal conditions of oxygenation such a concentration is harmless. The anoxic tissue thus seems sensitive to an increase in osmotic pressure. (*e*) After 5 h without O_2 the enzymatic activity of the LDH is decreased; the fall in activity of the SDH or the GOT is much smaller. (*f*) When testing the incubation medium for an activity of the LDH one finds that the enzymatic activity lost from the tissue can be found in the solution. At the same moment the activity of the SDH and the GOT is almost non-existent and increases only much later (Dolivo *et al.*, 1967). This difference can be explained by the fact that the LDH is located in the cytoplasm and the SDH in the mitochondria (De Duve *et al.*, 1962).

2.3. Histology and electron microscopy

(*a*) Histochemistry reveals a decrease in enzymatic activity, confirming the biochemical observations. (*b*) It shows that the LDH can be seen in the axons themselves; moreover this can only be observed in these particular conditions of anoxia. (*c*) The SDH remains in the mitochondria. Normally the histochemical reaction also very intensively stains the external limits of the cell processes — never the axoplasm — as if the enzyme were located in the Schwann cells. During anoxia this localized staining disappears.

Electron microscopy shows a lesion, first located in the satellite cells and later in the neurons themselves. The altered cells are scattered in the ganglion, being both at the surface of the tissue and in the middle, and they present various degrees of alteration. Even after 8 h of anoxia some cells are in a quite normal state though others are almost destroyed. The alteration of the satellite cells begins with a densification of their nucleus and a vacuolization of the cytoplasm which later becomes fragmentated and degenerated. It may even appear as emptied of its contents (Fig. 3). These findings show that the cells are more or less sensitive to anoxia, whatever their location in the tissue. It explains why an electrophysiological response can still be recorded after 5 h of anoxia, but it explains nothing about the reasons for the particular resistance of some neurons to the lack of oxygen. There are two types of neuron in the sympathetic ganglion, larger and smaller ones. It is impossible to tell at present if the smaller neurons better resist the lack of oxygen than the larger ones. The lesion of the satellite cells appearing earlier than of the neurons themselves, might explain the increased flow of cytoplasm in the axons, revealed by the staining of the LDH: it could well be the result of a dilatation of axons having lost their sheath of Schwann cells.

In contradiction with the consequences of the lack of glucose which mainly alters the presynaptic endings, these same endings remain uninjured even after 8 h of oxygen deprivation (Fig. 4). Moreover many observations on their ultrastructure suggest that undamaged endings make synapses with degenerating dendritic processes (Nicolescu *et al.*, to be published).

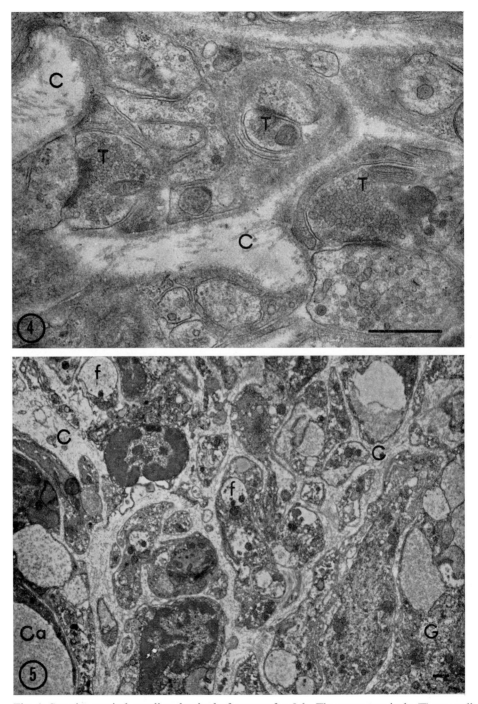

Fig. 4. Superior cervical ganglion deprived of oxygen for 8 h. The nerve terminals (T) are well preserved and the synaptic vesicles are numerous. Magnification 20 000 ×.

Fig. 5. Superior cervical ganglion kept for 19 h in 5 atm. oxygen, but at a normal p_{CO_2}. Severe necrosis of the nervous tissue. Ca, capillary. Magnification 4 300 ×.

The question may be raised whether the observed lesions are due to the tissue having to draw all its energy from anaerobic glycolysis, and to the change in pH, lowered intracellulary by production of lactic acid. Two observations might be brought against this hypothesis. When the pH is lowered to 6.8 in the medium (by increasing the p_{CO_2} to 132 mm Hg in presence of a concentration of bicarbonate of 16.19 mmoles/l), transmission is maintained for almost 40 h (Matthieu, to be published). Moreover, the maximal amount of lactate produced in the tissue in aerobic conditions is 8.2 mg/g dry weight/h, at a pH of 7.4 obtained by keeping the p_{CO_2} at 31.6 mm Hg and the amount of bicarbonate at 34.6 mmoles/l. In this last condition the time during which transmission is maintained reaches 46 h (Matthieu, to be published). Nevertheless these two observations do not completely rule out the hypothesis of a lesion caused by the lowering of the pH during anoxia, as it is very difficult to estimate the intracellular pH.

3. High oxygen pressure

This is a third situation in which a well-defined modification of the metabolic conditions of incubation results in a loss of the action potential transmitted through the synapses of the ganglion. In these experiments only the pressure of oxygen has been raised, correction being made to keep CO_2 at the usual pressure.

3.1. Electrophysiological response

(a) In contrast to the previous situations, the loss of function is slow: at 5 atm. the synaptic transmission is lost only after 7 h. At lower pressures this delay is longer. (b) Once more the synaptic transmission appears to be the most delicate mechanism, failure of the preganglionic nerve appearing within the time observed when the tissue is kept at the usual p_{O_2}. (c) As shown after glucose deprivation, the tissue is still able to give a response to acetylcholine added to the medium after transmission has been lost. (d) But contrasting with the situation after glucose withdrawal there is no spontaneous activity or depolarization of the tissue at the time when transmission is being lost. (e) In presence of eserine in the medium, one cannot observe the usual long asynchronous discharge following a short repetitive stimulation, though there is still a response to the electrical stimulation of the presynaptic fibers. (f) Repetitive stimulation results in an early reversible loss of transmission.

This last observation and others (Rossier, to be published) indicate that the synthesis or the release of acetylcholine may be impaired under conditions of high oxygen pressure.

3.2. Metabolic data

(a) The loss of function is no doubt due to the increased O_2 pressure as shown by the fact that keeping the p_{O_2} at a normal value but increasing the pressure with helium does not shorten the length of time during which synaptic transmission is possible *in vitro*. Thus neither compression nor decompression harms the tissue, and the reason for the failure of the transmission is a metabolic one (Rossier *et al.*, 1968). (b) Contrasting with the situation of glucose deprivation is the observation that refrigerating the tissue at 2° does not protect it from the effects of high O_2 pressure. Ganglia exposed to this same temperature and the same pressure but with helium, show a normal response after having been warmed again and for as long a time as in the standard conditions. (c) By increasing the amount of glucose in the solution one can prolong the time before failure of synaptic transmission due to high oxygen pressure by more than 5 h, at 5 atm. ($p_{O_2} = 4425$ mm Hg). The question arises whether this improvement is connected with an increased gradient helping the glucose to cross a membrane that became less permeable, or brings a better supply to a tissue using more glucose when put under a high pressure of O_2. The answer can partly be given by the observation that under these conditions the tissue very quickly uses the glycogen that it has accumulated before being put under high oxygen pressure; on the other hand it does not synthesize glycogen when under high oxygen pressure, even if all the other required conditions for this synthesis are realized.

MORPHOLOGY

After the tissue has been kept from 12 to 19 h under high oxygen pressure, it shows, at the phase-contrast microscopy regions where the structure is well maintained, and close to these, areas where the neurons are seriously injured. There is no region where damaged or intact cells are located specifically — in particular there is no difference between the periphery and the middle of the ganglion.

Electron microscopy (Rouiller et al., to be published) reveals in the injured regions that the components of the nervous tissue in the whole are degenerated (Fig. 4). In the less damaged regions, the structure of the neurons, fibers and satellite cells is more or less altered. Again, cells and fibers very well preserved can be seen in the neighborhood of cells whose protoplasm is degenerating, and of swollen and optically emptied fibers. When ganglia are kept under the same pressure (5 atm.) obtained by using helium and at a normal p_{O_2} and p_{CO_2}, there are no alterations of the ultrastructure except for the matrix of the mitochondria which appears somewhat clearer than usual, the neurons, the satellite cells and the fibers being undamaged (Figs. 6 and 7).

After 7 h under oxygen pressure at 5 atm., the observed lesions are a mixture of the specific lesion seen in the glucose lack situation and others affecting, by contrast, the neurons themselves. This helps us to understand why the electrophysiological results are different from those recorded in the absence of any substrate.

From these observations, and the inability of the tissue to synthesize glycogen, though able to use very quickly the amount previously stored, and that it greatly profits from an increase in the concentration of glucose in the solution, one may conclude that the neurons under high oxygen pressure probably suffer from a progressive lack of glucose. The very first failure in transmission might be an impairment in the production (or release) of acetylcholine, as shown by the electrophysiology (Rossier, to be published). Only later does a situation develop that is similar to the deprivation of glucose, and it results in the same lesions.

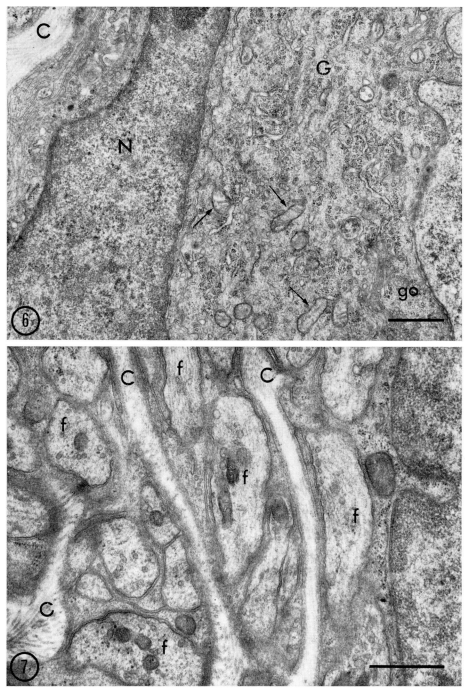

Fig. 6. Superior cervical ganglion kept for 19 h at 5 atm. helium, but at a normal p_{O_2} and p_{CO_2}. The ganglionic cell (G) is well preserved. The only visible modification is a slight mitochondrial swelling (arrows). N, satellite cell nucleus. Magnification 15 200 ×.

Fig. 7. Superior cervical ganglion kept for 19 h at 5 atm. helium, but at a normal p_{O_2} and p_{CO_2}. The cell processes (f) are well preserved. Magnification 21 000 ×.

SUMMARY AND CONCLUSIONS

We have studied the electrophysiological response and the ultrastructure of the superior cervical ganglion of the rat, kept *in vitro* in three well-defined metabolic conditions: deprivation of glucose, anoxia, and high oxygen pressure.

In the first of these conditions, the presence of O_2 allows the tissue to use internal substrates such as glycogen, lipids or amino acids. The neurons are thereby able to maintain their functional and morphological properties for more than 30 h. Nevertheless transmission is irreversibly lost after 2 h, as a consequence of a very specific lesion of the presynaptic endings.

In the absence of O_2, the tissue has to cover all its metabolic requirements through anaerobic glycolysis and therefore has to draw out of the solution up to 55 mg glucose/g (dry weight)/h (18.7 mg/g dry weight/h in aerobic conditions). Transmission is lost very early (in the first 15 min), but complete recovery is possible even after 3 h of anoxia. After the 5th hour without O_2 cytoplasmic enzymes are lost. The observed lesions of the ultrastructure are different from those seen in glucose lack: the satellite cells and the neurons are affected very early, the presynaptic fibers being still normal.

In the third condition, high oxygen pressure, function is lost much later, but irreversibly as it is after glucose deprivation. An increase in the amount of glucose in the solution prolongs the time during which transmission is possible. In this condition there appear to be both a lesion of the neurons and one of the presynaptic fibers.

Thus synaptic transmission is always lost first, but for different reasons in these three situations where the supply and use of glucose is impaired: (*a*) in glucose lack the presynaptic terminals are destroyed; (*b*) in anoxia, release of acetylcholine and the postsynaptic structures are first damaged; and (*c*) under high oxygen pressure the synthesis of acetylcholine is impaired and later the presynaptic fibers are injured, not enough glucose being available to maintain the integrity of these structures.

ACKNOWLEDGEMENT

The authors wish to thank Mrs. G. Kenel for much help in preparing the manuscript.

REFERENCES

BARKA, T., AND ANDERSON, P. J., (1963); *Histochemistry*, Hoeber, Harper, New York, p. 313.

BERGER, J.-P., AND DOLIVO, M., (1966); Lésion métabolique précoce par irradiation β du tissu nerveux *in vitro*. *Helv. physiol. pharmacol. Acta*, **24**, C8–C9.

DE DUVE, C., WATTIAUX, R., AND BAUDHUIN, P., (1962); Distribution of enzymes between subcellular fractions in animal tissues. *Advanc. Enzymol.*, **24**, 291–358.

DE PERROT, E., (1962); Relations entre l'activité de quelques enzymes et la fonction du tissu nerveux. *Helv. physiol. pharmacol. Acta*, **20**, 59–72.

DE RIBAUPIERRE, F., (1968); Localisation, synthèse et utilisation du glycogène dans le ganglion sympathique cervical du rat. *Brain Res.*, **11**, 42–64.

DE RIBAUPIERRE, F., ROUILLER, CH., AND DOLIVO, M., (1968); unpublished observation.

DOLIVO, M., (1966); Esquisse des relations entre le métabolisme et le fonctionnement du tissu nerveux isolé des vertébrés. *J. Physiol. (Paris)*, **58**, 127–194.

DOLIVO, M., FOROGLOU-KERAMEUS, CH., NICOLESCU, P., ROCH-RAMEL, F., AND ROUILLER, CH., (1965); Effet du manque de glucose sur la fonction et l'ultrastructure du ganglion sympathique cervical isolé du rat. *J. Physiol. (Paris)*, **57**, 602–603.

DOLIVO, M., LECHAIRE, F., AND DUNANT, Y., (1966); La libération d'acétylcholine par le ganglion sympathique cervical isolé du rat au cours de la privation de glucose. *Helv. physiol. pharmacol. Acta*, **24**, C80–C82.

DOLIVO, M., FOROGLOU-KERAMEUS, CH., KOCSIS, M., NICOLESCU, P., AND ROUILLER, CH., (1967); Altération et fonctionnement du tissu nerveux au cours de l'anoxie *in vitro*. *J. Physiol. (Paris)*, **59**, 393.

DUNANT, Y., (1967); Organisation topographique et fonctionnelle du ganglion cervical supérieur chez le rat. *J. Physiol. (Paris)*, **59**, 17–38.

DUNANT, Y., AND DOLIVO, M., (1968a); Presynaptic recording in excised sympathetic ganglion of the rat. *Brain Res.*, **10**, 268–270.

DUNANT, Y., AND DOLIVO, M., (1968b); Plasticity of synaptic function in the excised sympathetic ganglion of the rat. *Brain Res.*, **10**, 271–273.

FOROGLOU-KERAMEUS, C., AND DOLIVO, M., (1968); unpublished observation.

FORSSMANN, W. G., (1965); Eine Variation der Bichromat–Osmiumsäure-Fixation für das Nervensystem. *Experientia (Basel)*, **21**, 358–359.

KARNOVSKY, M. J., (1961); Simple method for staining with lead at high pH in electron microscopy. *J. biophys. biochem. Cytol.*, **11**, 729–732.

LARRABEE, M. G., (1958); Oxygen consumption of excised sympathetic ganglia at rest and in activity. *J. Neurochem.*, **2**, 81–101.

LARRABEE, M. G., (1961a); Conduction, transmission and metabolism in sympathetic ganglia excised from rats. In J. H. QUASTEL (Ed.), *Methods in Medical Research*, Year Book Medical Publishers, Chicago, pp. 241–247.

LARRABEE, M. G., (1961b); Glucose metabolism in ganglia and nerves. *Biophysics of Physiological and Pharmacological Actions*, American Association for the Advancement of Science, Washington, pp. 199–213.

LARRABEE, M. G., HOROWICZ, P., STEKIEL, W., AND DOLIVO, M., (1957); Metabolism in relation to function in mammalian sympathetic ganglia. In D. RICHTER (Ed.), *Metabolism of the Nervous System*, Pergamon, Oxford, pp. 208–220.

LUFT, J. H., (1961); Improvements in epoxy resin embedding methods. *J. biophys. biochem. Cytol.*, **9**, 409–414.

MILLONIG, G., (1961); Advantages of a phosphate buffer for OsO_4 solutions in fixation. *J. appl. Physiol.*, **32**, 1637–1639.

MUMENTHALER, M., AND ENGELS, N. K., (1961); Cytological localization of cholinesterase in developing chick embryo skeletal muscle. *Acta anat. (Basel)*, **47**, 274–299.

NICOLESCU, P., DOLIVO, M., ROUILLER, C., AND FOROGLOU-KERAMEUS, C., (1966); The effect of deprivation of glucose on the ultrastructure and function of the superior cervical ganglion of the rat *in vitro*. *J. Cell Biol.*, **29**, 267–285.

PEARS, A. G. E., (1961); *Histochemistry, Theoretical and Applied*. Churchill, London.

ROCH-RAMEL, F., AND DOLIVO, M., (1967); Activité de quelques enzymes et survie fonctionnelle du ganglion sympathique isolé du rat. *Helv. physiol. pharmacol. Acta*, **25**, 40–61.

ROSSIER, B., DOLIVO, M., DE RIBAUPIERRE, M., AND ROUILLER, C., (1968); Effet toxique de l'oxygène sous pression sur la conduction et la transmission dans le ganglion sympathique cervical isolé du rat. *Helv. physiol. pharmacol. Acta*, **26**, C241–C243.

RYTER, A., AND KELLENBERGER, ED., (1958); L'inclusion au polyester pour l'ultramicrotomie. *J. Ultrastruct. Res.*, **2**, 200–214.

WINCKLER, G., (1959); A propos de la technique de l'imprégnation argentique de Marschand, Glees et Erikson. *Arch. Anat. (Strasbourg)*, **42**, 233–241.

Effect of Preganglionic Stimulation Upon RNA Synthesis in the Isolated Sympathetic Ganglion of the Rat[*]

V. GISIGER AND A.-C. GAIDE-HUGUENIN

Department of Physiology, University of Lausanne (Switzerland)

Neuronal activity influences the synthesis of RNA and proteins in the nervous tissue (Pevzner, 1966; Hydén, 1960). The purpose of our work was to investigate the effect of precisely controlled preganglionic stimulation upon RNA synthesis in isolated ganglia. In this preliminary report we shall show that preganglionic stimulation is followed by an increased synthesis of RNA mainly during the post-activation period.

MATERIAL AND METHODS

The techniques of incubation in Eagle's medium and of the extraction of RNA with hot phenol have already been described (Gisiger *et al.*, 1967). Medium without choline was used in order to prevent an effect of this precursor of acetylcholine (Dunant, personal communication). The labeling with tritiated uridine (specific activity 20 C/mmole) was carried out for 1 h using a concentration of 10 μC/ml. The ganglia were incubated in a teflon chamber, in which 10 ganglia could be stimulated at the same time under identical conditions, while each individual action potential could be recorded. The chamber was placed in a water-saturated CO_2–O_2 incubator. A more detailed description of this chamber will be published later. The ganglia were placed on the electrodes in the chamber, their response to stimulation was tested, and they were kept at rest for a period of 2–3 h of preincubation. At the time of activation, 5 ganglia received supra-maximal shocks, while the other 5 remained at rest and were used as a control.

RESULTS

Labeling during activation

The ganglia were stimulated for 4 h at the following frequencies: 1, 2, 4, 8, 16 and 32/sec (Fig. 1). The labeling took place during the last hour of activation. Fig. 1A shows that the specific activity of RNA increased when the ganglia were stimulated

---

[*] This work was supported by grant 4795 of the Swiss National Foundation for Scientific Research.

References p. 129

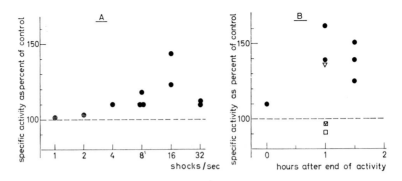

Fig. 1. Influences of preganglionic stimulation upon RNA specific activity of sympathetic ganglia. (A) The ganglia were activated for 4 h at the frequencies indicated. The labeling (conc. 10 μC/ml for 1 h) took place during the last hour of activation. (B) The ganglia were labeled immediately or half-an-hour after the end of an activation of 3 h at 32/sec. $\triangledown$, activation in the presence of atropine sulfate (2 μg/ml); $\square$, activation in the presence of mecamine (30 μg/ml).

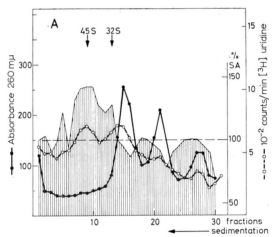

Fig. 2. Sucrose-gradient analysis of the RNA extracted from ganglia activated at 16/sec for 4 h. The shaded area represents the difference in specific activity, calculated fraction by fraction from the activated ganglia and the controls. The RNA was layered on top of a sucrose gradient (5–20% sucrose in a buffer containing NaCl 0.05 M, MgCl$_2$ 10^{-4}M, CH$_3$COONa 0.01 M, polyvinyl sulfate 20 μg/ml, pH 5.1). The tubes were centrifuged in Spinco model L$_2$-65 B, rotor SW 65 at 50 000 rev./min for 2.0 h. After the centrifugation, fractions of two drops were collected.

at 16/sec. The incorporation of tritiated uridine rose only slightly when 4, 8 and 32 shocks/sec were applied.

Fig. 2 shows a sedimentation analysis on a sucrose gradient of the total RNA from ganglia stimulated at 16/sec. The shaded area represents the difference in specific activity, calculated fraction by fraction from the activated ganglia and the controls. The maximal effect on RNA synthesis lies in the area of the 45 and 32 S fractions which include the preribosomal RNA. The ratios of the specific activity of the peaks at 45 and 32 S *versus* that of 18 S are greater as compared with the ratios of the controls

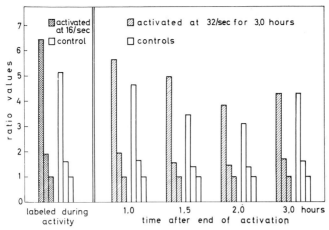

Fig. 3. Ratios of the specific activity of the RNA from the peaks at 45 S and 32 + 28 S *versus* that from the peak at 18 S. The specific activity of the peaks was determined by computing the values for the absorbance at 260 mμ and ^{3}H radioactivity obtained by sedimentation analysis.

(Fig. 3). This observation makes it rather unlikely that the increased specific activity is due to modifications of the intracellular pool size of uridine. Thus, preganglionic stimulation seems to activate the synthesis of preribosomal RNA. The sedimentation analysis of the RNA from ganglia stimulated at 8 or 32 shocks/sec sometimes showed smaller but similar modifications. In other experiments, no significant difference compared with the controls could be detected. We have as yet no clues to explain why specific activity of the RNA failed to increase significantly in ganglia stimulated at 32 shocks/sec.

Labeling after activation

The ganglia were incubated in the presence of tritiated uridine for 1 h at different intervals after the end of a 3-h activation period at 32 shocks/sec. Fig. 1B shows an increase in specific activity of 50% on an average when labeling was done immediately after the end of activation, and of 40% on an average when labeling was done from 30 to 90 min after the end of activation. The specific activity was still enhanced by about 20% 3 h after the end of activation. The specific activity of ganglia labeled during the hour following the end of an activation of 3 h at 16 shocks/sec showed an increase of 30%.

The sedimentation analysis of the RNA of ganglia labeled during the post-activation period showed a pattern similar to that of ganglia labeled during the stimulation at 16 shocks/sec. The increase of specific activity in the area of 45 and 32 S was most evident during the first hour after the end of stimulation. It declined with time, although an increased specific activity of the total RNA persisted for at least 3 h (Fig. 3).

In the sympathetic cervical ganglion of the rat, "nicotinic" and "muscarinic" synaptic junctions have been described. Mecamine blocks the "nicotinic" junctions (Dunant, 1968) and atropine blocks the "muscarinic" junctions (Dunant and Dolivo, 1967). When ganglia were stimulated after transmission had been completely blocked by mecamine (30 μg/ml), no increase in specific activity appeared during the post-activation period. On the other hand, the blockade of "muscarinic" receptors by atropine sulfate (2 μg/ml) failed to influence the increase in specific activity (Fig. 1B).

Preganglionic stimulation at 32 shocks/sec during 3 h represents a very heavy activation. However, when the ganglia were stimulated for 1 h only, the specific activity was nevertheless 30% greater than that of the control, whereas the increase was reduced to 14 or 12%, if the ganglia were activated for 30 or 15 min.

The localization of the radioactivity in the ganglia was studied with autoradiographs*. These show that almost the total amount of the grains were spread on the neurons and the neuroglia only. The labeled RNA remained in the nuclei after 1 h of labeling. There was no essential difference in the distribution of the grains between the stimulated ganglia and the controls.

DISCUSSION AND CONCLUSION

The preliminary results reported here are compatible with the well-known hypothesis, first proposed by the histologists Nissl (1892), Hydén (1960) and Altman (1966), that activation of the neurons stimulates the synthesis of Nissl's substance, which is composed of ribonucleoproteins.

The increase in RNA synthesis can take place during the activation, but it is enhanced more strongly at the end of the activation and lasts several hours. The increased synthesis is not influenced by the blockade of the "muscarinic" junctions responsible for the slow synaptic potentials (Dunant and Dolivo, 1967). On the other hand, the blockade of the "nicotinic" junctions, leading to the disappearance of the action potential, prevents the stimulation of RNA synthesis. From the results obtained it is impossible to decide whether this lack of enhanced synthesis is due to the absence of transmitter action on the synaptic membrane or to the lack of depolarization of the neurons.

SUMMARY

(*1*) The influence of the preganglionic stimulation on the RNA metabolism of the sympathetic cervical ganglion of the rat has been studied by radioactive labeling.

(*2*) A significant increase in the RNA-specific activity was observed· (*a*) during the activation at 16/sec for 4 h; and (*b*) during the period that follows the end of an activation at 32/sec and 16/sec for 3 h.

(*3*) The increase in the specific activity was greatest immediately after the end of activation.

(*4*) Blockade of the "nicotinic" junctions prevented the increase in the specific activity.

---

* The autoradiographs were kindly prepared in the Department of Cellular Biology ISREC, Lausanne.

ACKNOWLEDGEMENTS

We are grateful to Prof. M. Dolivo and Drs. Y. Dunant, K. Scherrer and B. Hirt for many useful suggestions and stimulating discussion. The technical assistance of Miss. M.-H. Conus is gratefully acknowledged.

REFERENCES

ALTMAN, J., (1966); Behavioral influences on the utilization of H³-leucine by the brain. In H. PEETERS (Ed.), *Protides of the Biological Fluids*. Elsevier, Amsterdam, pp. 127–136.

DUNANT, Y., (1968); Presynaptic spike and excitatory postsynaptic potential in sympathetic ganglion. Their modifications by pharmacological agents. In: K. AKERT AND P. G. WASER (Eds.), *Progress in Brain Research, Vol. 31, Mechanisms of Synaptic Transmission*, Elsevier, Amsterdam, pp. 131–139.

DUNANT, Y., AND DOLIVO, M., (1967); Relations entre les potentiels synaptiques lents et l'excitabilité du ganglion sympathique chez le rat. *J. Physiol. (Paris)*, **59**, 281–294.

GISIGER, V., DUNANT, Y., HUGUENIN, A.-C., AND DOLIVO, M., (1967); L'incorporation d'uridine tritiée à l'acide ribonucléique du ganglion sympathique du rat, incubé *in vitro*. *Helv. physiol. pharmacol. Acta*, **25**, CR 415–417.

HYDÉN, H., (1960); In J. BRACHET AND A. E. MIRSKY, (Eds.), *The Neuron. The Cell*. Vol. 4, Academic Press, New York, pp. 215–323.

NISSL, F., (1892); Über die Veränderungen der Ganglienzellen am Facialiskern des Kaninchens nach Ausreissung der Nerven. *Allg. Z. Psychiat.*, **48**, 197–198.

PEVZNER, L. Z., (1966); Nucleic acid changes during behavioral events. In J. GAITO (Ed.), *Macromolecules and Behavior*. North-Holland, Amsterdam, pp. 43–70.

Presynaptic Spike and Excitatory Postsynaptic Potential in Sympathetic Ganglion
Their Modifications by Pharmacological Agents[*]

Y. DUNANT[**]

Institute for Physiology, University of Lausanne (Switzerland)

An action potential derived from the activity of the presynaptic nerve endings (Dunant, 1968; Dunant and Dolivo, 1968a) can be recorded from the sympathetic ganglion of the rat. The object of this work is to demonstrate the precise relationship of this presynaptic spike with the excitatory postsynaptic potential (EPSP).

METHODS

The superior cervical ganglia of Wistar rats weighing 200–400 g were excised under urethane anesthesia and mounted on glass electrodes. The preparation bathed during the whole experiment in Krebs' solution remained usable for several hours (Dunant, 1967). To record presynaptic spikes, the transmission must be completely blocked either by *d*-tubocurarine or by a ganglion-blocking agent. We used mecamine (Mecamylamine, Merck Sharp and Dohme) at the concentration of 20 μg/ml. By stimulating the preganglionic nerve a small action potential was obtained if the recording electrode was placed precisely on the superior pole of the ganglion. Under these conditions the height of the presynaptic spike was about 20–50 μV, *i.e.* 1–5% of the amplitude of the ganglionic action potential before the transmission had been blocked. When the record was made on the superior extremity of the ganglion the presynaptic spike was small and monophasic, while, at a lower level it was larger and diphasic.

Identification of this action potential as a response from the presynaptic nerve endings is based on evidence which has been presented in a previous communication (Dunant, 1968).

Partial blockade of the transmission can also be achieved by smaller doses of mecamine (5 μg/ml). Ganglia so treated show both the presynaptic spike and the EPSP. This was the case for most of the experiments described in this paper. During the first 2–3 h of observation *in vitro* the amplitude of the presynaptic spike remains

[*] This work was supported by Grant 3893 from the Fonds National Suisse de la Recherche Scientifique.
[**] Present address: Department of Pharmacology, Downing Street, University of Cambridge (Great Britain).

stable, then it diminishes. The EPSP amplitude decreases in a regular way when the ganglion is placed in Krebs' solution (Fig. 3). Atropine sulfate (0.5 μg/ml) was added to the solution in a number of experiments to eliminate the influence of the slow synaptic potentials (Dunant and Dolivo, 1967).

RESULTS

Presynaptic spike and EPSP as recorded in these experiments are compound potentials integrating numerous unitary presynaptic spikes and numerous unitary EPSPs. However, there exists a simple ratio between the numbers of corresponding pre-synaptic and postsynaptic elements. This can be illustrated by stimulating the cervical trunk with shocks of increasing intensity thus activating more and more preganglionic B_2 fibers. As a consequence, the presynaptic spike increases in size and at the same time the EPSP increases proportionately to it (Fig. 1).

(1) Modifications of presynaptic spike and EPSP by a single conditioning volley

If double-shock stimulation is applied to the preganglionic nerve, the first one modifies the response to the second one in the following manner: The presynaptic spike is enlarged when the interval between the two shocks is less than 100 msec, then it returns to its control value, as for the EPSP, it is briefly facilitated in the beginning and then greatly depressed. It will not recover its initial amplitude for one or two minutes (Dunant and Dolivo, 1968b; Fig. 1).

The release of a bigger quantity of transmitter due to this increase in the pre-synaptic spike (Takeuchi and Takeuchi, 1962) can explain the homosynaptic facilitation described in the non-blocked ganglion (Dunant, 1967). The amplitude of the axonal action potential recorded on the preganglionic nerve itself is not increased after one volley. These findings represent the first difference between the properties of pre-synaptic terminals and axons of the same neurons.

(2) Modifications of presynaptic spike and EPSP after repetitive conditioning stimuli

Short term effects. The conditioning consists of a series of supramaximal shocks, *e.g.* 50/sec for 10 sec. Initially, *i.e.* during the first seconds following the conditioning train, the presynaptic spike was facilitated. Its amplitude increases proportional to the frequency of repetitive stimulation (Fig. 2). The EPSP itself was depressed after low-frequency conditioning and potentiated after intensive conditioning. Responses recorded on the same preparation after trains at different frequency show that increases in size of the EPSP were a logarithmic function of those of the presynaptic spike (Fig. 2, records). This relation is valid within certain limits only: The time interval should be 2–5 sec after the conditioning.

Long term effects. 5 min after a single conditioning stimulation (50/sec for 10 sec), the height of the EPSP attains about 150% of its control value. Afterwards, this facilitation decreases but remains apparent for more than 30 min (Fig. 3, line 1).

If trains of 10-sec duration are repeated every 5 min and the EPSP tested 5 min

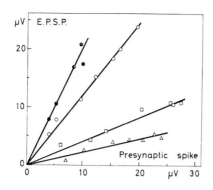

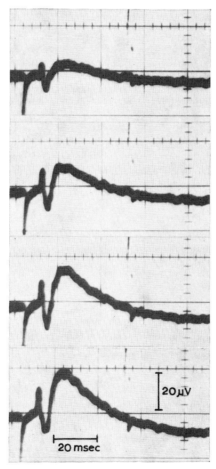

Fig. 1. Presynaptic spike and EPSP in response to preganglionic stimulation of increasing intensity. Mecamine 5 μg/ml. Above: Relative increases of the presynaptic spike and of the EPSP for four ganglia. The relation is linear for each ganglion. The different slopes are due to anatomical factors and to different recording conditions. Below: Responses of a preparation to four stimulating shocks of increasing intensity.

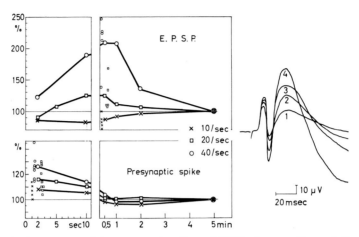

Fig. 2. Short-lasting changes of the presynaptic spike and EPSP after repetitive activity. Mecamine 5 μg/ml and atropine sulphate 0.5 μg/ml. Supramaximal stimulation of the preganglionic nerve. At left: Trains of 10-sec duration at the frequency indicated are given every 5 min. When the long-lasting facilitation has reached a steady state (usually after 3 trains), test shocks are delivered after each train at intervals indicated on the graph. The measured amplitude of the EPSP and of the pre-synaptic spike are expressed as percent of a control response checked just before every train. The lines are drawn through the means, but the individual measurements are also shown in the figure. At right: Superimposed drawings of the presynaptic spikes and of the EPSPs recorded on the same preparation. The first trace (1) is the record obtained after a long period of rest. The second trace (2) is the response recorded 2 sec after the end of a train of stimuli of 10/sec lasting for 10 sec. Traces 3 and 4 show presynaptic spikes and EPSPs recorded after the end of similar trains in which the frequency was raised to 20/sec (3) and 40/sec (4).

later, its amplitude progressively reaches a steady state (see Dunant and Dolivo, 1968b; Fig. 2). By increasing the stimulating frequency of the conditioning trains, the height of the EPSP increases once more towards a new steady state. On the contrary if this frequency is reduced, the EPSP decreases and stabilises itself at a lower value. The long-lasting facilitation could then be regulated to a higher or a lower level by changing the frequency of the conditioning trains.

The presynaptic spike does not participate in these long-lasting changes. Since 30 sec after the conditioning it has returned to its initial amplitude. The action po-tential of an unblocked ganglion is subject to the same modifications when it is sub-mitted to similar conditions. But the relative variations of its amplitude are smaller (Fig. 3, bottom).

These plastic properties of transmission in the sympathetic ganglion are not due to a change in the postsynaptic sensitivity to acetylcholine. 5 min after repetitive activation the response of the ganglion to acetylcholine applied directly is not in-creased, but is in fact decreased after more intensive stimulation (50/sec for 30 sec).

Importance of external calcium for the long-lasting facilitation. Long-term facilitation elicited by a single train of 20/sec for 10 sec is rather weak (Fig. 3, line 3). However, if the same conditioning train is given to a ganglion bathed in a calcium-rich solution and the preparation is washed soon after by a standard solution to test the EPSP in normal medium, the long-term facilitation is enhanced (Fig. 3, line 2). By repeating trains of same duration and frequency in the presence of different calcium concentra-

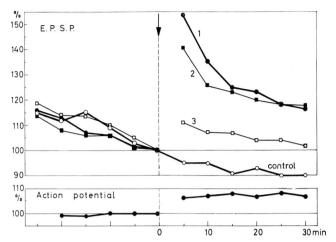

Fig. 3. Very long-lasting facilitation in the sympathetic ganglion. Upper part: Amplitude of the EPSP in a preparation blocked by mecamine (5 μg/ml). Control (open circles): regular decrease of the EPSP checked every 5 min. (1) (filled circles): At the time indicated by arrow the preparation was given a preganglionic stimulation of 50/sec for 10 sec. Half an hour later the EPSP is still facilitated. Standard Krebs' solution. (2) (filled squares): The ganglion had been placed in a modified solution containing 4.4 mM CaCl₂ and 0.6 mM MgCl₂ just before a train of 20/sec for 10 sec. Just after this conditioning the preparation is put again in a standard solution and the EPSP tested every 5 min. (3) (open squares): The same conditioning is given in a standard solution (2.2 mM CaCl₂ and 1.2 mM MgCl₂). The long-lasting facilitation is bigger when the conditioning has been effected in a calcium-rich solution. Lower part: Amplitude of the action potential of an unblocked preparation bathed in standard Krebs' solution without mecamine. Conditioning train of 50/sec for 10 sec.

tions, one observes that the amount of calcium at the moment of conditioning determines the size of an EPSP tested 5 min later in a standard Krebs' solution (see Dunant and Dolivo, 1968b; Fig. 2).

Therefore, calcium seems not only to permit an immediate release of transmitter but also to increase the quantity of transmitter available for a prolonged period of time. Both effects are antagonistically influenced by magnesium.

(3) Action of pharmacological agents on the presynaptic spike

Acetylcholine (perchlorate) decreases the amplitude of the EPSP in doses which block the transmission by depolarizing the postsynaptic structures (Dunant, to be published). These concentrations leave the presynaptic spike intact (Fig. 4). Acetylcholine does not therefore depolarize the presynaptic terminals of the sympathetic ganglion of the rat. This argues against the hypothesis that it is a trigger for an extra release of the transmitter (Volle and Koelle, 1961; Koketsu and Nishi, 1968).

Hemicholinium (HC-3) is known to have some blocking action in the first stages necessary for the synthesis of acetylcholine by presynaptic structures (Bhatnagar and MacIntosh, 1967). This substance does not modify the amplitude of the presynaptic spike in doses ($2 \cdot 10^{-4}$ mole/l) which suffice to make the EPSP disappear after repetitive activation.

Ouabain blocks the transmission very probably by depolarization of the pre-

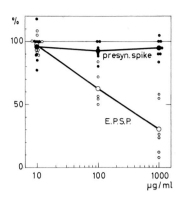

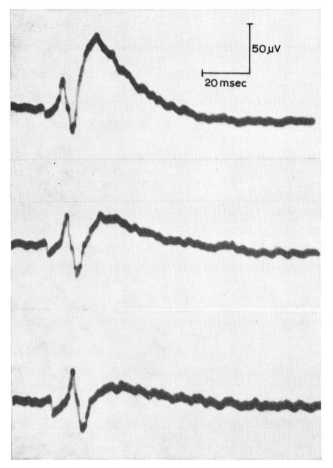

Fig. 4. Effect of acetylcholine on the presynaptic spike and on the EPSP. Mecamine 5 μg/ml. The amplitude of presynaptic spike and EPSP have been tested 5 min after adding acetylcholine (perchlorate) to the solution. Above: Means and individual measurements. Below: Three records from the same preparation. At top, control. In the middle, acetylcholine 100 μg/ml. Bottom, acetylcholine 1000 μg/ml. The EPSP is depressed by acetylcholine, the presynaptic spike remains unaltered.

synaptic terminals. At the concentration of $5 \cdot 10^{-4}$ mole/l it reduces the amplitude of the presynaptic spike and causes a massive spontaneous release of transmitter as shown by the appearance of a burst of postganglionic action potentials, which were abolished by *d*-tubocurarine (De Ribaupierre *et al.*, 1969).

Caesium chloride. When the external potassium was replaced by caesium a marked increase in both excitatory and inhibitory postsynaptic potentials of the crustacean neuro-muscular junction is observed (Gainer *et al.*, 1967). In the rat ganglion the presynaptic potential increases in size considerably and the EPSP increments are approximatively a logarithmic function of those of the presynaptic spike.

Metabolic conditions. If the ganglion was incubated in a solution without glucose, the presynaptic spike disappeared irreversibly during the period when the specific presynaptic lesions develop as Nicolescu *et al.* (1966) showed with the electron microscope (see also Dolivo and Rouiller, this Symposium, p. 111).

Oxygen lack also affects the amplitude of the presynaptic spike but this effect is partly reversible (M. Kocsis, personal communication).

DISCUSSION

The synaptic efficiency can be affected in 3 ways: (*1*) Modifications of the quantity of the transmitter available (by changing the uptake, the synthesis or the mobilisation of the transmitter), (*2*) Modifications of the amount of the transmitter released by presynaptic nerve impulse, (*3*) changes in the postsynaptic response to the transmitter.

The long-lasting facilitation, the depression of EPSP after single activity and the effect of hemicholinium, all belong to the first category.

Calcium ions are known to be a co-factor for the release of the transmitter (Katz and Miledi, 1967) but after preganglionic stimulation they also affect the quantity of the transmitter available later.

Unfavourable metabolic conditions and the effect of ouabain seem to belong to both the first and the second category, very probably by lowering the resting potential of the presynaptic nerve terminals. That peculiar sensitivity of the presynaptic endings should be stressed. It is related to their big surface to volume ratio and their high metabolic needs depending on an external energy supply.

The early facilitation after activity and the effect of caesium chloride potentiate the transmission by increasing the size of the presynaptic spikes. In those instances amplitude of EPSP's appear as a logarithmic function of those of the presynaptic spikes. This agrees with the observations made in numerous synapses in vertebrates and invertebrates (Liley, 1956; Takeuchi and Takeuchi, 1962; Katz and Miledi, 1967), and is consistent with the notion that the presynaptic spike signals the activity of nerve endings to the site, or very near the site, where the transmitter is released.

SUMMARY

(*1*) The action potential of the presynaptic nerve endings (presynaptic spike) and the excitatory postsynaptic potential (EPSP) were recorded simultaneously on the excised superior cervical ganglion of the rat.

(2) In response to preganglionic stimulation of increasing intensity the amplitudes of the presynaptic spike and of the EPSP are linearly related.

(3) After a single supramaximal shock the presynaptic spike is briefly facilitated, the EPSP is first facilitated then depressed.

(4) Brief repetitive stimulation produces changes of short duration and changes of very long duration. A few seconds after the conditioning train, the presynaptic spike is facilitated. The EPSP is depressed after trains of low frequency and potentiated after trains of high frequency. The amplitudes of the EPSP are within limits a logarithmic function of those of the presynaptic spike. The long-lasting changes affect the EPSP only. A facilitation persists as long as half an hour after a single train of 50/sec for 10 sec. This long-lasting facilitation can be modified by changing stimulation frequency of successive conditioning trains of the same duration. Calcium concentration in the solution at the time of the conditioning plays an essential role in long-lasting changes.

(5) Acetylcholine and hemicholinium block the transmission without modifying the presynaptic spike. Ouabain and unfavourable metabolic conditions block the transmission by decreasing the presynaptic spike. Caesium chloride potentiates the transmission by increasing the presynaptic spike.

ACKNOWLEDGEMENT

Many thanks are due to Miss G. Schwering for her excellent technical assistance. I am grateful to Prof. M. Dolivo, Mrs. C. Foroglou-Kerameus and A.-C. Gaide-Huguenin, Miss F. Léchaire, Messrs. J. Delèze, V. Gisiger, M. Kocsis, F. de Ribaupierre and B. Rossier for stimulating discussions and particularly to Dr. A. W. Cuthbert for help with the manuscript.

REFERENCES

BHATNAGAR, S. P., AND MACINTOSH, F. C., (1967); Effects of quaternary basis and inorganic cations on acetylcholine synthesis in nervous tissue. *Canad. J. Physiol. Pharmacol.*, **45**, 249–268.
DE RIBAUPIERRE, F., DUNANT, Y., DOLIVO, M., AND FOROGLOU-KERAMEUS, C., (1969); L'action présynaptique de l'ouabaïne sur le ganglion sympathique. *J. Physiol. (Paris)*, in the press.
DUNANT, Y., (1967); Organisation topographique et fonctionnelle du ganglion cervical superieur chez le rat. *J. Physiol. (Paris)*, **59**, 17–38.
DUNANT, Y., (1968); L'activité présynaptique dans le ganglion sympathique du rat. *J. Physiol. (Paris)*, **60**, suppl. I, 243.
DUNANT, Y., AND DOLIVO, M., (1967); Relations entre les potentiels synaptiques lents et l'excitabilité du ganglion sympathique chez le rat. *J. Physiol. (Paris)*, **59**, 281–294.
DUNANT, Y., AND DOLIVO, M., (1968a); Presynaptic recording in excised sympathetic ganglion of the rat. *Brain Res.*, **10**, 268–270.
DUNANT, Y., AND DOLIVO, M., (1968b); Plasticity of synaptic functions in the excised sympathetic ganglion of the rat. *Brain Res.*, **10**, 271–273.
GAINER, H., REUBEN, J. P., AND GRUNDFEST, H., (1967); The augmentation of postsynaptic potentials in crustacean muscle fibers by cesium. A presynaptic mechanism. *Comp. Biochem. Physiol.*, **20**, 877–900.
KATZ, B., AND MILEDI, R., (1967); A study of synaptic transmission in the absence of nerve impulses. *J. Physiol. (Lond.)*, **192**, 407–436.

KOKETSU, K., AND NISHI, S., (1968); Cholinergic receptors at sympathetic preganglionic nerve terminals. *J. Physiol. (Lond.)*, **196**, 293–310.

LILEY, A. W., (1956); The effects of presynaptic polarization on the spontaneous activity at the mammalian neuromuscular junction. *J. Physiol. (Lond.)*, **134**, 427–443.

NICOLESCU, P., DOLIVO, M., ROUILLER, C., AND FOROGLOU-KERAMEUS, C., (1966); The effect of deprivation of glucose on the ultrastructure and function of the superior cervical ganglion of the rat *in vitro*. *J. Cell Biol.*, **29**, 267–285.

TAKEUCHI, A., AND TAKEUCHI, N., (1962); Electrical changes in pre- and postsynaptic axons of the giant synapse of *Loligo*. *J. gen. Physiol.*, **45**, 1181–1193.

VOLLE, R. L., AND KOELLE, G. B., (1961); The physiological role of acetylcholinesterase in sympathetic ganglia. *J. Pharmacol. exp. Ther.*, **133**, 223–240.

Electron Microscopy of Excitatory and Inhibitory Synapses: A Brief Review

E. G. GRAY

Department of Anatomy, University College, London (Great Britain)

In this brief review attention will be confined to three well known categories of morphological configuration of neuro-neuronal and neuro-muscular synapses that have come to be recognised by electron microscopists during the past two decades. These configurations are best recognised in vertebrates (especially mammals). Such a classification is often more difficult to apply to invertebrates, where the distinction between axon and dendrite is often by no means clear.

CATEGORY 1. NON-SERIAL CLEFT SYNAPSES

These are simple (*i.e.* 2-component) contacts (Figs. 1–6), which might be either axo-dendritic, axo-somatic or axo-IS (initial segment). Most neuromuscular junctions can also be included in this category. Such synapses contain a presynaptic knob with synaptic vesicles thought to contain the transmitter substance. The vesicles often form aggregations near the synaptic cleft. The synaptic cleft is about 200–300 Å across or 600 Å or more at motor end-plates of vertebrates. Dense proteinaceous material usually lines and lies within the synaptic cleft. The material is often distributed asymmetrically (see below) in a manner related to the direction of transmission (Gray and Guillery, 1966). The function of the material remains unknown. It may be related, for example, to the transmission mechanism, mechanical adhesion of the synapse, or contact formation during ontogeny. The cleft of synapses in this category is always open along its full extent and never fused to form a tight junction. Synapses in this category are usually considered to have a chemical post-synaptic (see 3rd category) mode of excitatory or inhibitory transmission.

CATEGORY 2. NON-SERIAL SYNAPSES WITH TIGHT JUNCTIONS

These are also simple (*i.e.* 2-component) contacts. In vertebrates they may be axo-dendritic or axosomatic (or axo-axonal in some fishes, Bennett *et al.*, 1967a, b, c, d). No axo-IS contacts with tight junctions have yet been described. Synapses in this second category have not yet been described in mammals (with the possible exception of Dieters' nucleus; Sotelo and Palay, 1967), but are common in other vertebrates and less common in some invertebrates (axo-axonal). These synapses have

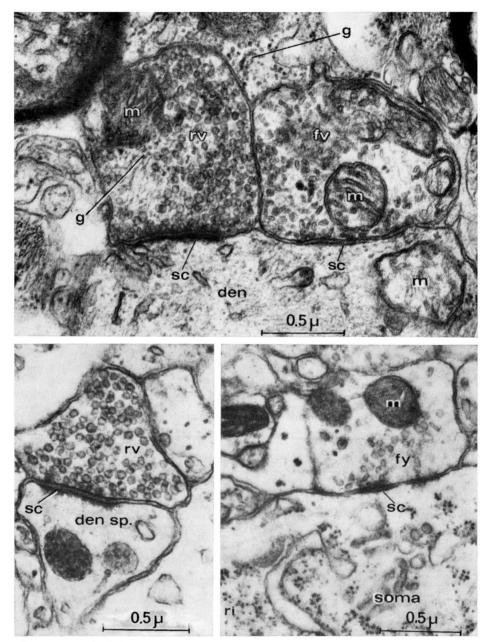

Fig. 1. Two axodendritic synapses on a dendrite of the goldfish ventral horn.

Fixation and staining. Figs. 1–7 aldehyde initial fixation. Figs. 8–10 osmium tetroxide initial fixation. Figs. 2 and 3 lead stained; Fig. 8 block PTA stain; others dark stained with block uranyl acetate and lead citrate on the section.

Abbreviations, used in all figures: a, b, c and d, see text; den, dendrite; den p, dendritic processes; den sp, dendritic spine; fv, flat synaptic vesicles; g, glycogen granules; Go, Golgi ending; m, mitochondrion; mo, mossy ending; my, myelin sheath; nf, neurofilaments; ri, ribosomes; rv, round vesicles; sc, synaptic cleft; sv, synaptic vesicles; tj, tight junction (region of presumed fusion of synaptic membranes).

Fig. 2. A dendrite (Type 1) spine synapse in the cerebral cortex of the cat with round vesicles.

Fig. 3. An axosomatic (Type 2) synapse from the cerebral cortex of the cat with flat vesicles. (Figs. 2 and 3 from Colonnier, 1968, by kind permission of the author.)

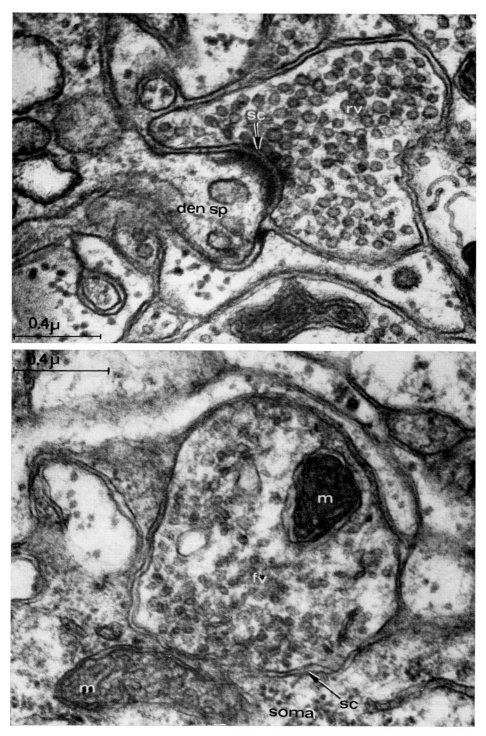

Fig. 4. A parallel fibre synapse on a dendritic spine of a Purkinje cell. Goldfish.
Fig. 5. A basket synapse on the soma of a Purkinje cell. Goldfish.

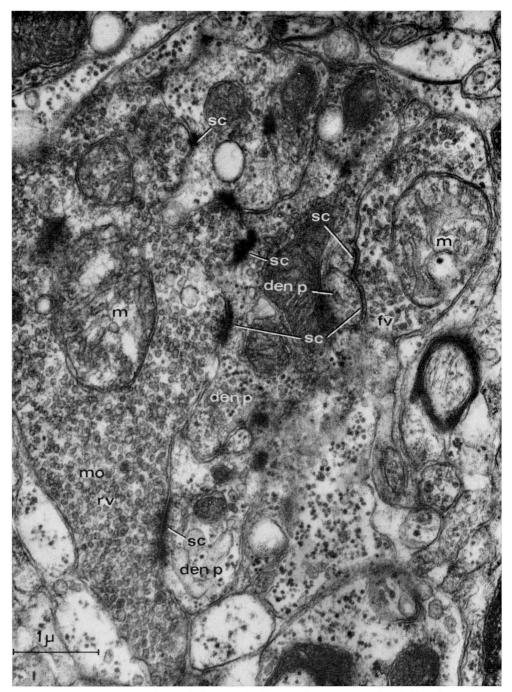

Fig. 6. Glomerulus of goldfish cerebellar granular layer. A large mossy ending (left) and a smaller
Golgi ending (right) contacting granule cell dendritic apices.

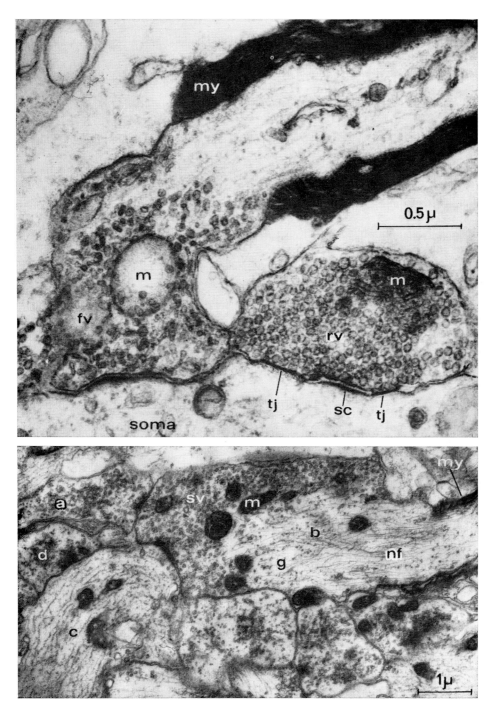

Fig. 7. Two axosomatic synapses in the ventral horn of tench cord.
The right contact has two tight junctions.
Fig. 8. An axonal knob (b) contacting a dendrite (c). (b) is contacted by axonal knob (a). (c) is also
contacted by another knob (d). Frog spinal cord (from Charlton and Gray, 1966).

one or more zones of the synaptic cleft closed by membrane "fusion" to form tight junctions (Fig. 7, right). Such synapses can often be shown physiologically to have an electrical mode of post-synaptic excitatory transmission. Synaptic vesicles and membrane thickenings (Fig. 7, right) may often be present, but in these synapses, which thus have in part the morphology of chemically transmitting synapses, chemical transmission has yet to be demonstrated physiologically.

CATEGORY 3. SERIAL SYNAPSES WITH NO TIGHT JUNCTIONS

Configurations in this category involve three components. In the vertebrates axo-axo-dendritic (Fig. 8) or axo-axo-somatic contacts have been described in various parts of the CNS (Kidd, 1961, 1962; Gray, 1962; Gray and Guillery, 1966; Szentá-gothai, 1968) and in the invertebrates similar serial arrangements have been observed in octopus brain (Gray and Young, 1964) and in certain crustacean muscles axo-axo-muscular junctions have been described (Dudel and Kuffler, 1961a, b; Atwood, 1968). At least some of these vertebrate and crustacean serial synapses are thought to be involved in the phenomenon of presynaptic inhibition (Frank and Fuortes, 1957; Dudel and Kuffler, 1961a, b; Eccles, 1964). The first synaptic knob influences the second knob to reduce the output of the second knob's excitatory transmitter and hence reduce or block the excitation of the third component of the serial arrangement.

THE THREE CATEGORIES IN TISSUE FIXED INITIALLY WITH ALDEHYDE

Initial fixation of the CNS by perfusion with buffered aldehyde solutions, formalde-hyde (best prepared from paraformaldehyde, Pease, 1964) or glutaraldehyde or a mixture of both has several advantages and is in general use nowadays (see Millonig and Marinozzi, 1968 for details). Post-fixation with buffered osmium tetroxide solution is usually carried out. Uchizono (1965) pointed out that electron microscopy of aldehyde-fixed mammalian cerebellum showed that excitatory parallel fibre presynaptic knobs contained round vesicles whereas the inhibitory basket axonal knobs contained flat vesicles. (The term 'flat' is used for convenience; 'polymorphic', 'elongated', 'ellipsoidal', 'ovoid' and 'tubular' profiles have been used by various authors; Gray, 1969). However, the morphology of the 'flat' vesicle as it occurs in the section is far from understood and is being studied at present by stereoelectron microscopy (Gray and Willis, 1968).

If, as Uchizono suggests, it is possible to distinguish excitatory from inhibitory terminals, even to a limited extent, simply on the difference of round or flat vesicles after aldehyde fixation, then this, of course, could be an enormous step forward in our understanding of the organisation of the CNS. In any event, so little is known about the origin and detailed morphology of the synaptic vesicle that studies on the flattening effect only on certain populations of vesicle after aldehyde fixation may well yield valuable cytological information (Walberg, 1966).

Following Uchizono's (1965) initial publication of mammalian material, I set out

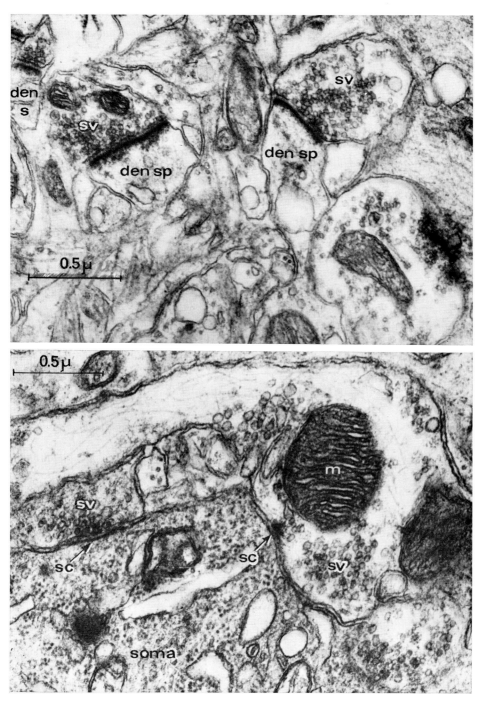

Fig. 9. Dendritic spine synapses in the occipital region of the cerebral cortex of the rat.
Fig. 10. Two axosomatic synapses in the occipital region of the cerebral cortex of the rat.

to pursue the problem on various regions of quite a different group of vertebrates, the teleost fishes. Observations were made on various regions of the CNS of the goldfish (*Carassius auratus* L.) and tench (*Tinca tinca* L.) after aldehyde perfusion. They will only be mentioned briefly here (see Gray, 1969 for details). The present paper is more concerned with a general review of the work of various authors.

Category 1

In the fish CNS aldehyde fixation reveals a dramatic and easily distinguishable difference in axonal knobs with round and those with flat vesicles (Fig. 1, in the ventral horn of the spinal cord). The left knob has round vesicles and pronounced synaptic thickening whilst the right knob has flat vesicles. The two sorts of ending occur in approximately equal proportions in the goldfish ventral horn. Bodian (1966a, b) made similar observations on the ventral horn of monkey cord. Uchizono (1966) found a 3 : 2 flat to round ratio on the motor neuron surface of cat ventral horn cells. These observations do not implicate specific synapses with excitation or inhibition, of course, for unfortunately it is not possible at present to examine a specific ventral horn synapse first physiologically then electron microscopically.

Observations on the fish cerebellar cortex support those of Uchizono (1965) on the mammalian cerebellum. The excitatory presynaptic knobs of the granule cell axons (parallel fibres) that contact the Purkinje spines (Gray, 1961) are clearly in the round-vesicle class (Fig. 4) whilst the inhibitory basket knobs that contact the Purkinje cell soma (Fig. 5) are in the flat (or polymorphic) class. The excitatory mossy terminals in the glomeruli of the granular layer (Gray, 1961) are clearly in the round-vesicle class. These contact the dendritic tips of the granule cells. The inhibitory Golgi knobs that lie at the periphery of the glomeruli and also contact the granule cell dendritic tips are clearly in the flat-vesicle class (Fig. 6). During the course of these observations (see Gray, 1969, for full details) similar conclusions on the mammalian cerebellum were published by Hirata (1966), Larramendi and Victor (1967), Larramendi *et al.* (1967) and Uchizono (1968). The climbing-fibre synapses will be mentioned in the DISCUSSION.

Other evidence for functional and morphological correlation of synapses in this category comes from observations on a special region of synaptic contact, the axonal initial segment. Westrum (1966) has shown that in the cerebral cortex flat-vesicled endings predominate on the IS, and points out that this region is strategically favourable for inhibitory contacts (Eccles, 1964). My own observations (Gray, 1969) on the IS of 13 motor cells in the ventral horn of the fish cord strongly support this view. Here, as Westrum showed, in the cortex, synaptic contacts occur right up to the point of entry of the axon into its myelin. Over 90% of the contacts were of the flat-vesicled class.

Other contacts that can be considered in this first category include the vertebrate motor endplate. These neuromuscular contacts are indisputably chemically excitatory and with aldehyde fixation the synaptic vesicles are clearly of the round type (Miledi, 1967).

In certain crustacean muscles there is good evidence for both chemically exciting and inhibiting contacts (Fatt and Katz, 1953a, b; Dudel and Kuffler, 1961a) and in correlation two classes of ending with round and flat vesicles respectively can be seen (Uchizono, 1967; Atwood, 1968). In the crustacean stretch receptor the dendrite of the receptor neuron has exclusively chemical inhibitory endings (Kuffler and Eyzaguirre, 1955) and Uchizono (1967) has shown clearly that they are of the flat-vesicled type. The stretch receptor muscle only has chemical excitatory contacts and Uchizono finds that these contacts are all of the round-vesicle type.

Recent work on the axo-dendritic synapses formed by the giant Mauthner axon collaterals in the teleost fish cord, which exert a powerful excitatory effect on the ipsilateral primary motor neurons (see Diamond and Yasargil in this volume, p. 201) shows that their axon terminals contain round vesicles (see Gray, 1969 for details).

Category 2

In the ventral horn of the teleost-fish cord axosomatic and axodendritic synapses with tight junctional zones at the synaptic cleft are a common occurrence (Fig. 7, right) (Charlton and Gray, 1966). Such contacts were first described by Pappas and Bennett at a Neuroscience Research Program in Boston 1964 (Pappas and Bennett, 1966a).

After aldehyde fixation, in the fish ventral horn, endings with tight junctions always have round vesicles (Fig. 7, right). Endings with flat vesicles (left) have never been observed to have tight junctions.

Such endings (in regions other than the ventral horn) have been shown to be electrically excitatory (Pappas and Bennett, 1966; Bennett *et al.*, 1967a–d) but there is apparently no evidence for chemical excitation. If so, then an anomaly exists. 'Round vesicles' is correlated with excitatory action, but if the synaptic vesicles contain transmitter substance then their presence seems superfluous. In the fish ventral horn (and frog cord) the endings with tight junctions also exhibit the morphological features of known chemically transmitting cleft synapses (category 1), in particular the asymmetric synaptic thickenings and related aggregations of (round) vesicles (Charlton and Gray, 1966). This is shown in Fig. 7 (sc) (see review of Gray and Guillery, 1967). Bennett *et al.* (1967d) have discussed the occurrence of these morphological features in synapses which might have no functional chemical mode of transmission.

My observation that tight junctions are associated exclusively with round vesicles in aldehyde preparations has not been confirmed in other sites in the fish cord with similar contacts (Pappas and Bennett, 1966b). Differences in preparative technique may possibly be responsible for this discrepancy.

Aldehyde-fixed synapses with tight junctions need investigation at other sites and in other groups of animals (for example those in the frog cord described by Charlton and Gray, 1966). Robertson *et al.* (1963) used aldehyde fixation for some of their observations on the club endings of the fish Mauthner neuron. These have tight junctions and 'synaptic' vesicles and are electrically excitatory, and, as yet, there seems to be no evidence for an additional chemical mechanism (Furshpan, 1964). Robertson *et al.* were not concerned with the distribution of round and flat vesicles, although they described endings (other than clubbed ones) with flat vesicles (their Fig. 14 — aldehyde fixed). Scrutiny of their Fig. 31, a section through an aldehyde-fixed club ending shows, however, that the vesicles are essentially of the round type. The shape of the vesicle in other sorts of synapse with tight or closely apposed synaptic membranes, for example the electrically transmitting crayfish synapse (Furshpan and Potter, 1959; Hama, 1961; Robertson, 1964) seems not yet to have been reported.

It is perhaps worth mentioning that the 'synaptic' vesicles when present are possibly not involved in electrical transmission for cells with this mechanism *e.g.* cardiac and smooth muscle and epithelia (Furshpan, 1964) have tight junctions, which are devoid of clusters of vesicles.

Category 3

Serial synapses occur in the mammalian spinal cord (Gray, 1962, 1963) and in the frog cord (Charlton and Gray, 1966). Fig. 8 shows an example of a presumed axo-axo-dendritic contact. Synaptic axonal knob (b), identified as such by the terminal region of its myelin sheath makes contact with dendrite (c). Knob (b) is itself contacted by knob (a). This morphological configuration agrees with that postulated by Eccles (1964) to account for the phenomenon of presynaptic inhibition (Frank and Fuortes, 1957), whereby one axonal knob excites a second knob with a lowering of its resting potential (hence the term presynaptic) resulting in a decrease or abolition of output of its excitatory transmitter. Hence the net result is inhibition without (in mammals) the intervention of an inhibitory transmitter. However, Granit (1968) has questioned this physiological interpretation and should be consulted.

The presence of serial contacts, *e.g.* in the mammalian and frog cord (Gray, 1962; Charlton and Gray, 1966) and the cuneate nucleus (Walberg, 1965) and crustacean muscle (Atwood, 1968 — see below) are all regions where presynaptic effects have been recorded; and important negative evidence comes from observations on the cerebral and cerebellar cortices. Here there are no serial synapses nor is there any evidence for presynaptic inhibition in these regions.

One serious criticism, however, has been the failure to demonstrate serial synapses on the surface of mammalian ventral horn cells where the group 1a afferents (Eccles, 1964) should on physiological evidence be involved in presynaptic inhibition (Conradi and Skoglund, 1968; Granit, 1968, Szentágothai, 1968). This criticism has now been countered, however, by a description of serial synapses (axo-axo-somatic) by Khattab (1968 and see below) on cat ventral-horn motor cells. Sampling is always a problem with electron microscopy and for this reason they may have been missed in the past, although much more work is needed on this point. For further details the review by Szentágothai (1968) should be referred to.

Now most of the observations on serial synapses so far have been on material initially fixed with osmium tetroxide (for example, Fig. 8), which, as we have seen, does not differentiate between round and flat-vesicled endings. It is of obvious importance to examine serial synapses after aldehyde fixation. Thus in the mammalian cord the axo-axonal contacts thought to be involved in presynaptic inhibition should both be chemically excitatory and both should have round vesicles. Now this is exactly as described by Khattab (1968), who shows in an aldehyde preparation a large ventral-horn bouton with round vesicles contacted by two smaller endings both with round vesicles. A second interesting example is the serial synapse in crustacean muscle (Atwood, 1968), the morphology of which fits the earlier physiological evidence of Dudel and Kuffler (1961b). Here the excitatory synapses (with glutamic acid the transmitter) on the muscle have round vesicles and at this synapse the first component (synaptic knob) of the serial arrangement liberates not an excitatory transmitter but an inhibitory one, GABA, which lowers the amplitude of voltage change by increasing the Cl^- conductance. In correlation Atwood (1968) has shown that this knob has the flattened type of vesicle, while the one it contacts, and which is directly excitatory to the muscle fibre, has round vesicles. Atwood (1968) should be consulted for further details and relevant references.

In other situations where serial synapses have been implicated in one way or another, interpretation of observations is less clear. Walberg (1966) and Mugnaini and Walberg (1967) report that endings of the cuneate fasciculus in the cuneate nucleus have elongated vesicles. These, however, were only identified because they were (experimentally) degenerating and we still need to know the shape of the vesicle in the normal terminals.

Also, the situation in the lateral geniculate nucleus, where serial synapses have been described (Szentágothai, 1962; Colonnier and Guillery, 1964) is far from clear. In aldehyde preparations the optic terminals can be identified and shown to have round vesicles and in correlation there is physiological evidence that they are chemically excitatory (see Maekawa and Rosina in this volume, p. 259). These optic terminals make direct contact with LGN neurons but they also contact other axonal knobs with flat vesicles and (if our anatomical criteria are correct) these in turn synapse with LGN neurons (Saavedra and Vaccarezza, 1968). These authors suggest that since the optic axons are the first components in the serial arrangement they might directly excite the LGN cells and also indirectly excite them by disinhibition, *i.e.* presynaptically bringing about a reduction of inhibitory transmitter from the flat vesicled endings. The theory is intriguing, and, of course, requires physiological confirmation. The fact that the optic axons are not post-synaptic to other axon knobs suggests that the optic endings are not themselves subjected to presynaptic inhibition (Saavedra and Vaccarezza, 1968). Physiological investigations have suggested presynaptic inhibition (see Saavedra and Vaccarezza, 1968, for references), but the evidence is open to other interpretations (Guillery, 1968).

TYPE 1 AND TYPE 2 CONTACTS

Some years ago (Gray, 1959) I described two sorts of synaptic contact based on the dense material and other features associated with the synaptic cleft. This classification was meant to apply only to the mammalian cerebral cortex and to material fixed initially in osmium tetroxide and stained with PTA. Although the distinction can be drawn in other regions of the CNS there are many situations where it cannot, and so the use of the epithets Type 1 and Type 2 in these regions, often on material subjected to different preparative and experimental techniques from those of my original description, has tended to cause some confusion in the literature.

PTA staining has certain disadvantages and so block staining with uranyl acetate followed by lead on the section (Westrum, 1965; Colonnier, 1968) has been used here to illustrate the two types in the occipital cortex of the rat. Fig. 9 shows Type 1 contacts on three dendritic spine profiles and Fig. 10 two Type 2 axosomatic contacts. In the former the postsynaptic membrane has a prominent postsynaptic thickening which extends along the full length of the cleft, whilst in the latter type the synaptic thickenings are localised and there is no prominent postsynaptic dense material.

In the hippocampus the axosomatic contacts known to be inhibitory have Type 2 contacts and dendritic spine synapses known to be excitatory have Type 1 contacts (see Walberg, 1968, for details and references). In the cerebellar cortex the parallel fibre-spine contacts are Type 1 and the axo-somatic basket contacts are Type 2 (Walberg, 1968). From these and other investigations Eccles (1964) concluded that there might well be a relationship between Type 1 and excitation and Type 2 and inhibition. If so, then one might expect a relationship between Type 1 contacts and round vesicles and Type 2 contacts and flat ones. Such a relationship has in fact been demonstrated by Uchizono (1965) in the cerebellar cortex and by Lund and Westrum (1966) in the olfactory cerebral cortex and superior colliculus of the rat. More recently Colonnier (1968) has discussed this relationship in detail in his work on the cerebral cortex. He suggests a new nomenclature, which in some respects might well prove more suitable than the Type 1–Type 2 nomenclature. Figs. 2 and 3 taken from Colonnier (1968) show the relationship in the cerebral cortex. In my aldehyde-fixed material there is often, but not invariably, a relationship between round vesicle/ pronounced synaptic thickening and flat vesicle/minimal synaptic thickening (*e.g.* Figs. 1, 4, 5 and 6).

However, the analysis of this problem is really only in its infancy. If Palay's (1967) identification of the climbing fibres in the cerebellum are correct then according to him they have Type 2 contacts, although they have a powerful postsynaptic excitatory action (Eccles, 1964). However, other authors (Larramendi and Victor, 1967; Uchizono, 1967) claim that climbing fibres make spine contacts (in conflict with Palay) which from their micrographs are Type 1 and they have round vesicles in aldehyde-fixed material. However, Gobel (1968) claims that Larramendi and Victor (and presumably Uchizono) have misidentified the climbing fibres.

CONCLUDING REMARKS

It is generally supposed that, on the assumption that the transmitter substance is enclosed within the synaptic vesicle, treatment with aldehyde affects the vesicles containing excitor in one way and inhibitor in another. This may be caused by tonicity changes or molecular changes in the vesicle wall or a combination of both due to the aldehyde reaction. One could then go on to argue that only certain excitatory or inhibitory transmitters produce the round or flat vesicle effect (respectively), and where the morphology failed to fit the physiology the transmitters involved were refractory to the aldehyde treatment. Two categories of vesicle cannot be detected in aldehyde fixed mollusc brain for example.

However, these ideas must remain highly speculative at present. Our knowledge of the cytoplasmic organisation of the presynaptic knob is really rudimentary. Aldehyde might be reacting with cytoplasmic factors, for example, and the resulting products might thus secondarily influence the shape of the vesicle. We know nothing of the presynaptic factors that influence the recognition involved in the laying down of specific connections in the ontogeny of the nervous system. It could be that excitatory endings all have one factor for connection recognition and inhibitory ones another, and it is these factors that respond to aldehyde fixation secondarily to affect the vesicle or directly if these factors are bound to the wall of the vesicle. Thus the aldehyde reaction could be explained without directly implicating the transmitter substance.

REFERENCES

ATWOOD, H. L., (1968); Peripheral inhibition in crustacean muscle. *Experientia (Basel)*, **24**, 753–763.

BENNETT, M. V. L., NAKAJIMA, Y., AND PAPPAS, G. D., (1967a); Physiology and ultrastructure of electrotonic junctions: I. Supramedullary neurons. *J. Neurophysiol.*, **30**, 161–179.

BENNETT, M. V. L., PAPPAS, G. D., ALJURE, E., AND NAKAJIMA, Y., (1967b); Physiology and ultrastructure of electrotonic junctions: II. Spinal and medullary electromotor nuclei in Mormyrid fish. *J. Neurophysiol.*, **30**, 180–208.

BENNETT, M. V. L., NAKAJIMA, Y., AND PAPPAS, G. D., (1967c); Physiology and ultrastructure of electrotonic junctions: III. Giant electromotor neurons of *Malapterurus electricus. J. Neurophysiol.*, **30**, 209–235.

BENNETT, M. V. L., PAPPAS, G. D., GIMENEZ, M., AND NAKAJIMA, Y., (1967d); Physiology and ultrastructure of electrotonic junctions: IV. Medullary electromotor nuclei in Gymnotid fish. *J. Neurophysiol.*, **30**, 236–300.

BODIAN, D., (1966a); Electron microscopy: two major synaptic types on spinal motoneurons. *Science*, **151**, 1093–1094.

BODIAN, D., (1966b); Synaptic types of spinal motoneurons: an electron microscope study. *Bull. Johns Hopk. Hosp.*, **119**, 16–45.

CHARLTON, B. T., AND GRAY, E. G., (1966); Comparative electron microscopy of synapses in the spinal cord. *J. Cell Sci.*, **1**, 67–80.

COLONNIER, M., AND GUILLERY, R. W., (1964); Synaptic organisation in the lateral geniculate nucleus of the monkey. *Z. Zellforsch.*, **62**, 333–355.

COLONNIER, M., (1968); Synaptic patterns on different cell types in the different laminae of the cat visual cortex. An electron microscope study. *Brain Res.*, **9**, 268–287.

CONRADI, S., AND SKOGLUND, S., (1968); Ultrastructural observations on the spinal cord after dorsal root section. In C. VON EULER *et al.* (Eds.), *Structure and Function of Inhibitory Neural Mechanisms*. Pergamon, Oxford, pp. 61–70.

DUDEL, J., AND KUFFLER, S. W., (1961a); The quantal nature of transmission and spontaneous miniature potentials at the crayfish neuromuscular junction. *J. Physiol. (Lond.)*, **155**, 514–519.

DUDEL, J., AND KUFFLER, S. W., (1961b); Presynaptic inhibition at the crayfish neuromuscular junction. *J. Physiol. (Lond.)*, **155**, 543–562.

ECCLES, J. C., (1964); *The Physiology of Synapses*, Springer, Berlin.

FATT, P., AND KATZ, B., (1953a); Distributed 'end-plate potentials' of crustacean muscle fibres. *J. exp. Biol.*, **30**, 433–439.

FATT, P., AND KATZ, B., (1953b); The effect of inhibitory nerve impulses on a crustacean muscle fibre. *J. Physiol. (Lond.)*, **121**, 374–389.

FOX, C. A., HILLMAN, D. E., SIEGESMUND, K. A., AND GUTTA, C. R., (1967); In C. A. FOX AND R. S. SNIDER (Eds.), *The Cerebellum (Progress in Brain Research*, Vol. 25), Elsevier, Amsterdam, pp. 174–225.

FRANK, F. K., AND FUORTES, M. G. S., (1957); Presynaptic and postsynaptic inhibition of monosynaptic reflexes. *Fed. Proc.*, **16**, 39–40.

FURSHPAN, E. J., (1964); "Electrical" transmission at an excitatory synapse in a vertebrate brain. *Science*, **144**, 878–880.

FURSHPAN, E. J., AND POTTER, D. D., (1959); Transmission at the giant synapses of the crayfish. *J. Physiol. (Lond.)*, **145**, 326–335.

GOBEL, S., (1968); Electron microscopical studies of the cerebellar molecular layer. *J. Ultrastruct. Res.*, **21**, 430–446.

GRANIT, R., (1968); The case for presynaptic inhibition by synapses on the terminals of motor neurons. In C. VON EULER *et al.* (Eds.), *Structure and Function of Inhibitory Neuronal Mechanisms.* Pergamon, Oxford, pp. 183–195.

GRAY, E. G., (1959); Axosomatic and axodendritic synapses of the cerebral cortex: an electron microscope study. *J. Anat. (Lond.)*, **93**, 420–433.

GRAY, E. G., (1961); The granule cells, mossy synapses and Purkinje spine synapses of the cerebellum: light and electron microscope observations. *J. Anat. (Lond.)*, **94**, 345–356.

GRAY, E. G., (1962); A morphological basis for presynaptic inhibition? *Nature (Lond.)*, **193**, 82–83.

GRAY, E. G., (1963); Electron microscopy of presynaptic organelles of the spinal cord. *J. Anat. (Lond.)*, **97**, 101–106.

GRAY, E. G., (1967); Round and flat vesicles in the goldfish CNS (abstract), in *3rd Conf. Anatomists and Histologists in Bulgaria, Plovdiv*, Medical and Physical Culture Publishing House, Sofia.

GRAY, E. G., (1969); Round and flat vesicles in the fish CNS, in S. H. BARONDES (Ed.), *Cellular Dynamics of the Neuron*, J.S.C.B. Symposium, Paris.

GRAY, E. G., AND GUILLERY, R. W., (1966); Synaptic morphology in the normal and degenerating nervous system. *Int. Rev. Cytol.*, **19**, 111–182.

GRAY, E. G., AND WILLIS, R. A., (1968); Problems of electron stereoscopy of biological tissues. *J. Cell Sci.*, **3**, 309–326.

GRAY, E. G., AND YOUNG, J. Z., (1964); Electron microscopy of synaptic structures of *Octopus* brain. *J. Cell Biol.*, **21**, 87.

GUILLERY, R. W., (1968); personal communication.

HAMA, K., (1961); Some observations on the fine structure of the giant fibres of the crayfishes with special reference to the synapses. *Anat. Rec.*, **141**, 275–293.

HIRATA, Y., (1966); Occurrence of cylindrical synaptic vesicles in the central nervous system perfused with buffered formalin. *Arch. histol. Jap.*, **26**, 269–279.

KHATTAB, F. I., (1968); A complex synaptic apparatus in spinal cord of cats. *Experientia (Basel)*, **24**, 690–691.

KIDD, M., (1961); Electron microscopy of the inner plexiform layer of the retina. *Proc. Anat. Soc.*, *Cytology of Neurons Tissue*, Taylor and Francis, London, pp. 88–91.

KIDD, M., (1962); Electron microscopy of the inner plexiform layer of the retina in the cat and pigeon. *J. Anat. (Lond.)*, **96**, 179–187.

KUFFLER, S. W., AND EYZAGUIRRE, C., (1955); Synaptic inhibition in an isolated nerve cell. *J. gen. Physiol.*, **39**, 155–184.

LARRAMENDI, L. M. H., FICKENSCHER, L., AND LEMKEY-JOHNSTON, N., (1967); Synaptic vesicles of inhibitory and excitatory terminals in the cerebellum. *Science*, **156**, 967.

LARRAMENDI, L. M. H., AND VICTOR, T., (1967); Synapses on the Purkinje cell spines in the mouse. An electron microscope study. *Brain Res.*, **5**, 15–30.

LUND, R. D., AND WESTRUM, L. E., (1966); Synaptic vesicle differences after primary formalin fixation. *J. Physiol. (Lond.)*, **185**, 7–9.

MILEDI, R., (1967); personal communication.

MILLONIG, G., AND MARINOZZI, V., (1968); Fixation and embedding in electron microscopy, in R. BARER AND V. E. COSSLETT (Eds.), *Advances in Optical and Electron Microscopy*, Vol. 2, Academic Press, New York, pp. 253–341.

MUGNAINI, E., AND WALBERG, F., (1967); An experimental electron microscopical study on the mode of termination of Purkinje axons in Deiters' nucleus. *Exp. Brain Res.*, **4**, 212–236.

PALAY, S. L., (1967); Principles of cellular organisation in the nervous system, in G. C. QUARTON *et al.* (Eds.), *The Neurosciences*, Rockefeller University Press, pp. 24–31.

PAPPAS, G. D., AND BENNETT, M. V. L., (1966a); Specialised sites involved in electrical transmission between neurons. *Ann. N.Y. Acad. Sci.*, **137**, 495–508.

PAPPAS, G. D., AND BENNETT, M. V. L., (1966b); The fine structure of vesicles associated with excitatory and inhibitory junctions. *Biol. Bull.*, **131**, 381.

PEASE, D. C., (1964); *Histological Techniques for Electron Microscopy*. 2nd ed., Academic Press, New York.

ROBERTSON, J. D., (1964); Unit membranes: A review with recent new studies of experimental alterations and a new subunit structure in synaptic membranes, in M. LOCK (Ed.), *Cellular Membranes in Development*, Academic Press, New York, pp. 1–81.

ROBERTSON, J. D., BODENHEIMER, T. S., AND STAGE, D. E., (1963); The ultrastructure of Mauthner cell synapses and nodes in goldfish brains. *J. Cell Biol.*, **19**, 159–199.

SAAVEDRA, J. P., AND VACCAREZZA, O. C., (1968); Synaptic organisation of the glomerular complexes in the lateral geniculate nucleus of Cebus monkey. *Brain Res.*, **8**, 389–393.

SOTELO, C., AND PALAY, S. L., (1967); The fine structure of the lateral vestibular nucleus of the rat 1. Neurons and glia. *J. Cell Biol.*, **36**, 151–180.

SZENTÁGOTHAI, J., (1962); Anatomical aspects of junctional transformation, in R. W. GERARD AND J. DUYFF (Eds.), *Information Processing in the Nervous System*, Excerpta Medica, Amsterdam.

SZENTÁGOTHAI, J., (1968); Synaptic structure and the concept of presynaptic inhibition, in C. VON EULER *et al.* (Eds.), *Structure and Function of Inhibitory Neural Mechanisms*, Pergamon, Oxford, pp. 15–32.

UCHIZONO, K., (1965); Characteristics of excitatory and inhibitory synapses in the central nervous system of the cat. *Nature (Lond.)*, **207**, 642–643.

UCHIZONO, K., (1966); Excitatory and inhibitory synapses in cat spinal cord. *Jap. J. Physiol.*, **16**, 570–575.

UCHIZONO, K., (1967); Inhibitory synapses on the stretch receptor neurone of the crayfish. *Nature (Lond.)*, **214**, 833–834.

UCHIZONO, K., (1968); Inhibitory and excitatory synapses in vertebrate and invertebrate animals, in C. VON EULER *et al.* (Eds.), *Structure and Function of Inhibitory Neural Mechanisms*, Pergamon, Oxford, pp. 33–60.

WALBERG, F., (1965); Axoaxonal contacts in the cuneate nucleus, a probable basis for presynaptic depolarization. *Exp. Neurol.*, **125**, 205–222.

WALBERG, F., (1966); The fine structure of the cuneate nucleus in normal cats and following interruption of afferent fibres. *Exp. Brain Res.*, **2**, 107–128.

WALBERG, F., (1968); Morphological correlates of postsynaptic inhibitory processes, in C. VON EULER *et al.* (Eds.), *Structure and Function of Inhibitory Neuronal Mechanisms*, Pergamon, Oxford.

WESTRUM, L. E., (1965); A combination staining technique for electron microscopy. 1. Nervous tissue. *J. Microscop.*, **4**, 275–278.

WESTRUM, L. E., (1966); Synaptic contacts on axons in the cerebral cortex. *Nature (Lond.)*, **210**, 1289–1290.

Electronmicroscopic and Autoradiographic Studies of Normal and Denervated Endplates

P. G. WASER AND ELVIRA NICKEL

Department of Pharmacology, University of Zürich (Switzerland)

Denervation separates the trophic part of a neuron from the conducting pathway. The distal axonal part then soon degenerates. In our research programme denervation is a tool for separating presynaptic nerve elements from the postsynaptic muscle fibre in the endplate. By this technique it is possible to divide the synapse in the synaptic cleft and functionally to split the degenerating presynaptic membrane from the post-synaptic membrane in the biological preparation.

For several years we have been interested in the fixation of radioactive molecules on the endplate of mouse diaphragms. Using this technique we hope to elucidate the function, and action site, of acetylcholine and of blocking drugs. Some problems

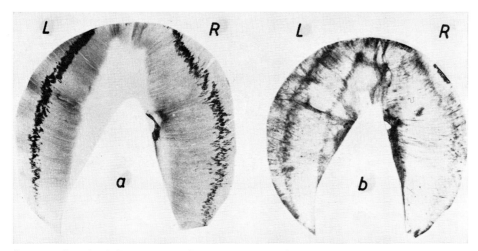

Fig. 1. Koelle stained diaphragm (a) of mouse with autoradiograph; (b) with [^{14}C]curarine 7 days after coagulation of left phrenic nerve (L). (R: normally innervated control side.)

Abbreviations for all figures

Af	axon fragment	Co	collagen
SVa	agglutinated synaptic vesicles	M	mitochondrion
Nt	nerve terminal	Jf	junctional folds
SC	Schwann cell	SN	soleplate nucleus
MC	muscle cell	prM	presynaptic membrane
SV	synaptic vesicle	BM	basement membrane
R	ribosome	poM	postsynaptic membrane

References p. 169

which are currently discussed concern the storage of acetylcholine in the presynaptic vesicles, the liberation and diffusion to the postsynaptic membrane, the formation and location of the acetyl- and pseudocholinesterases, the action site of the curare molecules and the nature of the cholinergic receptor. We have not yet been able to obtain electron-microscopic autoradiographs using these highly water-soluble compounds. In order to know more about the binding compartments for these drugs,

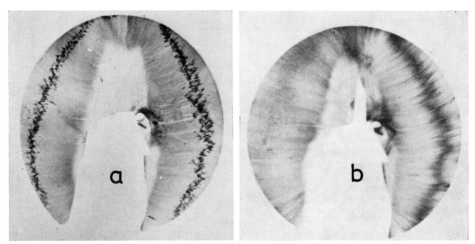

Fig. 2. Diaphragm of mouse 4 days after denervation on left side. Cholinesterase (a) is little diminished. Autoradiograph (b) with [¹⁴C]decamethonium shows increased spreading of radioactivity on to muscle fibres outside endplate region.

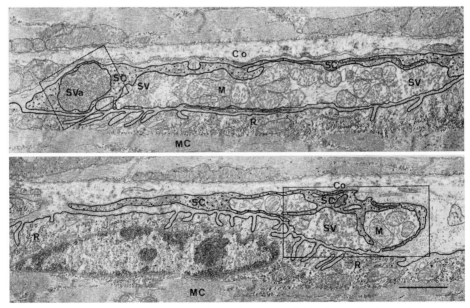

Fig. 3. Endplate region with the hypertrophying Schwann cell (darkly outlined) dividing the axon into fragments. 14 h after denervation.

we had to investigate the ultrastructure of endplates in normal diaphragms and at different stages after denervation.

For denervation, the thorax of an albino mouse under ether anaesthesia is opened by a small incision, and the left phrenic nerve is cut about 0.5 cm before entering the diaphragm. Within a few seconds the thorax is closed again by a previously prepared suture. Unilateral denervation has an important advantage because the subsequent

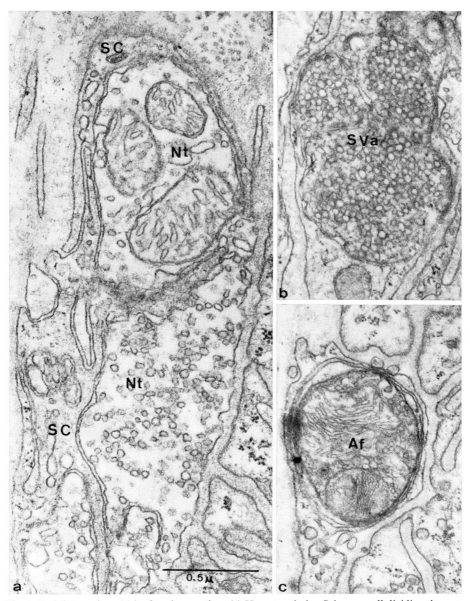

Fig. 4. Endplate regions 14 h after denervation. (a) Hypertrophying Schwann cell dividing the axon into fragments. Axon fragment filled with (b) agglutinated vesicles (honeycombs), (c) disintegrating vesicles and mitochondria.

degeneration process may be compared with the normal right side of the same diaphragm.

Early studies on the endplates of mouse diaphragms showed us that after denervation there was an increase of intravenously injected labelled curarine molecules
bound to the endplate (Fig. 1), and within 4 months simultaneously with the dimin-
ishing acetylcholinesterase, a slow decrease in radioactivity (Waser and Hadorn,
1961). On the other hand, it is well known to the electrophysiologist that denervation
results in an immediate spreading of the acetylcholine-sensitive area from the postsynaptic membrane in the endplate outward to the whole surface of the muscle
cell (Axelsson and Thesleff, 1959). We found with intravenously injected labelled
decamethonium a similar distribution in the mouse diaphragm (Fig. 2): these de-

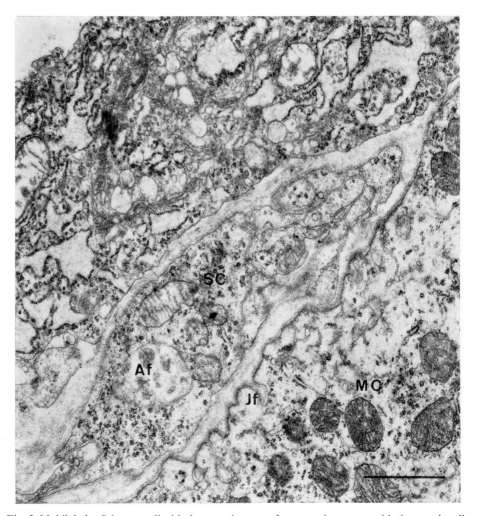

Fig. 5. Multilobular Schwann cell with degenerating axon fragments in contact with the muscle cell
2 days after denervation.

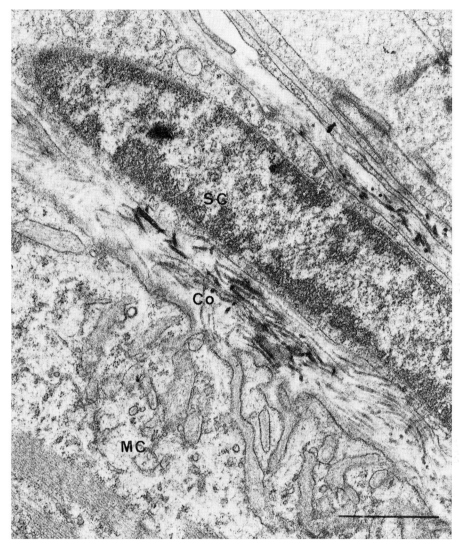

Fig. 6. Schwann cell separated by collagen fibrils from the muscle cell. 7 days after denervation. Note the swollen basement membrane on the postsynaptic membrane filling the junctional folds.

polarizing cholinergic molecules probably act at the same receptors of the muscle membrane (Waser and Truog, 1969).

The ultrastructural changes begin immediately after nerve sectioning (Nickel and Waser, 1968). The abnormal structures in the first stage are especially varied and complicated. In the same area, even in the same endplate, different forms of degeneration are observed. All three components of an endplate are affected by the degeneration process: the terminal axon, the Schwann cell and the muscle cell.

In the first stage (14 h after denervation), the terminal axon is divided into fragments by the hypertrophying Schwann cell processes (Fig. 3). These fragments of the same axon mostly show different forms of degeneration. Some are almost empty

(Fig. 4), containing a few scattered vesicles and swollen mitochondria. Others are filled with masses of agglutinated vesicles, the so-called honeycombs of Birks *et al.* (1960). In these honeycombs there are sometimes swollen mitochondria whose internal structures may be broken up or filled with dense material. At this stage the axon and the Schwann cell membranes are clearly visible and still distinct from each other.

During the further stages of degeneration the Schwann cell processes hypertrophy and extend into the primary synaptic cleft, so that the axon remnants are completely surrounded by the Schwann cell. The internal structure of the axon fragments has disintegrated. In some places between the Schwann cell and the axon only one of the two cell membranes is visible. The Schwann cell forms numerous vesicles, some of them coated, especially near the surrounding axon fragments. Furthermore, the number of ribosomes and the volume of ergastoplasm in the Schwann cell are increased compared with the normal undenervated endplate, an indication of a high Schwann cell activity. This disappearance of one membrane, presumably the axonal membrane, and the occurrence of numerous vesicles which might function in the uptake of axon material, lead us to conclude that the whole axon is absorbed by the Schwann cell.

The relations between Schwann cell and axon are often complicated and can only be clarified with the aid of a comparative time series (Fig. 5). Two days after denervation the axon has nearly disappeared. Only some degenerating axonal remnants are to be seen between the Schwann cell processes. After 3 days the axon has completely vanished, leaving one cell in contact with the folds of the muscle cell (Fig. 6). The identification of this cell as a Schwann cell is difficult because the normal characteristics have changed and the structural details alone are no longer sufficiently distinctive to differentiate it from other extraneous cells, for instance, fibroblasts and endothelial cells. One characteristic criterion is the presence of the Schwann cell basement membrane. Some times the increased number of ribosomes can also serve as a distinction. Later, when remnants of the Schwann cell are observed they no longer have direct contact with the muscle cell but are separated by collagen fibrils.

The process of degeneration occurs also in the muscle cell. 14 h after denervation the ribosomes have increased in the region of the junctional folds. Sole-plate nuclei, and also the junctional folds, do not undergo drastic changes. This is of practical use for locating endplates in a denervated muscle up to 4 months after denervation (Fig. 7). Sometimes the folds have an unusually wide lumen filled with fine granular material. The basement membrane appears to be thicker than in the normal endplate. The degeneration process leads to a complete lysis of the muscle cell structure, and within 6 months after denervation muscle fibres are replaced by collagen fibrils.

The acetylcholinesterase (Fig. 8), which is normally localized on the pre- and postsynaptic membranes, is still evident 4 weeks after denervation only on the postsynaptic membrane.

Further studies, with a zinc–iodide–osmium impregnation (ZIO) of Maillet (1962) and Jabonero (1964), reinforce our conclusion that the axon is absorbed by the Schwann cell (Nickel and Waser, 1969). In a normal motor endplate this stain seems to be specific for the synaptic vesicles, as Akert and Sandri (1968) have shown (Fig. 9). It

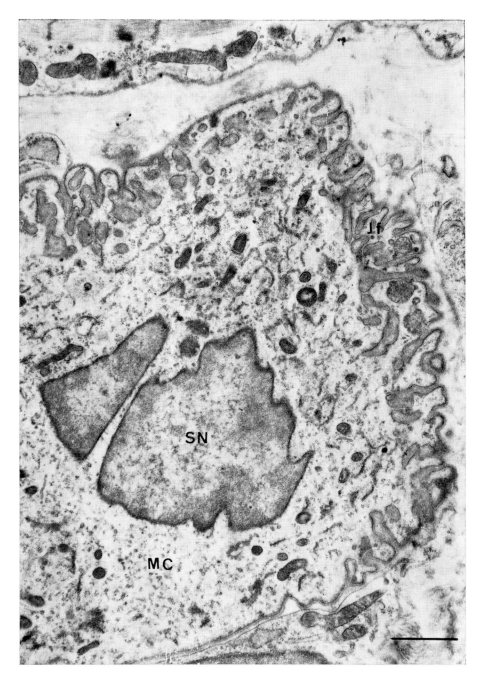

Fig. 7. Muscle cell 2 months after denervation. Soleplate nuclei and junctional folds are still visible. The basement membrane appears to be thicker than in the normal endplate.

is noticeable that there is no ZIO reaction in the junctional region, in the synaptic cleft, or in the Schwann cell.

After denervation a change in this staining pattern develops. Fourteen hours after

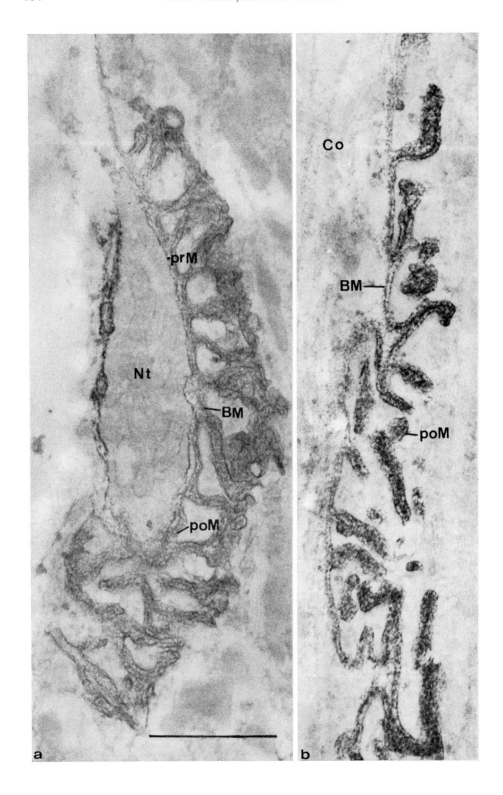

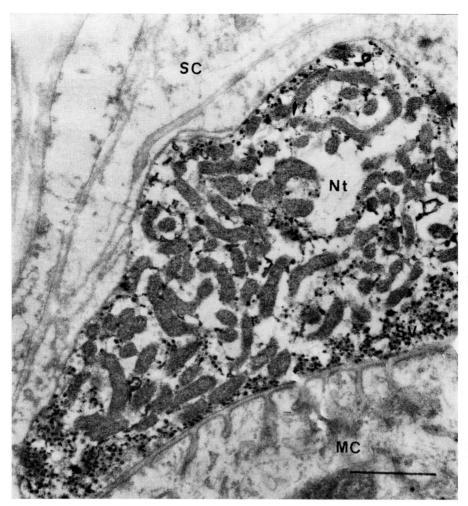

Fig. 9. Motor endplate after zinc–iodide–osmium (ZIO) impregnation with selective staining of synaptic vesicles.

denervation (Fig. 10) the whole nerve internal structure is stained with only the membranes of vesicles and mitochondria remaining unstained. This compact precipitate may originate from the disintegrating vesicular material diffusing into the axon cytoplasm. However, staining is still strictly limited to the terminal axon. No precipitate can be observed in the junctional region or in the Schwann cell.

One day after the sectioning of the nerve (Fig. 11) the hypertrophying Schwann cell has fragmented the axon. These axon fragments still appear densely stained, but at this stage dark precipitates also occur in vesicles of the Schwann cell. Their contents

Fig. 8. Motor endplate stained with the gold-thiolacetic method (Koelle). (a) Normal, (b) 28 days after denervation.

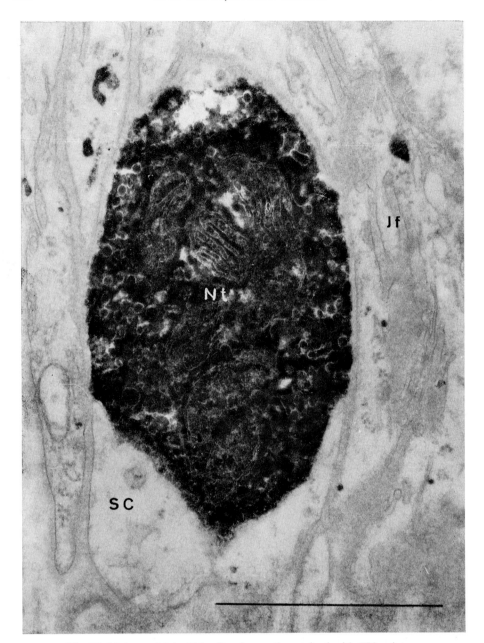

Fig. 10. Motor endplate 14 h after denervation stained with ZIO mixture.

are probably axonal material, as there is no other material in the endplate region which is specific for this ZIO stain.

Within 3 days after denervation in most cases the terminal axon has completely disappeared, leaving the empty Schwann cell on the junctional folds. In general, precipitates are no longer observed in the Schwann cell cytoplasm. From this we

conclude that the ingested axonal material is metabolized in the Schwann cell cytoplasm.

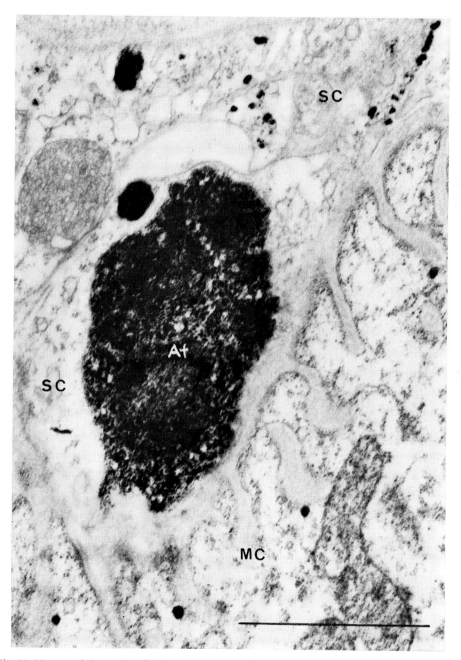

Fig. 11. Motor endplate 1 day after denervation with ZIO staining. Note the dark precipitates in the
Schwann cell cytoplasm.

CONCLUSIONS

Our investigations, combining different morphological techniques, have led to the following conclusions.

(*1*) Curarine, as a typical curare drug, is evidently concentrated 7–60 days after denervation on the postsynaptic membrane, the only remaining part of the synaptic membrane, since even the Schwann cell disappears after 7–10 days. The basement membrane of the postsynaptic membrane is thick and the junctional folds are full of granular material at the time when the most curare is present.

(*2*) The cholinesterase remains for a long time (30 days) on the postsynaptic membrane, but the depolarizing decamethonium molecules are bound mainly outside the endplate on the muscle cell surface.

(*3*) The preliminary results of our denervation experiments on the liberation, distribution and uptake of acetylcholine from the vesicles into the Schwann cell confirm earlier studies by Birks *et al.* (1960) and Miledi and Slater (1968). It seems possible that in frog sartorius Schwann cells take over acetylcholine-containing vesicles from the degenerating terminal nerve axon, thus being responsible for the miniature endplate potentials during the first 5 days. However, in the mouse diaphragm at later stages after denervation, there is no longer evidence that the low-rate spontaneous activity originates in the Schwann cell, as this cell disappears. Most promising for further studies will be the Jabonero or some other specific stain for acetylcholine.

SUMMARY

(*1*) The terminal nerve axon disintegrates within hours after denervation.

(*2*) The axonal material is taken up by the Schwann cell and may be recognized there for a few days.

(*3*) The Schwann cell seems to metabolize this material as indicated by increased ribosomal and endoplasmic reticulum activity.

(*4*) Some vesicles of the Schwann cell after denervation contain the same stained material as the normal nerve terminal, which might be acetylcholine.

(*5*) After 5–7 days collagen fibres separate the Schwann cell from the postsynaptic membrane, and the Schwann cell eventually disappears.

(*6*) The postsynaptic membrane of the endplate is the main binding compartment for curarizing molecules.

(*7*) The binding of depolarizing decamethonium molecules on the muscle fibre is independent of the cholinesterase in the postsynaptic membrane.

ACKNOWLEDGEMENT

We acknowledge the financial help of the Swiss National Foundation for Scientific Research (Project 5066).

REFERENCES

AKERT, K., AND SANDRI, C., (1968); An electron-microscopic study of zinc–iodide–osmium impregnation of neurons. I. Staining of synaptic vesicles at cholinergic junctions. *Brain Res.*, **7**, 286–295.

AXELSSON, J., AND THESLEFF, S., (1959); A study on supersensitivity in denervated mammalian skeletal muscle. *J. Physiol. (Lond.)*, **145**, 48–49P.

BIRKS, R., KATZ, B., AND MILEDI, R., (1960); Physiological and structural changes at the amphibian myoneural junction in the course of nerve degeneration. *J. Physiol. (Lond.)*, **150**, 145–168.

JABONERO, V., (1964); Über die Brauchbarkeit der Osmiumtetroxyd–Zinkjodid Methode zur Analyse der vegetativen Peripherie. *Acta neuroveg. (Wien)*, **26**, 184–210.

MAILLET, M., (1962); La technique de Champy à l'osmium–ioduré de potassium et la modification de Maillet à l'osmium–ioduré de zinc. *Trab. Inst. Cajal Invest. biol.*, **56**, 1–36.

MILEDI, R., AND SLATER, K. R., (1968); Electrophysiology and electronmicroscopy of rat neuromuscular junctions after nerve denervation. *Proc. Roy. Soc. B*, **169**, 289–306.

NICKEL, E., AND WASER, P. G., (1968); Elektronenmikroskopische Untersuchungen am Diaphragma der Maus nach einseitiger Phrenikotomie. I. Die degenerierende motorische Endplatte. *Z. Zellforsch.*, **88**, 278–296.

NICKEL, E., AND WASER, P. G., (1969); An electron microscopic study of denervated motor endplates after zinc–iodide–osmium impregnation. *Brain Res.*, **13**, 168–176.

WASER, P. G., AND HADORN, J., (1961); Relations of cholinergic receptors to acetylcholinesterase of endplates in denervated muscle. *Bibl. anat. (Basel)*, **2**, 155–160.

WASER, P. G., AND TRUOG, P., (1969); Einflüsse der Denervation von Muskelendplatten auf Acetyl cholinesterase und Bindung von Decamethonium. In preparation.

The Pharmacology of Spinal Postsynaptic Inhibition

D. R. CURTIS

Neuropharmacology Research Group, Department of Physiology, Australian National University, Canberra (Australia)

Although the ionic mechanism of spinal postsynaptic inhibition, and the various spinal inhibitory pathways, have been known for some years, it is only comparatively recently that evidence has been obtained for the probable nature of the inhibitory transmitter substance, primarily as a result of the investigations of Aprison, Werman and their colleagues (for review see Werman and Aprison, 1968). Following an analysis of the intraspinal distribution of glycine (Aprison and Werman, 1965), the action of this amino acid on spinal neurones was re-investigated, and, on the basis of a hyperpolarization of motoneurones by a membrane process similar to, or identical with, that occurring during synaptic inhibition, glycine was proposed as an inhibitory transmitter in the cord (Werman *et al.*, 1966a). These results have been confirmed in Canberra. In addition, γ-aminobutyric acid (GABA) has been shown to hyperpolarize spinal neurones, but the antagonism demonstrated between glycine and strychnine has added considerable weight to the proposal that this particular amino acid is a major spinal inhibitory transmitter.

SPINAL POSTSYNAPTIC INHIBITION

The postsynaptic inhibition of spinal neurones, observed as a temporary decrease of excitability, is accompanied by a membrane hyperpolarization, the inhibitory postsynaptic potential or IPSP (Fig. 1A, Eccles, 1964, 1966). The ionic mechanism of this process has been analysed by observing the effects of alterations of membrane potential, and of intracellular ion content, on the IPSP's of motoneurones generated by segmental afferent and antidromic impulses. IPSP's are increased in magnitude (Fig. 1E) when the membrane potential is lowered (depolarized), and reversed (Fig. 1G) when the membrane is hyperpolarized. The reversal potential (Fig. 1F) lies between the resting level of membrane potential and the equilibrium potential for potassium ions. Intracellular injections of a variety of anions and cations indicate that some convert hyperpolarizing IPSP's into depolarizations (Fig. 2B, E for chloride ion) whereas others fail to do so. These findings have led to the proposal that the inhibitory transmitter transiently increases the membrane permeability to cations and anions having a hydrated ion diameter less than approximately 1.14 times that of the potassium ion (Fig. 3; see Eccles, 1966). Under normal conditions there is a net efflux of potassium ions and a net influx of chloride ions (Fig. 1A).

References p. 186–189

INHIBITION

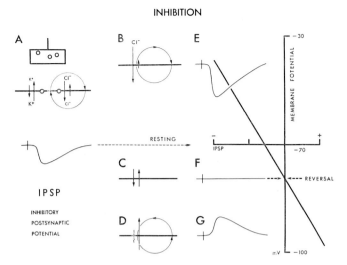

Fig. 1. The operation of inhibitory synapses. (A), Ion fluxes are indicated by arrows; the net outward movement of potassium ions and the inward movement of chloride ions induced by the transmitter released from an inhibitory terminal results in a membrane current (circle with arrows) which hyperpolarizes the membrane. The IPSP at the resting level of membrane potential is hyperpolarizing in direction. (B–D), The direction of movement of chloride ions at different membrane potentials. (B, E), Depolarization of the membrane enhances the ionic current and increases the amplitude of the IPSP. On the other hand, hyperpolarization reverses the direction of current flow and produces a depolarizing IPSP, (D, G). At the reversal potential, the net influx and efflux of ions participating in inhibition are equal (C, F).

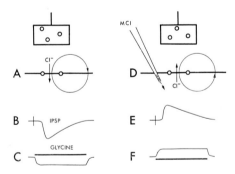

Fig. 2. Reversal of IPSP by intracellular chloride ion injection. (A–C), Under normal conditions the transmitter and glycine produce a net influx of Cl⁻, the membrane is hyperpolarized. (D–F), Elevation of the intracellular Cl⁻ concentration by electrophoretic administration from a micropipette containing a solution of a metallic chloride (MCl) reverses this influx to an efflux, and the membrane is depolarized by both the inhibitory transmitter and glycine.

A presynaptic "inhibitory" process has also been described in the spinal cord in which synaptic depolarization of presynaptic terminals diminishes the output of excitatory transmitter, and hence reduces the effectiveness of excitatory impulses (Eccles, 1964). The amplitude of intracellularly recorded excitatory postsynaptic

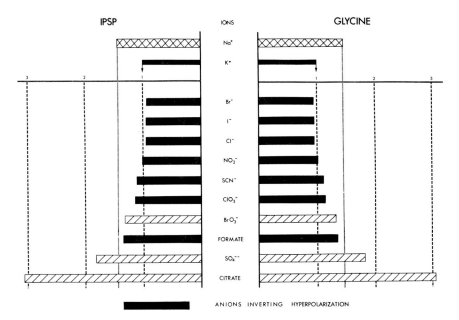

Fig. 3. Hydrated ion diameters, and the inversion of IPSP's and glycine hyperpolarizations. The lengths of the horizontal bands indicate ion sizes calculated from the limiting conductance in water, relative to that of K^+, broken vertical lines. The black bands are for ions which invert IPSP's and glycine hyperpolarizations into depolarizations, and the cross-hatched bands for anions which are ineffective. The upper criss–cross-hatched band and the dotted vertical lines indicate the size of Na^+, intracellular injection of which is assumed to result in changes in the levels of K^+ and Cl^-.

potentials (EPSP) is reduced in the absence of any alteration in the postsynaptic membrane potential, conductance or excitability (Frank and Fourtes, 1957; Frank, 1959; Eide *et al.*, 1968). Postsynaptic and presynaptic inhibition also differ pharmacologically: strychnine blocks postsynaptic inhibition (Curtis, 1963) but does not reduce presynaptic inhibition (Eccles *et al.*, 1963); in contrast intravenously administered picrotoxin reduces presynaptic inhibition but not postsynaptic inhibition. Although evidence has been provided for a picrotoxin-sensitive postsynaptic inhibition of lumbar motoneurones induced by stretching muscles (Kellerth, 1968), this inhibition is accompanied by depolarization of the terminals of the appropriate afferent fibres (Devanandan *et al.*, 1965a, b), and hence may be presynaptic in nature.

The various spinal postsynaptic inhibitory pathways which have been studied can be listed as follows:

(*1*) Afferent inhibition of spinal motoneurones by impulses in ipsi- and contralateral dorsal root fibres of both muscle and cutaneous origin. It is generally accepted that the primary afferent fibres are excitatory, and that inhibition results from the excitation of inhibitory interneurones, located predominantly in Rexed layers IV–VII, which send axons to motoneurones in the same segment, and in adjacent segments *via* short propriospinal fibres (Eccles, 1967; Lundberg, 1966). These fibres lie in both grey and white matters, particularly in the ventral and ventrolateral columns

References p. 186–189

adjacent to the ventral horn (Szentágothai, 1964); few fibres are located in the dorsal columns (Nathan and Smith, 1959).

(2) Afferent inhibition of spinal interneurones, including Renshaw cells, by impulses in ipsi- and contralateral afferent fibres of muscle and cutaneous origin (Lundberg, 1966; Wilson, 1966; Hongo et al., 1966).

(3) Recurrent inhibition of motoneurones (and interneurones) which follows excitation of Renshaw cells by impulses propagated antidromically into the spinal cord along ventral roots (Eccles et al., 1954; Wilson, 1966).

(4) "Descending" inhibition of spinal interneurones and motoneurones from supraspinal centres, including the cerebral cortex, red nucleus, reticular formation, vestibular nuclei, cerebellum and rostral spinal segments (Lloyd and McIntyre, 1948; Sasaki et al., 1962; Lundberg, 1966; Shapovalov, 1966; Engberg et al., 1968; Kubota et al., 1968). Again it is generally assumed that the descending tract fibres are excitatory, and have few or no direct terminations upon feline motoneurones (Nyberg-Hansen, 1966; Petras, 1967); inhibitory interneurones may be common to both segmental and supraspinal pathways. Spinal effects which result from stimulation of supraspinal structures are usually complex mixtures of inhibition and excitation, in part because of difficulties associated with the electrical stimulation of specific nuclei or tracts. Furthermore, presynaptic inhibition, resulting in disfacilitation of interneurones and motoneurones, may provide an additional complication.

The sites of termination on motoneurones of the various inhibitory pathways are of interest. Renshaw cell axons ramify as fine terminal fibres over the soma and dendrites (Szentágothai, 1958). Polarizing currents passed through an intracellular microelectrode readily influence spinal afferent and recurrent IPSP's (Coombs et al., 1955a), and detect the accompanying membrane impedance change (Smith et al., 1967). Hence the inhibitory synapses for these pathways are presumably located predominantly on the cell body. On the basis of similar evidence, the inhibition of extensor motoneurones evoked by stimulating the bulbar reticular formation (Llinas and Terzuolo, 1964; Jankowska et al., 1968), the inhibition of motoneurones elicited by stimulating the vestibular nuclei, the red nucleus, or the corticospinal tract (Shapo-valov, 1966), and the inhibition of lumbar motoneurones by stimulation of the fore-limb superficial radial nerve (Kubota et al., 1968), probably involve synapses located near the cell bodies. On the other hand, although not confirmed by recent experiments (Jankowska et al., 1968), the inhibition of flexor motoneurones from the bulbar reticular formation may be mediated via synapses located on motoneurone dendrites: the appropriate hyperpolarizations are accompanied by little or no conductance change as measured with an intracellular microelectrode, and the hyperpolarizations can only be reduced in amplitude, but not reversed in direction, by artificial hyper-polarization of the membrane or by elevation of the intracellular chloride ion con-centration (Llinas and Terzuolo, 1965). It may be difficult to distinguish by such tests postsynaptic inhibitory action on dendrites remote from the motoneurone soma, the usual site of microelectrode penetration, from a presynaptic inhibitory reduction of excitation (disfacilitation) which may also be recorded as a "hyperpolarization".

Although detailed analyses have not been made of the effects of alterations of membrane potential or intracellular ion content upon all of the various types of IPSP recorded from motoneurones, no evidence has been obtained which would suggest that different ionic mechanisms are associated with the activity of different spinal inhibitory synapses.

Both the "direct" and recurrent inhibition of spinal motoneurones are reversibly blocked by strychnine administered intravenously (Bradley *et al.*, 1953; Eccles *et al.*, 1954) or electrophoretically (Curtis, 1962). These inhibitions, each involving one interneurone between motoneurones and excitatory nerve terminals, can be observed uncomplicated by superimposed excitation. Other spinal and supraspinal inhibitions involve many interneurones, and the depressant effect of systemically administered strychnine is often not readily apparent. In the first place depression of strychnine-sensitive inhibitory synapses may modify the transmission of impulses through a polysynaptic network, apparently enhancing excitatory effects and perhaps also facilitating the final inhibitory interneurone. Secondly, again as a consequence of the action of strychnine on participating neurones, a volley descending from a supraspinal centre may be altered in nature. These difficulties can be overcome to some extent by administering strychnine electrophoretically close to a cell being inhibited by impulses in a particular inhibitory pathway, although further difficulties may arise from the non-uniform distribution of the alkaloid in the tissue. Receptors close to the point of administration will be influenced by higher concentrations of strychnine than receptors located further away. It is thus perhaps fortuitous that the majority of inhibitory synapses upon motoneurones appear to be located on the bodies of the cells, regions presumably most accessible to strychnine administered extracellularly from the drug-containing barrels of parallel or co-axial micropipettes. Nevertheless, the strychnine sensitivity of remote dendritic inhibitory synapses cannot be determined so readily.

With the possible exception of picrotoxin-sensitive postsynaptic inhibition induced by muscle stretch (Kellerth, 1968), all forms of motoneurone inhibition studied so far are reduced by strychnine, including those of spinal (Bradley *et al.*, 1953; Coombs *et al.*, 1955b; Eccles *et al.*, 1954; Curtis, 1959, 1962, 1963) and supraspinal origin (Shapovalov and Arushanyan, 1963, 1965; Kawai and Sasaki, 1964; Llinas, 1964; Shapovalov, 1966). For example, the inhibitory hyperpolarization recorded from a gastrocnemius motoneurone in response to stimulation of the peroneal nerve (Fig. 6A) was practically abolished (Fig. 6C) by strychnine diffusing from a 10 m*M* solution of strychnine hydrochloride in the "outer" barrel of a co-axial electrode assembly, yet the monosynaptic excitatory postsynaptic potential (gastrocnemius nerve stimulation) remained unaffected (Fig. 6B, D). Similarly, the inhibition of Renshaw cells by dorsal root volleys, or by stimulation of the medullary reticular formation, is blocked by strychnine, particularly when administered electrophoretically (Wilson and Talbot, 1963; Biscoe and Curtis, 1966; Curtis *et al.*, 1968a). A similar pharmacological study of the inhibition of spinal interneurones has yet to be carried out. Other substances with strychnine-like effects on spinal postsynaptic inhibition when administered electrophoretically include brucine, thebaine, morphine, diaboline,

Wieland–Gumlich aldehyde, 4-phenyl-4-formyl-N-methylpiperidine (1762 I.S.), 5,7-diphenyl-1,3-diazadamantan-6-ol (1757 I.S.), and hexahydro-2′-methylspiro-[cyclohexane-1,8′(6H)-oxazino(3,4-A)pyrazine] (C.O.P). Many of these substances are also effective intravenously, but all are less potent than strychnine as antagonists of spinal inhibition (Longo and Chiavarelli, 1962; Curtis, 1963; Kruglov, 1964). Coniine (Sampson, 1966; Sampson et al., 1966), and pilocarpine (Esplin and Zablocka, 1964), in relatively high doses, block a variety of spinal postsynaptic inhibitions, possibly because of chemical similarities to strychnine and strychnine-like compounds (Curtis, 1968).

Tetanus toxin, injected into a peripheral nerve or directly into the spinal cord, also blocks the postsynaptic inhibition of spinal motoneurones produced by impulses in spinal and supraspinal afferent fibres (Brooks et al., 1957; Curtis, 1959; Wilson et al., 1960). This toxin also blocks the inhibition of Renshaw cells by volleys in dorsal root fibres (Curtis and De Groat, 1968). As in the case of strychnine, the inhibitory interneurones of both the "direct" and recurrent inhibitory pathways are unaffected, and the toxin thus presumably has an action in the vicinity of inhibitory synapses.

The specific depression of spinal inhibition by strychnine and tetanus toxin, in the absence of an alteration in synaptic excitation, provides an explanation for the convulsant activity of these substances. Other convulsants, includung picrotoxin, pentamethylenetetrazol, β-methyl-β-ethylglutarimide, tubocurarine, and meperidine do not affect spinal postsynaptic inhibition (Curtis, 1959, 1963).

GLYCINE

Against this background summary of knowledge concerning the action of the spinal inhibitory transmitter, the varieties of spinal inhibitory pathways, and the effects of strychnine and tetanus toxin, it is now possible to discuss the evidence which suggests that the transmitter is probably glycine.

Distribution of glycine in spinal tissue

Glycine occurs free in the mammalian central nervous system (Tallan, 1962), and levels are higher in the cervical and lumbar enlargement of the spinal cord, and in the medulla, than in more rostral structures (Shaw and Heine, 1965; Aprison et al., 1968). The concentrations along the spinal cord parallel the amount of grey relative to white matter (Aprison et al., 1968), and within the cord the highest values occur in the ventral horn of the grey matter (Aprison and Werman, 1965; Graham et al., 1967; Davidoff et al., 1967a; Johnston, 1968). A diagrammatic cross section of the feline lumbar spinal cord (Fig. 4A) shows the approximate location of inhibitory interneurones on the "direct" and recurrent pathways, together with reported levels of glycine in the various white and grey segments (Graham et al., 1967). This distri-bution of glycine suggests at least two functions for the amino acid, one of general nature concerned with the metabolism of nervous tissue (white matter, dorsal and ventral roots, grey matter, perhaps of the order of 0.6 μmoles/g, possibly higher in cell bodies), the other a specific association with spinal interneurones. The

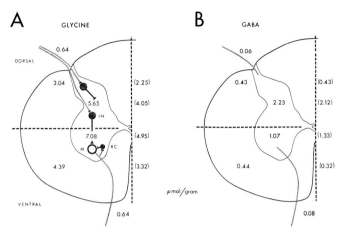

Fig. 4. The distribution of glycine (A) and GABA (B) in the spinal cord (μmoles/g, data of Graham *et al.*, 1967; Davidoff *et al.*, 1967b). Schematic hemisection of lumbar spinal cord showing dorsal and ventral roots, white and grey matter and the approximate location of interneurones (IN), motoneurones (M) and Renshaw cells (RC). The cord is divided into dorsal and ventral portions by a horizontal line through the central canal. The concentrations in brackets refer to values found after anoxic destruction of spinal interneurones (see text).

comparatively high levels within the columns of white matter may be associated with propriospinal fibres: concentrations are apparently very low in the dorsal columns and are highest in the ventrolateral region (Davidoff *et al.*, 1967a). A close association between spinal interneurones and glycine is further suggested by the significant correlation between the loss of spinal interneurones in the central portion of the cord and the reduction in dorsal and ventral grey matter glycine levels which follows temporary aortic occlusion (Davidoff *et al.*, 1966, 1967a, b). The related glycine levels are indicated in brackets to the right of Fig. 4A. In contrast, GABA is normally more concentrated in the dorsal grey matter than ventrally (Fig. 4B), and the levels are not significantly altered after anoxic destruction of interneurones. Although experiments such as these cannot establish a definite relationship between glycine and spinal *inhibitory* interneurones, such a relationship is strongly suggested by the inhibitory effect of the amino acid on spinal neurones, together with the high concentrations found in the ventral horn, the site of termination of inhibitory interneurones upon motoneurones, and probably the location of the majority of inhibitory synapses in the spinal cord.

In addition to glycine, other amino acids present in spinal tissue need to be considered as possible inhibitory transmitters because of their depressant effects on neurones (Curtis and Watkins, 1960; Curtis *et al.*, 1968b). These include cystathionine (Werman *et al.*, 1966b; Werman and Aprison, 1968; Johnston, 1968), α-alanine, serine and taurine (Johnston, 1968; see also Werman and Aprison, 1968), and are marked with an asterisk in Table I. The levels of α-alanine and serine are slightly higher in grey matter than elsewhere in the spinal cord (Werman and Aprison, 1968;

References p. 186–189

MICROELECTROPHORESIS

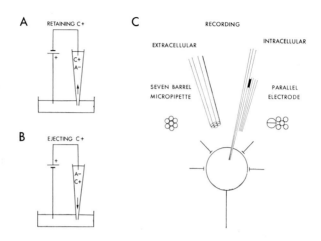

Fig. 5. The technique of microelectrophoresis (see text). (A, B), the retention and ejection of an active cation (C+) by an "anionic" and "cationic" current respectively. (C), types of multibarrel micropipette available for extracellular and intracellular recording of the cellular response to an extracellularly administered substance.

Johnston, 1968), and cystathionine appears to be evenly distributed (Johnston, 1968; but see Werman *et al.*, 1966b). The effects of spinal-cord anoxia on the levels of amino acids other than glycine and GABA have not been determined, but the importance of glycine as an inhibitory transmitter is perhaps indicated by its higher intraspinal concentrations and the greater potency as a depressant of spinal neurones.

The subcellular distribution of these amino acids may also provide additional support for a transmitter function (Whittaker, 1968), particularly if one, or several, of these substances are found to be present in synaptosomes containing flattened vesicles which are evidently characteristic of inhibitory synapses (Uchizono, 1968).

Central action of glycine

The effects of glycine and related amino acids have been determined by administering the substances electrophoretically into the immediate extracellular environment of single neurones, whilst simultaneously recording intra- or extracellular responses. This technique of microelectrophoresis is illustrated in Fig. 5: the amino acid cations (C+) are retained within (Fig. 5A), and ejected from (Fig. 5B), glass micropipettes by an electrical current passed between an aqueous solution of suitable pH within the pipette and the external medium (Curtis, 1964). Extracellular potentials are recorded by means of the centre barrel of five- or seven-barrel micropipettes (Fig. 5C) of overall tip diameter 4–8 μ. Intracellular records of resting, synaptic and action potentials, measurements of membrane conductance and excitability, and alterations of membrane potential and intracellular ion content are made with single- or double-

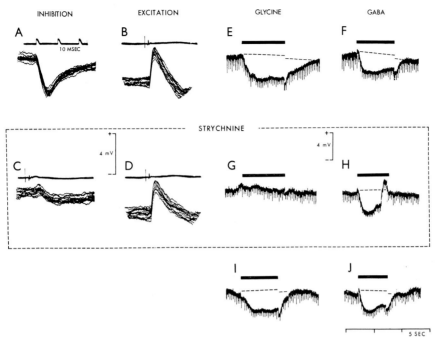

Fig. 6. Intracellular potentials recorded from two motoneurones (A–D and E–J) demonstrating the action of strychnine upon postsynaptic potentials. (A–D), gastrocnemius motoneurone, recorded with the central barrel of a co-axial electrode; (E–J), tibial motoneurone, recorded with parallel electrode. (A), inhibitory postsynaptic potential, stimulation of peroneal nerve. (B), excitatory postsynaptic potential, stimulation of gastrocnemius nerve. (C, D), the same responses after strychnine was allowed to diffuse from the outer barrel of a co-axial electrode for 3 min. (E), hyperpolarization induced by extracellularly administered glycine (30 nA), as signalled by the horizontal black bar, the fast vertical deflections are inhibitory postsynaptic potentials evoked by stimulation of the sural nerve. The horizontal broken lines provided a base line from which the amount of hyperpolarization can be measured. (F), hyperpolarization induced by GABA (60 nA). (G, H), the same responses during the extracellular electrophoretic administration of strychnine from one barrel of the five-barrel micropipette of a parallel electrode. (I, J), recorded several minutes after the termination of the strychnine administration. *Calibration*, voltage, 4 mV for A–D and E–J, hyperpolarizations recorded as downward deflections. Time, 10 msec for A–D and 5 sec for E–J.

barrel micropipettes (tip diameter less than 1 μ) cemented to, and projecting beyond, the orifices of a single- (Werman *et al.*, 1968) or a five-barrel (Curtis *et al.*, 1968b) micropipette (parallel electrode, Fig. 5C). Suitable tests can be carried out to demonstrate that the effects induced by the amino acids are independent of the pH of the solution, and the current used to administer the ion (Curtis and Watkins, 1960; Curtis, 1964; Werman *et al.*, 1968).

When administered electrophoretically from the extraneuronal barrel of parallel micropipettes, glycine hyperpolarises the large majority of motoneurones (Werman *et al.*, 1966a, 1967, 1968; Curtis *et al.*, 1967a, b, 1968b). The variations in the sensitivity of different cells to glycine, and the differing time courses of the hyperpolarization, presumably reflect to a large extent interference to glycine diffusion by structures between the orifice of the micropipette and the surface membrane of the impaled

References p. 186–189

neurone. The hyperpolarization attains a maximum level within a few seconds, the dose (current)–response curve is typically sigmoid in shape, the peak response for any one current often fades to a lower level (Curtis et al., 1968b), and recovery after termination of the glycine ejecting current is rapid (Fig. 6E). Evidence that the hyperpolarization is accompanied by an increased membrane conductance is provided by the following observations: direct measurement of the membrane conductance and excitability; reduction in amplitude of E- and IPSP's; reduction in the sensitivity of the neurone to electrophoretically administered excitant amino acids; and a blockage of invasion by antidromically propagated impulses. When the membrane potential of the neurone is reduced by passing current through the intracellular microelectrode, the hyperpolarization produced by a given quantity of glycine is increased. In contrast, the glycine effect can be reduced, and even reversed to a depolarization, by hyperpolarization of the membrane. A strict comparison of the equilibrium potentials of the ionic events associated with IPSP's and the effects of glycine entails uniform polarization of the membrane activated by the transmitter and the amino acid. Such uniform polarization is unlikely to be obtained by passing current through an intracellular microelectrode, but the "reversal" potential of the glycine hyperpolarization is very close to that of IPSP's in some cells, and at a slightly less hyperpolarized level in others. Hence it seems very likely that glycine and the spinal inhibitory transmitter induce the same change in the ionic permeability of the motoneurone membrane (Werman et al., 1968; Curtis et al., 1968b). Further confirmation is provided by experiments in which intracellular ion concentrations are altered by passing potassium, sodium, chloride and other anions from an intracellular microelectrode. The alterations in intracellular potassium and chloride ion concentration subsequent upon Na, K or Cl injections (Eccles, 1964) produce identical alterations in IPSP's and glycine hyperpolarizations. For example, intracellular injection of chloride ions converts both inhibitory and glycine hyperpolarizations into depolarizations (Fig. 2, D–F). Similar alterations occur after intracellular potassium and sodium injections (Curtis et al., 1968b). The intracellular injection of a series of different anions (Fig. 3) shows that only those which invert IPSP's convert glycine hyperpolarizations into depolarizations. Consequently, the membrane "pores" associated with the increased membrane conductance produced by glycine presumably have the same mean diameter as those associated with spinal IPSP's. Glycine does not hyperpolarize intraspinal axons, and its action is most probably confined to inhibitory synapses. The other neutral amino acids, GABA (Fig. 6F) and β-alanine, also hyperpolarize motoneurones and have the same effect on the membrane as glycine (Curtis et al., 1968b).

The hyperpolarizing action of these and related amino acids readily explains the depressant effects upon interneurones and Renshaw cells (Curtis and Watkins, 1960, 1965; Werman et al., 1968; Curtis et al., 1968a). In general, glycine is more effective than either GABA or β-alanine in hyperpolarizing motoneurones, and in depressing the firing of interneurones (Table I). On the other hand, glycine and GABA are approximately equally effective depressants of the firing of Renshaw cells (Curtis et al., 1968a). The other amino acids found free in spinal tissue, α-alanine, serine, cystathionine and taurine are relatively weak depressants of interneurones (Table I).

TABLE I

DEPRESSANT AMINO ACIDS

The activity of amino acids as depressants of spinal interneurones relative to that of GABA (– – –), a reduction or increase in the number of symbols indicates a significant reduction or increase respectively in depressant activity. Antagonism by strychnine of this depression is indicated by Yes, No or NT (not tested). Amino acids marked with an asterisk are found free in spinal tissue.

Compound	Action	Strychnine antagonist
α-Amino acids		
★ Glycine	– – – –	Yes
★ L-α-Alanine	– –	Yes
★ L-Serine	–	Yes
D-Serine	(–)	Yes
DL-, DL-*allo*-Cystathionine	–	Yes
★ L-Cystathionine	(–)	NT
Aminomethane sulphonic acid	0	
β-Amino acids		
β-Alanine	– – –	Yes
DL-β-Amino-isobutyric acid	– –	Yes
★ Taurine	– –	Yes
γ-Amino acids		
★ γ-Aminobutyric acid	– – –	No
γ-Amino-β-hydroxybutyric acid	– –	No
3-Aminopropane sulphonic acid	– – – – –	No
Higher ω-amino acids		
δ-Aminovaleric acid	– –	No
ε-Aminocaproic acid	–	No

Some spinal neurones however, have been reported to be more sensitive to cystathionine than to either glycine or GABA (Werman *et al.*, 1966b).

Glycine antagonists

The identification of a compound as the transmitter at particular synapses gains considerable support from the demonstration that postsynaptic antagonists of synaptic action also block the effects of the compound when artificially administered. Thus the effects of strychnine and tetanus toxin on the action of amino acids upon spinal neurones are of considerable interest.

When administered electrophoretically strychnine reversibly abolishes the hyperpolarizing action of glycine (Fig. 6E, G, I) but not that of GABA (Fig. 6F, H, J); similar results are observed when the alkaloid is administered intravenously (Curtis *et al.*, 1967a, b, 1968a, b). Antagonism between strychnine and various amino acids is most readily determined in experiments in which extracellular action potentials are recorded from interneurones or Renshaw cells (Curtis *et al.*, 1968a). Furthermore, comparisons can be made between the effects of strychnine on the synaptic inhibition of the spontaneous or chemically induced firing of Renshaw cells, and the depression of firing resulting from the administration of neutral amino acids. On the basis of

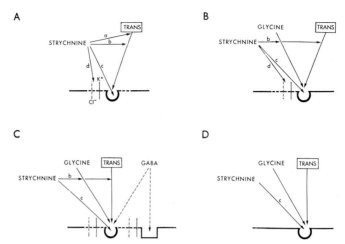

Fig. 7. The postsynaptic action of strychnine at spinal inhibitory synapses (see text). The simplest postulate to explain the experimental findings is illustrated in D: the interaction between the transmitter (glycine) and inhibitory receptors is prevented by strychnine.

antagonism by strychnine these amino acids have been divided into two groups (Table I): "glycine-like" (α and β) amino acids and "GABA-like" (γ and higher ω) amino acids. All of the other alkaloids and synthetic substances which depress postsynaptic inhibition also block the effects of "glycine-like" amino acids, and the relative potencies of these substances in blocking these two actions are similar (Curtis *et al.*, 1968a).

Prior to these experiments four explanations were offered for the effect of strychnine at spinal inhibitory synapses (Fig. 7A): (*a*), a reduction in the amount of inhibitory transmitter released; (*b*), chemical combination with the released transmitter; (*c*), competitive antagonism at subsynaptic receptors, and (*d*), interference with the movement of ions through activated inhibitory membrane (Araki, 1965). The postsynaptic action of artificially administered glycine is blocked by strychnine, hence if glycine be the transmitter, the effect of the alkaloid on synaptic inhibition is unlikely to be the result of a reduction of transmitter release (Fig. 7B). Furthermore, both glycine and GABA produce the same alteration in ionic permeability by interaction with the same or different receptors, yet the action of glycine, but not that of GABA, is prevented by strychnine. Hence it appears improbable that concentrations of strychnine specifically suppressing synaptic inhibition interfere with the movement of potassium or chloride ions at inhibitory synapses (Fig. 7C). Interaction between glycine-like amino acids and all of the compounds which block both spinal inhibition and the postsynaptic action of the amino acids appears an unlikely explanation of the observed phenomena, particularly in view of the relatively low concentrations of these compounds required for antagonism. Hence strychnine most probably suppresses spinal inhibition at the receptor level, preventing the access of the transmitter to inhibitory receptors (Fig. 7D). This argument presupposes that glycine receptors are identical with those activated by the inhibitory transmitter, a postulate which most simply explains the experimental findings.

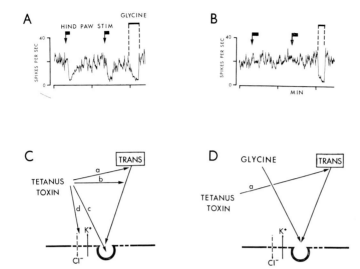

Fig. 8. The action of tetanus toxin upon the synaptic inhibition and the depression by glycine of a Renshaw cell. (A, B), the firing frequency of a Renshaw cell before (A) and 49 min after (B) the pressure injection of tetanus toxin 80–100 μ from the cell. Firing was induced by the continuous ejection of acetylcholine in A, and was of "spontaneous" origin in B. The horizontal bars and arrows indicate stimulation of the ipsilateral hind paw by a mechanically applied "squeeze"; the horizontal bars and vertical broken lines indicate the electrophoretic ejection of glycine (0.5 M solution, pH 3, 2 nA). (C), the possible modes of action of tetanus toxin. (D), the reduction in the release of inhibitory transmitter by tetanus toxin (see text).

It is of considerable interest that tetanus toxin blocks spinal postsynaptic inhibition by an entirely different mode of action. Renshaw cells are inhibited by volleys in afferent nerves from the hind limb (Wilson *et al.*, 1964), and this inhibition can be demonstrated as a reduction in firing rate which follows squeezing of the ipsilateral hind paw (Fig. 8A). Both this afferent inhibition and the depressant effect of electrophoretically administered glycine are blocked by strychnine (Biscoe and Curtis, 1966; Curtis *et al.*, 1968a). The injection of tetanus toxin by pressure into the environment of a Renshaw cell is followed by progressive reduction, and finally abolition of synaptic inhibition (Fig. 8B), yet the inhibitory action of glycine (and GABA) remains unreduced (Curtis and De Groat, 1968). Again, assuming that glycine is the inhibitory transmitter, the simplest explanation of these observations is that tetanus toxin acts at a presynaptic site (Fig. 8D), and reduces the amount of transmitter released from inhibitory terminals. The process is apparently specific for inhibitory synapses as the synaptic excitation of motoneurones (Brooks *et al.*, 1957) and Renshaw cells (Brooks *et al.*, 1957; Curtis and De Groat, 1968) remains unaffected. The finding that glycine levels in the spinal cord are not altered by tetanus toxin may indicate that the toxin prevents transmitter release rather than hinders synthesis (G. A. R. Johnston, W. C. de Groat and D. R. Curtis, unpublished observations).

The convulsants pentamethylene tetrazole and picrotoxin do not block the depressant effects of either glycine or GABA on spinal neurones. The latter substance has been administered both electrophoretically (Curtis *et al.*, 1968a) and by pressure (from a saturated solution of picrotoxin in 165 m*M* NaCl) near single neurones (D. R. Curtis and W. C. de Groat, unpublished observations). A similar lack of antagonism has been observed between glycine and GABA and a large series of analogues structurally related to these amino acids (Curtis *et al.*, 1968a), many of which are weak depressants.

Glycine synthesis, inactivation and release

Metabolic pathways in which glycine participates are complex (Weinhouse, 1955; Meister, 1965), and few studies upon nervous tissue have been reported. Following the suppression of spinal inhibition at a presynaptic site by tetanus toxin, there is a significant increase in the amount of free aspartic acid in the spinal cord, glycine and GABA levels remaining unaltered (G. A. R. Johnston, W. C. de Groat and D. R. Curtis, unpublished observations). Thus aspartic acid may be involved as a glycine precursor, but further studies are obviously required as the increased levels of aspartic acid may merely reflect the association of this amino acid with the increased activity of spinal excitatory interneurones (Davidoff *et al.*, 1967a).

On the assumption that the brief duration of the conductance change associated with the "direct" inhibition of motoneurones reflects the time course of the change of concentration of transmitter in the synaptic cleft, the transmitter concentration falls to a very low level within 1–2 msec of the beginning of the IPSP (Eccles, 1964). It appears probable that the duration of transmitter action at other spinal inhibitory synapses is similarly very brief, and that prolonged IPSP's result from repetitive firing of interneurones and temporal dispersion of inhibitory volleys. Transmitters are assumed to be removed from the synaptic cleft by diffusion, by extracellular enzymatic inactivation, and also by uptake into cells and nerve endings. Although simple diffusion may account for the brief time course of transmitter action (Eccles and Jaeger, 1958), the close proximity of synapses on the same and adjacent neurones probably excludes this as the only mechanism for transmitter removal. Both enzymes and active transport systems may be susceptible to antagonism, and it may thus be possible to establish similarities between an administered compound and a released transmitter if the effects of both can be potentiated in a specific fashion.

The inhibitory action of glycine upon spinal neurones ceases rapidly after the termination of the ejecting electrophoretic current, and the effectiveness of this amino acid can be neither enhanced nor prolonged by the simultaneous electrophoretic administration of a series of glycine analogues or inhibitors of enzymes possibly associated with glycine metabolism (Curtis *et al.*, 1968a). The enzyme inhibitors tested include hydroxylamine, amino-oxyacetic acid, thiosemicarbazide, hydroxyethylhydrazine, kojic acid, *p*-aminobenzoic acid, *p*-aminohippuric acid and aminopterin. Only with *p*-hydroxymercuribenzoate was a significant increase obtained of the depressant action of glycine. Considerable technical difficulties were experienced in these experiments (Curtis *et al.*, 1968a), in which little or no enhancement was observed of the depressant action of GABA. However, in more recent experiments, the related mercurial, *p*-chloromercuriphenylsulphonic acid, increased the effectiveness of glycine, and to a lesser extent also that of GABA, β-alanine, L- and D-α-alanine. Furthermore, both mercurials ($10^{-4}M$) inhibit the uptake of glycine and GABA ($10^{-3}M$) by brain slices (D. R. Curtis, A. W. Duggan and G. A. R. Johnston, unpublished observations). These results suggest that the mercury derivatives may interfere with amino acid transport mechanisms rather than inhibit specific enzymes associated with glycine inactivation, although the participation of extracellular enzymes which inactivate glycine cannot be fully excluded. A variety of structurally specific amino acid uptake systems have been described in brain slices (Levi *et al.*, 1967; Blasberg and Lajtha, 1966), but the processes studied *in vitro* may not be directly applicable to those occurring in central nervous tissue *in vivo*, particularly in view of the complex metabolic and ionic requirements of this tissue. Nevertheless, since elevation of the *intra*cellular glycine content does not inhibit spinal neurons, cellular uptake, followed by subsequent enzymatic modification, could account for the rapid reversibility of the depressant action of extracellularly administered glycine. It is possible that enzyme inhibitors administered locally for a relatively brief period may not gain access to intracellularly located enzyme systems in concentrations adequate to produce detectable effects, particularly if a considerable excess of enzyme is present and the major rate-limiting step in amino acid removal is transport across the cellular membrane. The antagonism demonstrated between glycine and strychnine, and the failure of strychnine to modify the uptake of glycine by spinal and cortical slices (G. A. R. Johnston, unpublished results; A. Lajtha, personal communication), indicates that the amino acid transport system *per se* is unlikely to be directly associated with the hyperpolarizing action of glycine.

Little success has been achieved in experiments relating drug-induced alterations in the time course of action of glycine (and GABA) to the enhancement and prolongation of inhibitory synaptic action in the spinal cord.

The high efficiency of processes removing glycine from the vicinity of neurones, and the absence of a substance which blocks these processes in a specific fashion, will probably render difficult attempts to detect a release of glycine from spinal tissue related to the firing of inhibitory interneurones. No results have been published of the release of glycine from the surface of the spinal cord, into the venous effluent or into a tissue space created by a "push-pull" cannula.

CONCLUSIONS

The evidence which favours the participation of glycine as the transmitter at strychnine-sensitive hyperpolarizing spinal inhibitory synapses can be summarized as follows:

(*1*) The intraspinal distribution of this amino acid is compatible with its presence in inhibitory interneurones in amounts higher than those required for general "metabolic" purposes.

(*2*) Glycine hyperpolarizes spinal neurones, and the associated alteration in membrane permeability appears to be identical to that produced by the synaptically released inhibitory transmitter.

(*3*) Strychnine and a series of related alkaloid and synthetic compounds, all of which block spinal postsynaptic inhibition, block the effects of glycine, most probably by interfering with the access of the amino acid to subsynaptic receptor sites.

(4) Electrophoretically administered glycine is removed very rapidly from the extraneuronal space, probably by cellular uptake, and it has not been possible to enhance or prolong its action, or that of the spinal inhibitory transmitter, in a specific fashion.

Assuming that glycine is the inhibitory transmitter, the suppression of spinal inhibitory transmission by tetanus toxin probably results from a reduction in the amount of transmitter released by presynaptic impulses.

As neither strychnine nor picrotoxin block the hyperpolarization of spinal neurones by GABA, an interpretation of the effects of this amino acid in terms of an action at particular inhibitory synapses must await the finding of a specific antagonist.

ACKNOWLEDGEMENTS

It is a pleasure to acknowledge the collaboration of my colleagues Drs. G. A. R. Johnston, L. Hösli, J. C. Watkins, W. C. de Groat and A. W. Duggan in this investigation. Mrs. A. Daday, Mrs. H. Walsh and Mr. B. Maher provided invaluable technical assistance.

REFERENCES

APRISON, M. H., SHANK, R. P., DAVIDOFF, R. A., AND WERMAN, R., (1968); The distribution of glycine, a neurotransmitter suspect in the central nervous system of several vertebrate species. *Life Sci.*, **7**, 583–590.

APRISON, M. H., AND WERMAN, R., (1965); The distribution of glycine in cat spinal cord and roots. *Life Sci.*, **4**, 2075–2083.

ARAKI, T., (1965); The effects of strychnine on the postsynaptic inhibitory action. *Lectures and Symposia, XXIII Int. Cong. Physiol. Sci.*, pp. 96–97.

BISCOE, T. J., AND CURTIS, D. R., (1966); Noradrenaline and inhibition of Renshaw cells. *Science*, **151**, 1230–1231.

BLASBERG, R., AND LAJTHA, A., (1966); Heterogeneity of the mediated transport systems of amino acid uptake in brain. *Brain Res.*, **1**, 86–104.

BRADLEY, K., EASTON, D. M., AND ECCLES, J. C., (1953); An investigation of primary or direct inhibition. *J. Physiol. (Lond.)*, **122**, 474–488.

BROOKS, V. B., CURTIS, D. R., AND ECCLES, J. C., (1957); The action of tetanus toxin on the inhibition of motoneurones. *J. Physiol. (Lond.)*, **135**, 655–672.

COOMBS, J. S., ECCLES, J. C., AND FATT, P., (1955a); The specific ionic conductances and the ionic movements across the motoneuronal membrane that produce the inhibitory postsynaptic potential. *J. Physiol. (Lond.)*, **130**, 326–373.

COOMBS, J. S., ECCLES, J. C., AND FATT, P., (1955b); The inhibitory suppression of reflex discharges from motoneurones. *J. Physiol. (Lond.)*, **130**, 396–413.

CURTIS, D. R., (1959); Pharmacological investigations upon the inhibition of spinal motoneurones. *J. Physiol. (Lond.)*, **145**, 175–192.

CURTIS, D. R., (1962); The depression of spinal inhibition by electrophoretically administered strychnine. *Int. J. Neuropharmacol.*, **1**, 239–250.

CURTIS, D. R., (1963); The pharmacology of central and peripheral inhibition. *Pharmacol. Rev.*, **15**, 333–364.

CURTIS, D. R., (1964); Microelectrophoresis. In W. L. NASTUK (Ed.), *Physical Techniques in Biological Research*, Vol. 5, Academic Press, New York, pp. 144–190.

CURTIS, D. R., (1968); Pharmacology and neurochemistry of mammalian central inhibitory processes. In C. VON EULER, S. SKOGLUND AND U. SÖDERBERG (Eds.), *Structure and Function of Inhibitory Mechanisms*, Pergamon, Oxford, pp. 429–456.

CURTIS, D. R., AND DE GROAT, W. C., (1968); Tetanus toxin and spinal inhibition. *Brain Res.*, **10**, 208–212.

CURTIS, D. R., HÖSLI, L., AND JOHNSTON, G. A. R., (1967a); The inhibition of spinal neurones by glycine. *Nature (Lond.)*, **215**, 1502–1503.

CURTIS, D. R., HÖSLI, L., AND JOHNSTON, G. A. R., (1968a); A pharmacological study of the depression of spinal neurones by glycine and related amino acids. *Exp. Brain Res.*, **6**, 1–18.

CURTIS, D. R., HÖSLI, L., JOHNSTON, G. A. R., AND JOHNSTON, I. H., (1967b); Glycine and spinal inhibition. *Brain Res.*, **5**, 112–114.

CURTIS, D. R., HÖSLI, L., JOHNSTON, G. A. R., AND JOHNSTON, I. H., (1968b); The hyperpolarization of spinal motoneurones by glycine and related amino acids. *Exp. Brain Res.*, **5**, 238–262.

CURTIS, D. R., AND WATKINS, J. C., (1960); The excitation and depression of spinal neurones by structurally related amino acids. *J. Neurochem.*, **6**, 117–141.

CURTIS, D. R., AND WATKINS, J. C., (1965); The pharmacology of amino acids related to gamma-aminobutyric acid. *Pharmacol. Rev.*, **17**, 347–392.

DAVIDOFF, R. A., GRAHAM JR., L. T., SHANK, R. P., WERMAN, R., AND APRISON, M. H., (1966); Interneuronal cell loss and amino acid concentration in cat spinal cord. *Physiologist*, **9**, 165.

DAVIDOFF, R. A., GRAHAM JR., L. T., SHANK, R. P., WERMAN, R., AND APRISON, M. H., (1967a); Changes in amino acid concentrations associated with loss of spinal interneurons. *J. Neurochem.*, **14**, 1025–1031.

DAVIDOFF, R. A., SHANK, R. P., GRAHAM JR., L. T., APRISON, M. H., AND WERMAN, R., (1967b); Association of glycine with spinal interneurones. *Nature (Lond.)*, **214**, 680–681.

DEVANANDAN, M. S., ECCLES, R. M., AND YOKOTA, T., (1965a); Depolarization of afferent terminals evoked by muscle stretch. *J. Physiol. (Lond.)*, **179**, 417–429.

DEVANANDAN, M. S., ECCLES, R. M., AND YOKOTA, T., (1965b); Muscle stretch and the presynaptic inhibition of the group Ia pathway to motoneurones. *J. Physiol. (Lond.)*, **179**, 430–441.

ECCLES, J. C., (1964); *Physiology of Synapses*, Springer, Berlin.

ECCLES, J. C., (1966); The ionic mechanisms of excitatory and inhibitory synaptic action. *Ann. N.Y. Acad. Sci.*, **137**, 473–494.

ECCLES, J. C., (1967); Functional organization of the spinal cord. *Anesthesiology*, **28**, 31–45.

ECCLES, J. C., FATT, P., AND KOKETSU, K., (1954); Cholinergic and inhibitory synapses in a pathway from motor-axon collaterals to motoneurones. *J. Physiol. (Lond.)*, **126**, 524–562.

ECCLES, J. C., AND JAEGER, J. C., (1958); The relationship between the mode of operation and the dimensions of the junctional regions at synapses and motor end-organs. *Proc. Roy. Soc. B*, **148**, 38–56.

ECCLES, J. C., SCHMIDT, R. F., AND WILLIS, W. D., (1963); Pharmacological studies on presynaptic inhibition. *J. Physiol. (Lond.)*, **168**, 500–530.

EIDE, E., JURNA, I., AND LUNDBERG, A., (1968); Conductance measurements from motoneurons during presynaptic inhibition. In C. VON EULER, S. SKOGLUND AND U. SÖDERBERG (Eds.), *Structure and Function of Inhibitory Neuronal Mechanisms*, Pergamon, Oxford, pp. 215–219.

ENGBERG, I., LUNDBERG, A., AND RYALL, R. W., (1968); Reticulospinal inhibition of transmission in reflex pathways. *J. Physiol. (Lond.)*, **194**, 201–223.

ESPLIN, D. W., AND ZABLOCKA, B., (1964); Pilocarpine blockade of spinal inhibition in cats. *J. Pharmacol. exp. Ther.*, **143**, 174–180.

FRANK, K., (1959); Basic mechanisms of synaptic transmission in the central nervous system. *I.R.E. Trans. Med. Electron.*, **ME-6**, 85–88.

FRANK, K., AND FUORTES M. G. F., (1957); Presynaptic and postsynaptic inhibition of monosynaptic reflexes. *Fed. Proc.*, **16**, 39–40.

GRAHAM JR., L. T., SHANK, R. P., WERMAN, R., AND APRISON, M. H., (1967); Distribution of some synaptic transmitter suspects in cat spinal cord: glutamic acid, aspartic acid, γ-aminobutyric acid, glycine and glutamine. *J. Neurochem.*, **14**, 465–472.

HONGO, T., JANKOWSKA, E., AND LUNDBERG, A., (1966); Convergence of excitatory and inhibitory action on interneurones in the lumbosacral cord. *Exp. Brain Res.*, **1**, 338–358.

JANKOWSKA, E., LUND, S., LUNDBERG, A., AND POMPEIANO, O., (1968); Inhibitory effects evoked through ventral reticulospinal pathways. *Arch. ital. Biol.*, **106**, 124–140.

JOHNSTON, G. A. R., (1968); The intraspinal distribution of some depressant amino acids. *J. Neurochem.*, **15**, 1013–1018.

KAWAI, I., AND SASAKI, K., (1964); Effects of strychnine upon supraspinal inhibition. *Jap. J. Physiol.*, **14**, 309–317.

KELLERTH, J.-O., (1968); Aspects on the relative significance of pre- and postsynaptic inhibition in the spinal cord. In C. VON EULER, S. SKOGLUND AND U. SÖDERBERG (Eds.), *Structure and Function of Inhibitory Neuronal Mechanisms*, Pergamon, Oxford, pp. 197–212.

KRUGLOV, N. A., (1964); Effect of the morphine-group analgesics on the central inhibitory mechanisms. *Int. J. Neuropharmacol.*, **3**, 197–203.

KUBOTA, K., KIDOKORO, Y., AND SUZUKI, J., (1968); Postsynaptic inhibitions of trigeminal and lumbar motoneurons from the superficial radial nerve in the cat. *Jap. J. Physiol.*, **18**, 198–215.

LEVI, G., KANDERA, J., AND LAJTHA, A., (1967); Control of cerebral metabolic levels. I. Amino acid uptake and levels in various species. *Arch. Biochem. Biophys.*, **119**, 303–311.

LLINAS, R., (1964); Mechanisms of supraspinal actions upon spinal cord activities. Pharmacological studies on reticular inhibition of alpha extensor motoneurones. *J. Neurophysiol.*, **27**, 1127–1137.

LLINAS, R., AND TERZUOLO, C. A., (1964); Mechanisms of supraspinal actions upon spinal cord activities. Reticular inhibitory mechanisms on alpha-extensor motoneurons. *J. Neurophysiol.*, **27**, 579–591.

LLINAS, R., AND TERZUOLO, C. A., (1965); Mechanisms of supraspinal actions upon spinal cord activities. Reticular inhibitory mechanisms upon flexor motoneurons. *J. Neurophysiol.*, **28**, 413–422.

LLOYD, D. P. C., AND MCINTYRE, A. K., (1948); Analysis of forelimb–hindlimb reflex activity in acutely decapitated cats. *J. Neurophysiol.*, **11**, 455–470.

LONGO, V. G., AND CHIAVARELLI, S., (1962); Neuropharmacological analysis of strychnine-like drugs. In W. D. M. PATON (Ed.), *Pharmacological Analysis of Central Nervous Action*, Pergamon, Oxford, pp. 189–198.

LUNDBERG, A., (1966); Integration in the reflex pathway. In R. GRANIT (Ed.), *Muscular Afferents and Motor Control*, Almqvist and Wiksell, Stockholm, pp. 275–305.

MEISTER, A., (1965); *Biochemistry of the Amino Acids*, Vol. II, Academic Press, New York, pp. 636–673.

NATHAN, P. W., AND SMITH, M. C., (1959); Fasciculi proprii of the spinal cord in man. *Brain*, **82**, 610–668.

NYBERG-HANSEN, R., (1966); Functional organization of descending supra-spinal fibre systems to the spinal cord. Anatomical observations and physiological correlations. *Ergbn. Anat. EntwGesch.*, **39**, 1–48.

PETRAS, J. M., (1967); Cortical, tectal and tegmental fiber connections in the spinal cord of the cat. *Brain Res.*, **6**, 275–324.

SAMPSON, S. R., (1966); Mechanism of coniine-blockade of postsynaptic inhibition in the spinal cord of the cat. *Int. J. Neuropharmacol.*, **5**, 171–182.

SAMPSON, S. R., ESPLIN, D. W., AND ZABLOCKA, B., (1966); Effects of coniine on peripheral and central synaptic transmission. *J. Pharmacol. exp. Ther.*, **152**, 313–324.

SASAKI, K., TANAKA, T., AND MORI, K., (1962); Effects of stimulation of pontine and bulbar reticular formation upon spinal motoneurons of the cat. *Jap. J. Physiol.*, **12**, 45–62.

SHAPOVALOV, A. I., (1966); Excitation and inhibition of spinal neurones during supraspinal stimulation. In R. GRANIT (Ed.), *Muscular Afferents and Motor Control*, Almqvist and Wiksell, Stockholm, pp. 331–348.

SHAPOVALOV, A. I., AND ARUSHANYAN, E. B., (1963); Effect of strychnine on activity of motor and internuncial neurons of the spinal cord during stimulation of the anterior lobe of the cerebellum. *Byull. eksper. biol.*, **56**, No. 12, 3–10.

SHAPOVALOV, A. I., AND ARUSHANYAN, E. B., (1965); Effect of brain stem and motor cortex stimulation on the activity of spinal neurons. *Sechenov Physiol. J. (USSR)*, **51**, No. 6, 670–680.

SHAW, R. K., AND HEINE, J. D., (1965); Ninhydrin positive substances present in different areas of normal rat brain. *J. Neurochem.*, **12**, 151–155.

SMITH, T. G., WUERKER, R. B., AND FRANK, K., (1967); Membrane impedance changes during synaptic transmission in cat spinal motoneurons. *J. Neurophysiol.*, **30**, 1072–1096.

SZENTÁGOTHAI, J., (1958); The anatomical basis of synaptic transmission of excitation and inhibition in motoneurones. *Acta morph. Acad. Sci. Hung.*, **8**, 287–309.

SZENTÁGOTHAI, J., (1964), Propriospinal pathways and their synapses. In J. C. ECCLES AND J. P. SCHADÉ (Eds.), *Organization of the Spinal Cord (Progress in Brain Research*, Vol. 11*)*, Elsevier, Amsterdam, pp. 155–174.

TALLAN, H. H., (1962); A survey of amino acids and related compounds in nervous tissue. In J. T. HOLDEN (Ed.), *Amino Acid Pools*, Elsevier, Amsterdam, pp. 471–485.

UCHIZONO, K., (1968); Inhibitory and excitatory synapses in vertebrate and invertebrate animals. In C. VON EULER, S. SKOGLUND AND U. SÖDERBERG (Eds.), *Structure and Function of Inhibitory Neuronal Mechanisms*, Pergamon, Oxford, pp. 33–59.

WEINHOUSE, S., (1955); The synthesis and degradation of glycine. In W. D. MCELROY AND B. H. GLASS (Eds.), *Amino Acid Metabolism*, Johns Hopkins, Baltimore, pp. 637–657.

WERMAN, R., AND APRISON, M. H., (1968); Glycine: the search for a spinal cord inhibitory transmitter. In C. VON EULER, S. SKOGLUND AND U. SÖDERBERG (Eds.), *Structure and Function of Inhibitory Neural Mechanisms*, Pergamon, Oxford, pp. 473–486.

WERMAN, R., DAVIDOFF, R. A., AND APRISON, M. H., (1966a); Glycine and postsynaptic inhibition in cat spinal cord. *Physiologist*, **9**, 318.

WERMAN, R., DAVIDOFF, R. A., AND APRISON, M. H., (1966b); The inhibitory action of cystathionine. *Life Sci.*, **5**, 1431–1440.

WERMAN, R., DAVIDOFF, R. A., AND APRISON, M. H., (1967); Inhibition of motoneurones by iono-phoresis of glycine. *Nature (Lond.)*, **214**, 681–683.

WERMAN, R., DAVIDOFF, R. A., AND APRISON, M. H., (1968); Inhibitory action of glycine on spinal neurons in the cat. *J. Neurophysiol.*, **31**, 81-95.

WHITTAKER, V. P., (1968); The subcellular distribution of amino acids in brain and its relation to a possible transmitter function for these compounds. In C. VON EULER, S. SKOGLUND AND U. SÖDER-BERG (Eds.), *Structure and Function of Inhibitory Neuronal Mechanisms*, Pergamon, Oxford, pp. 487–504.

WILSON, V. J., (1966); Regulation and function of Renshaw cell discharge. In R. GRANIT (Ed.), *Muscular Afferents and Motor Control*, Almqvist and Wiksell, Stockholm, pp. 317–329.

WILSON, V. J., DIECKE, F. P. J., AND TALBOT, W. H., (1960); Action of tetanus toxin on conditioning of spinal motoneurones. *J. Neurophysiol.*, **23**, 659-666.

WILSON, V. J., AND TALBOT, W. H., (1963); Integration at an inhibitory interneurone: inhibition of Renshaw cells. *Nature (Lond.)*, **200**, 1325–1327.

WILSON, V. J., TALBOT, W. H., AND KATO, M., (1964); Inhibitory convergence upon Renshaw cells. *J. Neurophysiol.*, **27**, 1063–1079.

Comparative Microelectrophoretic Studies of Invertebrate and Vertebrate Neurones

F. A. STEINER AND L. PIERI

Department of Experimental Medicine, F. Hoffmann-La Roche & Co Ltd., Basle and Brain Research Institute, University of Zürich (Switzerland)

Comparative microelectrophoretic studies of invertebrate and vertebrate nerve cells seem of interest for the following two reasons: (*1*) Arthropods — specially insects — are known to contain high concentrations of substances which in vertebrates are thought to be neurotransmitters. (*2*) The lack of a well-defined blood–brain barrier in arthropods seems to be associated with a fundamentally different organisation and dimension of extracellular cerebral fluid space.

The effects of the following substances were investigated: acetylcholine, eserine (physostigmine), L-glutamic acid, γ-aminobutyric acid (GABA) and dopamine (3,4-dihydroxy-phenylethylamine = 3-hydroxy-tyramine).

In the first part neuronal effects in vertebrates (rat and cat) will be described, whereas the second part will be concerned with the effects of the same substances on neuronal activity in the ant brain.

METHODS

Animals and anaesthesia

Vertebrate experiments were carried out on cats and male rats anaesthetized with α-chloralose + urethane. Technical details have been previously described (Steiner, 1968; Steiner *et al.*, 1969). Invertebrate experiments were performed on the adult wood ant (*Formica lugubris* Zett.). The ant was immobilized with tackiwax under anaesthesia with CO_2. The chitin overlaying the protocerebrum was removed. The indifferent silver chloride electrode was fixed in a posterior lateral position within the cranial cavity.

Recording

The action potentials were monitored extracellularly through the central barrel of a five-barrelled microelectrode (tip diameter 1–3 μ), filled with a solution of 2 M NaCl to which a dye such as fast green (vertebrates) or methyl blue (arthropods) was added if the simultaneous marking of the microelectrode tip position was desired. This barrel was connected to a BAK cathode follower and the action potentials were displayed after adequate amplification on a cathode ray oscilloscope and through a

References p. 198–199

loudspeaker system. The signals were stored on magnetic tape and filmed when required.

Microelectrophoresis (Curtis, 1964; Salmoiraghi and Steiner, 1963)

The outer barrels of the multi-barrelled microelectrodes were filled with acetylcholine chloride (1–2 *M*), eserine (physostigmine) (0.5 *M*), sodium L-glutamate (1 *M*), γ-aminobutyric acid hydrochloride (1 *M*), dopamine hydrochloride (3,4-dihydroxy-phenylethylamine hydrochloride) (1 *M*). The pH of these solutions had been adjusted to values assuring a sufficient degree of ionization. One barrel was routinely filled with sodium chloride (1/6 *M*) for current control. Electrophoretic currents ranging from 5–120 nA (10^{-9} A) for vertebrates and 5–40 nA for arthropods were used for drug ejection. Since the amounts of ionized substances delivered in this way are proportional to the intensity of the ejecting current they are commonly expressed in the terms of nanoamperes (nA) per time unit.

Localization of the electrode tip

The localization of the electrode tip in the mammalian brain was marked according to Thomas and Wilson (1965) by electrophoretic ejection of fast green (12 μA, 5–10 min). At the end of the experiment the animals were sacrificed by an overdose of phenobarbital and perfused with saline followed by 4% formaline in saline. Fixed brains were embedded in paraffin (or celloidin). The position of the electrode tip was localized in serial sections (24 μ) by careful identification of the colour spot.

The exact localization of the electrode tip in the ant brain was marked by the same method, but methyl blue (5–8 μA, 8–10 min) was used instead of fast green. The ant brain was removed and fixed with glutaraldehyde in a phosphate buffer solution and embedded in paraffin. Serial sections of 8–10 μ were made.

OBSERVATIONS ON VERTEBRATE NEURONES

(1) Acetylcholine

Microelectrophoretically applied acetylcholine activates certain neurones in diverse brain regions such as brain stem, nucleus Deiters, hippocampus, lateral geniculate body, hypothalamus. The percentage of cells activated by acetylcholine in these regions varies. The discharge pattern of activated neurones is similar in most areas: The neurones are activated with a relatively long delay, *i.e.* a latency period of 2–20 sec. Only hippocampal neurones are activated with a relatively short delay, a latency period being less than 1 sec. In all regions the firing rate gradually subsided 2–30 sec after the end of microelectrophoresis. Fig. 1 shows the excitatory effect of acetylcholine on a single neurone located in the hypothalamus of the rat, anaesthetized with chloralose and urethane. The maximum increase of the rate of discharge is achieved after 3 sec. The activation outlasts the end of microelectrophoresis by at least 5 sec.

After microelectrophoresis of eserine (inhibitor of the acetylcholinesterase) the acetylcholine effect is enhanced. The discharge rate is higher, the delay is diminished

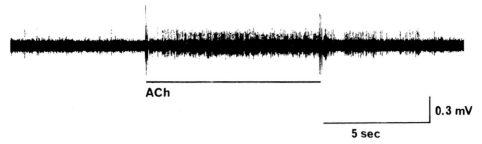

ACh

0.3 mV

5 sec

Fig. 1. Activation of a hypothalamic neurone (rat) by acetylcholine (ACh) (20 nA). Localization: zona incerta.

and after the end of microelectrophoresis the acetylcholine effect subsided very slowly. Eserine alone has a stimulating effect on many acetylcholine-sensitive cells.

Only a very small proportion of acetylcholine-sensitive cells (about 4–10%) is depressed.

(2) Amino acids

(a) *L-Glutamic acid.* L-Glutamic acid activates more or less all vertebrate neurones (cat and rat); spontaneously active as well as silent ones. The latency period is short, *i.e.* in the order of 100–200 msec. Almost immediately after termination of electrophoretic delivery of L-glutamate the initial rate of discharge is resumed. In addition with higher amounts of L-glutamate a diminution of the size of action potentials occurs which parallels the increase in the rate of discharge. Fig. 2 gives an example of the activation of a silent hippocampal neurone in the rat by L-glutamic acid (10 nA). Immediately after the end of microelectrophoretic delivery of L-glutamate the cell stops to fire.

(b) *γ-Aminobutyric acid.* γ-Aminobutyric acid consistently inhibits spontaneously active as well as glutamate-activated neurones (Fig. 3). The inhibitory effects of γ-aminobutyric acid in cat and rat are also rapid and confined to the time of microelectrophoresis of the drug. Almost immediately after the end of its electrophoretic delivery the spontaneous rate of discharge is resumed. The same conditions apply to L-glutamate-activated neurones.

(3) Dopamine (3,4-dihydroxy-phenylethylamine)

Dopamine strongly inhibits certain hypothalamic neurones (Fig. 4) (20%) and

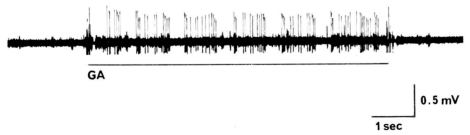

GA

0.5 mV

1 sec

Fig. 2. Activation of a silent neurone in the hippocampus (rat) by L-glutamic acid (GA) (10 nA).

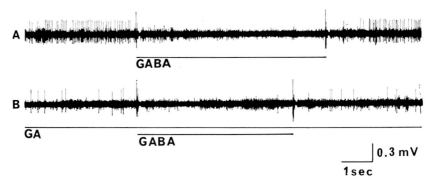

Fig. 3. Inhibition of a hypothalamic neurone (rat) by γ-aminobutyric acid (GABA): (A) of a spontaneous active neurone (20 nA); (B) of a L-glutamate(GA)-activated neurone (10 nA).

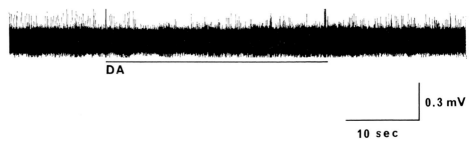

Fig. 4. Inhibition of a hypothalamic neurone (rat) by dopamine (DA) (30 nA).

neurones in the nucleus cuneatus and gracilis. The time course of inhibition with dopamine is very uniform. Neuronal activity is inhibited almost instantaneously after the onset of microelectrophoresis and the recovery time is also short (1–5 sec).

OBSERVATIONS ON INVERTEBRATE NEURONES

Fig. 5 illustrates the experimental situation during recording from the ant brain (protocerebrum).

(1) Acetylcholine

Acetylcholine has an excitatory effect in different regions of the ant brain (neuropile of the corpora pedunculata and neuropile of the β-lobe). Acetylcholine not only enhances the discharge rate of spontaneous active neurones but also stimulates silent neurones. In both instances the excitatory effect usually increases during the microelectrophoresis until a maximum is achieved. The neuronal discharge rate rises gradually during 3–10 sec. At the end of microelectrophoresis this activation subsides progressively after 3–10 sec. Fig. 6 demonstrates the enhancement of neuronal activity by acetylcholine in the ant protocerebrum, neuropile of the β-lobe. Occasionally very short latencies are seen for the onset of the drug effect as well as for its disappearance. In one case a clear inhibition of neuronal activity by acetylcholine was found.

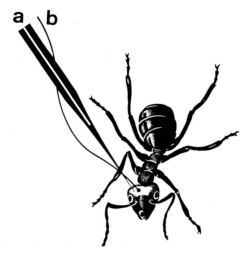

Fig. 5. Experimental situation for the recording in the ant brain. a, multibarrelled microelectrode; b, indifferent silver chloride electrode.

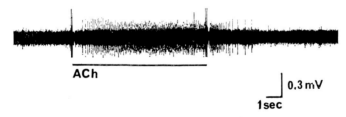

ACh

0.3 mV

1 sec

Fig. 6. Activation of a neurone in the ant brain (neuropile of the β-lobe) by acetylcholine (ACh) (20 nA).

(2) Eserine

Eserine — an acetylcholinesterase inhibitor — applied by microelectrophoresis also activates acetylcholine-sensitive neurones, but the gradual increase of activity is much slower than with acetylcholine alone. The latency period is clearly longer and the activation is less. At the end of the application eserine prolongs the recovery time. Fig. 7 illustrates the effect of acetylcholine after previous local delivery of eserine. It would appear that the previous administration of eserine enhances the activation by acetylcholine. These results, namely the activation of neurones by eserine and the enhancement of the acetylcholine effect by previous administration of eserine are remarkably similar to those obtained in vertebrates but less pronounced.

(3) Amino acids

(a) L-Glutamic acid. With L-glutamic acid an effect on spontaneously active neurones was found only in a few cases. With but one exception the effect was a small excitatory one. Only once a clear inhibition of spontaneous activity could be observed; this is a finding which was never encountered in vertebrates.

(b) γ-Aminobutyric acid. γ-Aminobutyric acid usually has a clear inhibitory

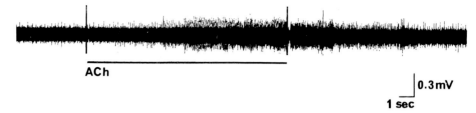

ACh

|0.3 mV
1 sec

Fig. 7. Activation of a neurone in the ant brain by acetylcholine (ACh) after locally applied eserine (20 nA).

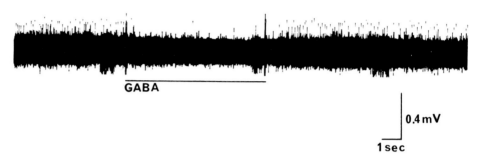

GABA

|0.4 mV
1 sec

Fig. 8. Inhibition of neuronal activity in the ant brain by γ-aminobutyric acid (GABA) (20 nA).

effect on single units in the ant brain. Two types of inhibitory effects have been observed: In the first case γ-aminobutyric acid silences the recorded neuronal activity completely with a short delay (Fig. 8) and immediately after termination of its micro-electrophoretic delivery the spontaneous rate of discharge is resumed. In the second type the inhibitory effect of γ-aminobutyric acid slowly increases after a short delay. At the end of microelectrophoretic delivery the spontaneous rate of discharge is gradually resumed, following a short delay. In insects the inhibition of central neurones has sometimes been less complete than in vertebrates. γ-Aminobutyric acid also inhibited acetylcholine-activated cells; this inhibition is a gradual one.

(4) Dopamine (3,4-dihydroxy-phenylethylamine)

Dopamine inhibits spontaneously active neurones. The inhibition starts almost immediately after the onset of the microelectrophoresis but is more progressive than in vertebrates. Fig. 9 demonstrates a more gradual suppression of neuronal activity. In vertebrates the inhibitory effect is always more or less immediate.

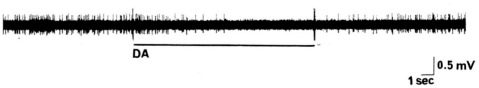

DA

|0.5 mV
1 sec

Fig. 9. Inhibition of a neurone in the ant brain by dopamine (DA) (20 nA).

DISCUSSION

This comparative analysis has shown remarkable similarities and a few dissimilarities between arthropods and vertebrates. With acetylcholine, activation and — in a few instances — inhibition were observed in both phyla. However, acetylcholine-sensitive neurones were less frequently encountered in the ant. In both experimental groups onset and disappearance of the acetylcholine effect were usually delayed by several seconds. Occasionally, these delays were shorter (less than 1 sec). Such rapid effects were seen in the ant as well as in hippocampal neurones (Steiner, 1968) and Renshaw cells of vertebrates (Curtis and Eccles, 1958).

Eserine, a cholinesterase inhibitor, has a similar excitatory effect as acetylcholine in arthropod and in vertebrate central nervous tissue. Furthermore eserine enhances the activation due to acetylcholine.

L-Glutamic acid, which invariably activates neurones in vertebrates, may exhibit the same effect in the ant brain, but to a markedly lesser extent. Rather surprisingly, inhibitory effects of L-glutamic acid were also unequivocally observed, in a few instances, in the ant. Further studies are necessary to decide whether these effects are direct or due to activation of an inhibitory pathway.

γ-Aminobutyric acid clearly inhibits neurones in the ant brain as well as in vertebrates. Two types of responses occur: in the first, the inhibition starts and ends with short latencies. A second type is particularly common in arthropod neurones: action potentials subside gradually during γ-aminobutyric acid microelectrophoresis, and neuronal recovery is likewise prolonged. Such neurones are only exceptionally found in vertebrates.

Dopamine produces a clear-cut and rapid inhibition in both vertebrates and arthropods. In the ant, the onset of the dopamine effect is sometimes more gradual; yet, eventually it is more marked.

From these results it would appear that in principle the same neurotransmitters are operational in both vertebrates and arthropods, but in a quantitatively or even qualitatively different manner.

Central nervous system responses to locally applied acetylcholine are less frequent in the ant. This finding may indicate a lack of sensitivity (possibly of the postsynaptic membrane) to acetylcholine. On the other hand, the cholinesterase activity of central nervous tissue of insects is high, and the presence of acetylcholinesterase in synapses of the corpora pedunculata has been demonstrated (Landolt and Sandri, 1966). Also, the cerebral concentration of acetylcholine itself is much higher in certain arthropod species (especially insects such as the cockroach) than in vertebrates (Treherne, 1966). The relative insensitivity of the insect central nervous system to locally applied acetylcholine might be a consequence of the very high content in acetylcholine and cholinesterase (Treherne, 1966). In spite of these strong indices for a role of acetylcholine in the central synaptic transmission of insects, the substance does not seem to be involved in impulse transmission at the peripheral (*i.e.* neuromuscular) level of arthropods (Harlow, 1958; Treherne, 1966). Therefore, caution must be used in the extrapolation of peripheral findings to central structures.

It is conceivable that in the course of evolution a progressive differentiation of acetyl-choline-sensitive neurones has taken place.

The amino acids of the arthropod nervous system have multiple roles: they serve as synaptic transmitters, they are involved in the maintenance of the osmotic equilibrium of nerve cells, they provide energy and they are incorporated into proteins. These factors may explain their high concentration (Treherne, 1966). The huge stores of γ-aminobutyric acid seem to be maintained by decarboxylation of glutamic acid; thus in homogenates of bee-brain the glutamic acid decarboxylase is 2.5 times more active than in mouse brain (Frontali, 1964). It is not known whether the partial in-efficiency of locally applied L-glutamic acid found in this study might be due to the increased presence of this enzyme concerned with its removal. Similarly, it cannot be decided whether the lesser activity of certain exogenous amino acids in insects is explainable by higher stores of endogenous material; conceivably, their local delivery by microelectrophoresis may not cause a sufficient increment over previous con-centrations.

The strong inhibitory effect of dopamine in parts of the central nervous tissue of the ant (e.g. the β-lobe of the corpora pedunculata) correlates well with the presence of catecholamine- containing nerve cells in the brain of the cockroach (Mancini and Frontali, 1968), but is at variance with findings of Gahery and Boistel (1965) on the abdominal ganglia of the species. These authors observed an excitatory rather than an inhibitory effect of topically applied dopamine. Here again, these discrepancies in responsiveness between peripheral and central nervous structures might reflect the appearance of certain synaptic mechanisms at different states of phylogenetic development.

SUMMARY

A comparative study between the central neurones of arthropods (ant) and of verte-brates (rat and cat) has shown remarkable similarities as well as a few dissimilarities. Acetylcholine activates and — in a few instances — inhibits central neurones in the ant and in vertebrates similarly, but acetylcholine-sensitive neurones are less frequently encountered in insects. γ-Aminobutyric acid inhibits neuronal activity in the central nervous tissue in the ant and in vertebrates similarly. In contrast L-glutamic acid which invariably activates neurones in vertebrates may exhibit the same effect to a markedly less extent in the ant brain, but it may also exceptionally inhibit central neurones in the latter. Dopamine inhibits some neurones of both arthropods and vertebrates.

REFERENCES

CURTIS, D. R., (1964); Microelectrophoresis. In W. L. NASTUK (Ed.), *Physical Techniques in Biological Research*. Vol. 5. *Electrophysiological Methods*, pt. A, Academic Press, London, pp. 144–190.
CURTIS, D. R., AND ECCLES, R. M., (1958); The excitation of Renshaw cells by pharmacological agents applied electrophoretically, *J. Physiol. (Lond.)*, **141**, 435–445.

FRONTALI, N., (1964); Brain glutamic acid decarboxylase and synthesis of γ-aminobutyric acid in vertebrate and invertebrate species. In D. RICHTER (Ed.), *Comparative Neurochemistry*, Pergamon, Oxford, pp. 185–192.

GAHERY, Y., AND BOISTEL, J., (1965); Study of some pharmacological substances which modify the electrical activity of the sixth abdominal ganglion of the cockroach, *Periplaneta americana*. In J. E. TREHERNE AND J. W. D. BEAMENT (Eds.), *The Physiology of the Insect Central Nervous System*, Academic Press, London, pp. 73–78.

HARLOW, P. A., (1958); The action of drugs on the nervous system of the locust (*Locusta migratoria*), *Ann. appl. Biol.*, **46**, 55–73.

LANDOLT, A. M., AND SANDRI, C., (1966); Cholinergische Synapsen im Oberschlundganglion der Waldameise (*Formica lugubris* Zett.), *Z. Zellforsch.*, **69**, 246–259.

MANCINI, G., AND FRONTALI, N., (1968); On the ultrastructural localization of catecholamines in the brain of cockroach, *Periplaneta americana*, *Proc. Fourth European Regional Conference on Electron Microscopy, Rome*, Vol. II, pp. 543–544.

SALMOIRAGHI, G. C., AND STEINER, F. A., (1963); Acetylcholine sensitivity of cat's medullary neurons, *J. Neurophysiol.*, **26**, 581–597.

STEINER, F. A., (1968); Influence of microelectrophoretically applied acetylcholine on the responsiveness of hippocampal and lateral geniculate neurones, *Pflügers Arch. ges. Physiol.*, **303**, 173–180.

STEINER, F. A., RUF, K., AND AKERT, K., (1969); Steroid sensitive neurones in rat brain: anatomical localization and responses to neurohumors and ACTH, *Brain Res.*, **12**, 74–85.

THOMAS, R. C., AND WILSON, V. J., (1965); Precise localization of Renshaw cells with a new marking technique, *Nature (Lond.)*, **206**, 211–213.

TREHERNE, J. E., (1966); *The Neurochemistry of Arthropods*, Cambridge University Press, Cambridge, pp. 80–147.

Synaptic Function in the Fish Spinal Cord: Dendritic Integration

J. DIAMOND AND G. M. YASARGIL

Department of Physiology, University College London (Great Britain) and Physiology Institute, University of Zürich (Switzerland)

Some results we have obtained on the Mauthner reflex in teleost fish can be generalised to give an interesting view of dendritic function in neurons. Our experimental preparations were lightly-anaesthetised goldfish and tench, and we used conventional techniques of stimulating and recording.

THE STARTLE-RESPONSE AND ITS INHIBITION

The system we have investigated is a spinal neuronal circuit, and it has the property of discriminating to a very precise extent between two signals (nerve impulses) which arrive along two identical inputs (the giant Mauthner axons which run on either side of the spinal cord, giving off numerous collaterals *en route*). On its own, a single Mauthner-axon impulse causes the mass discharge of a large population of motoneurons, which results in a sudden powerful tail flip to the side of the excited Mauthner axon (Fig. 1a, b). When two impulses, one in each Mauthner axon, are closer together than 0.15–0.20 msec, there is no ventral root output from either side of the system (Fig. 1c), which can be considered as two identical linked halves. A mutual crossed inhibition of the excitatory response on each side occurs. When the separation of the two Mauthner-axon spikes is greater than this time, there is a finite output in response to the earlier impulse but none to the later, unless this is delayed by at least 8–10 msec (Yasargil and Diamond, 1968).

THE CONSTANCY OF THE "DISCRIMINATION TIME"

This minimum separation of 0.15–0.20 msec between impulses which the system can resolve, is its "discrimination time", and it is remarkably constant, from fish to fish (goldfish or tench), and in the same fish in successive tests. The achievement of this discrimination time depends on the interval between the Mauthner impulse in a given cord segment, and the moment when (*a*) the motoneurons on the ipsilateral side fire, and (*b*) the inhibition of the *contralateral* motoneurons becomes effective. The crossed inhibition, when the two Mauthner impulses are synchronous, begins in the motoneurons just early enough to prevent the excitatory process from reaching thresh-

References p. 208–209

Mauthner Cell Spike   Trunk E.M.G.

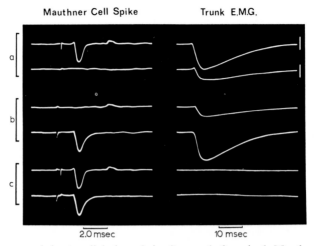

2.0 msec   10 msec

Fig. 1. Responses recorded extracellularly and simultaneously from both Mauthner cells in brain, and both right and left trunk muscle. Corresponding records are alongside each other. (Mauthner axons cross before descending in spinal cord, so an impulse from right cell propagates along left axon, which is ipsilateral to left muscle, and *vice versa*). Vertical calibrations alongside upper pair of EMG records are 2.0 mV for all right muscle and all M-cell records, and 1.25 mV for all left muscle records (the lower of each pair).

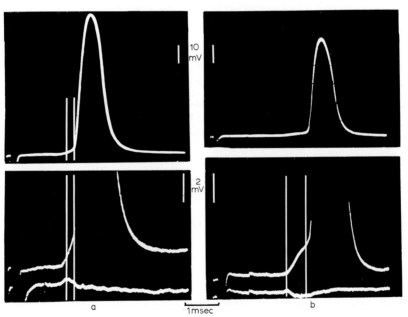

a   1msec   b

Fig. 2. Intracellular records of the activity in two different motoneurons. Each set of three traces shows: above, low-gain record of motoneuron spike caused by excitation of ipsilateral Mauthner axon; middle, same, at high-gain to show e.p.s.p. and inflexion point where spike fired (the spike rose too rapidly to be photographed in cell on left); below, high-gain record of response when *both* Mauthner axons were fired synchronously. The vertical lines are drawn through the points where (*1*) the e.p.s.p. reached the firing threshold in the absence of inhibition (right-hand line), and (*2*) the inhibitory process (due to the contralateral Mauthner-axon activity) cut off the e.p.s.p. shortly after it began to rise (left-hand line). The time interval between these two lines = the "discrimination time' for that motoneuron. It is 0.25 msec for the cell on the left, and 0.57 msec for that on the right,

old and firing a spike (Fig. 2). The inhibition is chemically transmitted and post-synaptic (though there may be a pre-synaptic component). The time between the onset of the crossed inhibition in the motoneuron, and the moment when the cell would otherwise reach threshold is the discrimination time of that cell. This means that if the impulse in the contralateral Mauthner axon is delayed by more than this time, then the inhibition of the motoneuron begins too late to prevent it from firing. Individual discrimination times vary from about 0.8–1.0 msec in some motoneurons to as little as 0.15–0.20 msec in others, this being also the minimum for the whole system (Fig. 2a, b). The effects of the *delayed* Mauthner-axon impulse are completely suppressed during a period which lasts for at least 8–10 msec after the impulse in the opposite Mauthner axon.

How is this unvarying and remarkable precision achieved? It might be expected that, as in most central neurons, there would be synaptic noise in the cells, which would preclude the establishment of the steady baseline conditions which would seem to be necessary. In fact, we find that the membrane potential in the units which are the first to be affected by the Mauthner-axon activity is sufficiently steady for a given excitatory process always to take a constant time to reach threshold, and an inhibitory one always to achieve a precisely timed cut-off of this response. This necessary stability seems to be assured by a functional isolation from the rest of the motoneuron of a special region with which the Mauthner-axon collateral makes synaptic contact, and where the earliest component of the crossing inhibition acts.

THE CIRCUITRY

The morphological situation is illustrated diagrammatically in Fig. 3, which also shows the correlation between our histological and physiological findings. The proposed high-resistance bridge between the special synaptic region and the main part of the motoneuron is shown as a special transitional region (Fig. 3c, which is based also on light and electronmicroscopic evidence to be reported elsewhere (Diamond, Gray and Yasargil, in preparation)). There are indications in the literature of some unusual morphological features here which support this (Tiegs, 1931; Barets, 1961). The evidence for this functional arrangements is as follows:

(*1*) The first units to be fired after the Mauthner-axon impulse show a clear excitatory post-synaptic potential (e.p.s.p.) and a spike. The e.p.s.p. begins abruptly about 0.5–0.6 msec after the steepest-rising portion of the ipsilateral Mauthner-axon spike in the same segment (at 12–15°) (Figs. 2, 5a).

(*2*) These units are located close to the Mauthner-axon, especially in the region of the junction between its dorsal collateral and the ventral dendrite of the primary motoneuron (from which the motoneuron axon takes off) (Fig. 3b).

(*3*) Distributed over a larger area, which is that where the cell bodies, ventral dendrites and initial axon-segments (IS) of these motoneurons occur (Fig. 3a), are units whose spikes *appear* to be excited by a two-step e.p.s.p., whose latency is the same as that of the simple e.p.s.p. in the unit described above (Figs. 4a, 5b, c).

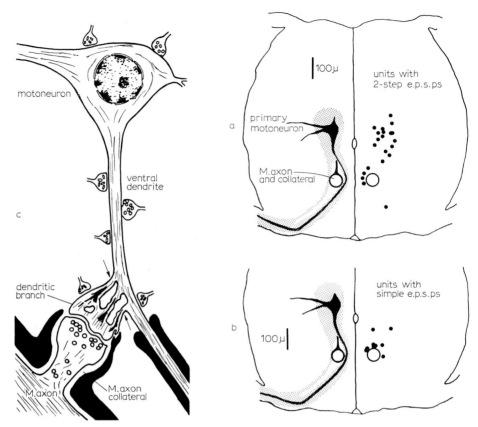

Fig. 3. (a) and (b) Diagrammatic cross-sections of teleost spinal cord, based on light-microscopic data, showing on left-hand side of sections, the relationship between Mauthner-axon collateral and primary motoneuron, and on the right-hand side the distribution of impaled units from various experiments. The dotted areas on the left side indicate the approximate variation in the position of the motoneuron soma, ventral dendrite and axon (the latter two sometimes run around the lateral side of the Mauthner axon). (a) units with 2-step "e.p.s.ps."; (b) units with simple e.p.s.ps. (c) is a diagram of an oblique section through the Mauthner axon and its collateral, showing a greatly simplified version of the region of synaptic contact with the dendrite branch, based on electron-microscopic data of E. G. Gray. The region between the arrows is the transitional zone referred to in the text.

(4) Antidromic spikes invade this second type of unit, but do not cause the two-step excitatory potential seen in the orthodromic records (Fig. 4).

(5) In the limited number of experiments where it could be investigated, no antidromic invasion of the first (junctional) unit occurred, but a very small potential was produced in it at about the time when the antidromic spike would have reached the ventral dendrite of the primary motoneuron. (This failure of invasion may, of course, have resulted from damage; these units were difficult to find and to record from satisfactorily.)

(6) The two-steps of the "e.p.s.p." of the second unit correspond very closely in time to the e.p.s.p. and spike in the first unit; this can be seen when records of the first and second type of unit from the same segment of the spinal cord are aligned

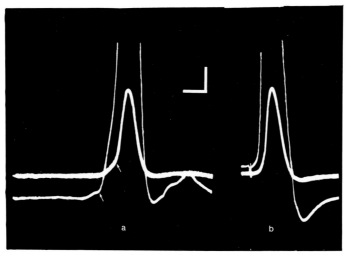

Fig. 4. Motoneuron responses recorded from main part of ventral dendrite. High- and low-gain records superimposed. (a) orthodromic excitation, due to Mauthner-axon stimulation. (b) antidromic excitation due to stimulation of ventral root. Arrows in (a) show the inflexion points of the 2-step "e.p.s.p.". The first step is visible only on the high-gain record. Calibrations, 20 mV and 1.25 mV; 1 msec.

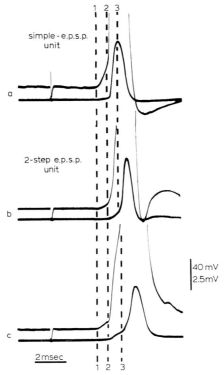

Fig. 5. Superimposed high- and low-gain records of responses recorded from the two types of unit in the same segment of the spinal cord. (a) unit of the simple e.p.s.p. type. (b) unit of the 2-step "e.p.s.p." type. (c) is same unit as (b), after deterioration had occurred. Dotted lines show (1) time of onset of responses, (2) beginning of second phase of response, and (3) beginning of third phase of response in the 2-step "e.p.s.p." unit. Further description in text.

vertically as in Fig. 5. (The Mauthner-axon spikes recorded simultaneously in each case, were made coincident in order to allow this comparison.)

The conclusion, which also incorporates the morphological findings, is that the first unit is not, as could be possible, a separate cell or fibre, but a branch of the main motoneuron dendrite (perhaps analogous to a dendritic spine); this is the part of the motoneuron which is chemically excited by the Mauthner-axon collateral (Fig. 3c). The branch is connected to the main part of the dendrite by a relatively high-resistance transitional region, which allows electrical excitation in the orthodromic direction (from junctional region to main part of motoneuron), but possibly not in the reverse direction. The inhibition due to excitation of the contralateral Mauthner axon was found to have a powerful action both on the special junctional branch, and on the main part of the motoneuron.

THE CIRCUIT STABILITY

The arrangement described above means that synaptic noise (and indeed possibly even an impulse), originating in the main part of the primary motoneuron will be attenuated to a negligible level by the time it has conducted electrotonically to the special synaptic region of the junctional branch; in this latter region, therefore, a relatively noise-free baseline condition is achieved. This condition is exactly what we have observed. Synaptic noise has, however, been recorded in the cell body/ ventral dendrite region of the primary motoneuron. Moreover, viewed from the synaptic region of the junctional branch, any post-synaptic inhibition of the main part of the motoneuron soma or ventral dendrite (but not of the branch itself) will be of the "dendritic remote inhibition" type, and be therefore relatively ineffective on the distal side of the transitional region (Diamond, 1968). The arrangement promotes the effectiveness of the Mauthner cell excitatory input to the motoneuron. It also ensures that the functionally important precise discrimination is achieved without interference from other excitatory or inhibitory activity impinging elsewhere on the motoneuron.

DENDRITIC INTEGRATION

Can this sort of arrangement be expected in other neurons? One analogous situation could well involve long dendrites. The distal parts of such dendrites may be often effectively isolated from other dendrites, and to a large extent from the cell soma, by their cable characteristics. We know that dendritic remote inhibition is one which can efficiently control excitation in its own vicinity without especially affecting excitation in the cell soma (Diamond, 1968). Excitatory activity at these distal regions is also "remote" from the soma and initial segment. However, it is known that in a number of neurons dendritic impulses occur. Evidence for these has now been obtained for motoneurons in the brain stem (Lorente de No, 1947) and spinal cord (Fatt, 1957; Nelson and Frank, 1964); pyramidal cells in the hippocampus (Cragg and Hamlyn, 1955; Andersen, 1960; Spencer and Kandel, 1961; Andersen and Jansen, 1961; Fujita and Sakata, 1962; Andersen *et al.*, 1966a); large cells in the cord dorsal horn (Wall, 1965); Dentate granule cells (Andersen *et al.*, 1966b); Purkinje cells in the cerebellum (Eccles *et al.*, 1966) and also cerebellar Golgi cells (Eccles *et al.*, 1967); for various types of crustacean mechanoreceptor neurons (Eyzaguirre and Kuffler, 1955; Grampp, 1966; Washizu and Terzuolo, 1966; Mendelson, 1963; Mellon and Kennedy, 1964); and finally for insect bipolar chemoreceptor cells (Morita, 1959; Hanson and Wolbarsht, 1962). It seems very likely, therefore, that out on a dendrite which is capable of generating a spike, the integration of the effects of local excitatory and inhibitory inputs can be considered almost solely in a local context; neither the resultant e.p.s.ps nor the inhibitory conductance changes need be of much immediate importance at any other site in the cell. With such an arrangement, the integrative activity of the cell should not be viewed simply as a single mass affair, with the soma/initial segment spike (or its prevention) as the overriding criterion of input effectiveness. Rather, the integration should be considered in at least two parts, dendritic integration, and the final somatic/IS integration.

The particular function which is exemplified by the present results relates to circuit discrimination of a sort which requires extremely stable conditions. The dendrite provides, from the point of view of pre-synaptic structures, a valuable site where *precise timing* of effects can be organised on a baseline which is effectively isolated and noise-free with respect to *other*, possibly unrelated, systems. The inputs to such a remote dendritic site have the role of determining the initiation of dendritic spikes, and it is here that we are concerned with dendritic integration. Once these dendritic impulses reach the soma a larger scale assessment is required, which must take account of influences from a variety of different sources. A single dendritic impulse, when it arrives at the soma, will very likely become a brief sub-threshold excitatory potential, since the current density across the expanded neuron membrane is unlikely to be adequate to reduce the membrane potential to threshold. The integration of such "failed-spike" potentials with synaptic activity will conform to the usual picture of somatic and initial-segment integration; this describes a situation which may not easily lend itself to a solution of the sort of timing problem described above for the fish spinal motoneuron, and it must be considered from a different viewpoint. Conceivably, however, if enough dendritic spikes were to arrive near-simultaneously at the soma, then a soma, or even an IS, spike *would* be initiated; the dendrites then may offer a useful time-discriminating system for controlling the neuron excitation.

This view of dendritic integration does not, of course, by any means exclude those aspects of dendritic function which depend upon the production of dendritic e.p.s.ps which, while they may not initiate dendritic spikes, are large enough to contribute to somatic/IS integration.

We have based this discussion on an example where a high degree of organisation is achieved at the level of the individual cell, but this seems likely to be quite common; it need not require the distinctive properties of the Mauthner cell–primary moto-neuron complex, which may be usefully regarded as a model system in this context.

References p. 208–209

The long dendrites of other neurons provide a substantially analogous situation (and possibly certain dendritic spines too may come into this category). This view seems worth stressing at a time when the role of the individual neuron is in danger of becoming neglected, in a view of neuronal organisation in which only populations of cells are sometimes regarded as the minimum functional entities in integrative activity. Dendritic integration, in dendrites which support spikes, provides opportunities particularly for precise timing arrangements, which are otherwise likely to be achieved only with the less economical provision of large numbers of neurons.

SUMMARY

The spinal circuitry involved in the startle-response in teleost fish is briefly described. The achievement of a very constant and precise time-discrimination, which is the important characteristic of the system, is shown to depend partly upon special properties of the 1st-activated synaptic region of the motoneuron. The initiation of the spike is determined by the integration, in this same region, of local synaptic activity. This is expressed as "dendritic integration". This concept is extended to neuron activity in general.

REFERENCES

ANDERSEN, P., (1960); Interhippocampal impulses, 11. Apical dendritic activation of CAI neurons. *Acta physiol. scand.*, **48**, 178–208.

ANDERSEN, P., AND JANSEN JR., J., (1961); The local cortical response in the hippocampus of rabbit. *Arch. ital. Biol.*, **99**, 349–368.

ANDERSEN, P., HOLMQUIST, B., AND VOORHOEVE, P. E., (1966a); Excitatory synapses on hippocampal apical dendrites activated by entorhinal stimulation. *Acta physiol. scand.*, **66**, 461–472.

ANDERSEN, P., HOLMQUIST, B., AND VOORHOEVE, P. E., (1966b); Entorhinal activation of dentate granule cells. *Acta physiol. scand.*, **66**, 448–460.

BARETS, A., (1961); Contribution à l'étude des systèmes moteurs "lent" et "rapide" du muscle latéral des téléostéens. *Arch. Anat. micr. Morph. exp.*, **50**, 91–187.

CRAGG, B. G., AND HAMLYN, L. H., (1955); Action potentials of the pyramidal neurons in the hippocampus of the rabbit. *J. Physiol. (Lond.)*, **129**, 608–627.

DIAMOND, J., (1968); The activation and distribution of GABA and L-glutamate receptors on goldfish Mauthner neurones: an analysis of dendritic remote inhibition. *J. Physiol. (Lond.)*, **194**, 669–723.

ECCLES, J. C., LLINAS, R., AND SASAKI, K., (1966); Parallel fibre stimulation and the response induced thereby in the Purkinje cells of the cerebellum. *Exp. Brain Res.*, **1**, 17–34.

ECCLES, J. C., SASAKI, K., AND STRATA, P., (1967); Interpretation of the potential fields generated in the cerebellar cortex by a mossy fibre volley. *Exp. Brain Res.*, **3**, 58–80.

EYZAGUIRRE, C., AND KUFFLER, S. W., (1955); Further study of soma, dendrites and axon excitation in single neurons. *J. gen. Physiol.*, **39**, 121–153.

FATT, P., (1957); Electric potentials occurring around a neurone during its antidromic activation. *J. Neurophysiol.*, **20**, 27–60.

FUJITA, Y., AND SAKATA, H., (1962); Electrophysiological properties of CAI and CA2 apical dendrites of rabbit hippocampus. *J. Neurophysiol.*, **25**, 209–222.

GRAMPP, W., (1966); Multiple-spike discharge evoking after-depolarisations in the slowly adapting stretch receptor neuron of the lobster. *Acta physiol. scand.*, **67**, 100–115.

HANSON, F. E., AND WOLBARSHT, M. L., (1962); Dendritic action potentials in insect chemoreceptors. *Amer. Zool.*, **2**, 528.

LORENTE DE NO, R., (1947); Action potential of the motoneurons of the hypoglossus nucleus. *J. cell. comp. Physiol.*, **29**, 207–288.

MELLON, D., AND KENNEDY, D., (1964); Impulse origin and propagation in a bipolar sensory neuron. *J. gen. Physiol.*, **47**, 487–499.

MENDELSON, M., (1963); Some factors in the activation of crab movement receptors. *J. exp. Biol.*, **40**, 157–169.

MORITA, H., (1959); Initiation of spike potentials in contact chemosensory hairs of insects, III. D.C. stimulation and generator potential of labellar chemoreceptor of Calliphora. *J. cell. comp. Physiol.*, **54**, 189- 204.

NELSON, P. G., AND FRANK, K., (1964); Orthodromically produced changes in motoneuronal extracellular fields. *J. Neurophysiol.*, **27**, 928–941.

SPENCER, W. A., AND KANDEL, E. R., (1961); Electrophysiology of hippocampal neurons, IV. Fast prepotentials. *J. Neurophysiol.*, **24**, 272–285.

TIEGS, O. W., (1931); A study of the neurofibril structure of the nerve cell. *J. comp. Neurol.*, **52**, 189–222.

WALL, P. D., (1965); Impulses originating in the region of dendrites. *J. Physiol. (Lond.)*, **180**, 116–133.

WASHIZU, Y., AND TERZUOLO, C. A., (1966); Impulse activity in the crayfish stretch receptor neuron. *Arch. ital. Biol.*, **104**, 181–194.

YASARGIL, G. M., AND DIAMOND, J., (1968); The startle-response in teleost fish: an elementary circuit for neural discrimination. *Nature (Lond.)*, **220**, 241–243.

The Nature of the Acetylcholine Pools in Brain Tissue

V. P. WHITTAKER

Department of Biochemistry, University of Cambridge (Great Britain) and Institute for Basic Research In Mental Retardation, Staten Island, N.Y. (U.S.A.)

It has been known for many years that when brain tissue is comminuted in iso-osmotic saline media most of the acetylcholine remains bound to particulate material. In this state it is unaffected by cholinesterase and is pharmacologically inactive until released by treatments destructive to the integrity of lipoprotein membrane structures. Hebb and Whittaker (1958) showed that the same is true of brain homogenized in iso-osmotic sucrose; even when an anticholinesterase is added to stabilize any free acetylcholine extracted, only about 20–25% of the total tissue acetylcholine can be detected pharmacologically; the remaining 75–80% remains particle-bound and pharmacologically undetectable until released (*e.g.* by heating at pH 4.0 and 100° for 10 min). On subcellular fractionation, the free acetylcholine of the homogenate, as would be expected, is recovered in the high-speed supernatant (cell sap) fraction (S_3): the bound acetylcholine, on the other hand, is found mainly in the crude mito-chondrial fraction (P_2) and, on further separation of this fraction on a density gradient (Whittaker, 1959) is mostly recovered in a particulate fraction denser than myelin and lighter than mitochondria, the other two main constituents of the fraction. This intermediate fraction (B) consists largely of detached nerve terminals (synapto-somes) (Gray and Whittaker 1960, 1962; Whittaker 1960); the bound acetylcholine present in it evidently represents the store of acetylcholine in the immediately pre-synaptic portions of cholinergic neurones which have become detached during homo-genization and which have been isolated along with other presynaptic nerve terminals by the subcellular fractionation procedure.

Further work (Whittaker, 1959; Whittaker *et al.*, 1964; Marchbanks, 1968) has shown that bound (*i.e.* synaptosomal) acetylcholine itself exists in more than one form. When synaptosomes are suspended in hypo-osmotic media, they burst and soluble cytoplasmic constituents rapidly diffuse out. A fraction of bound acetylcholine (the 'labile-bound' fraction of Whittaker, 1959) diffuses out, and, in the absence of an anticholinesterase, is destroyed by the cholinesterase in the preparation. This fraction behaves in all respects like any soluble cytoplasmic constituent (thus it exchanges with [^{14}C]acetylcholine added to the suspension medium) and its stability in intact synaptosomes in the absence of an anticholinesterase suggests that function-ally, cholinesterase is attached to the *outside* of the synaptosome. Subcellular distri-bution studies (Whittaker *et al.*, 1964) and histochemical evidence (Lewis and Shute,

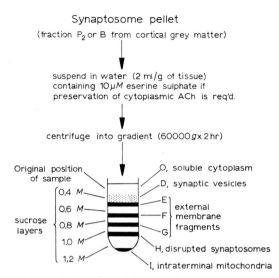

Fig. 1. Scheme summarizing technique for subfractionating osmotically ruptured synaptosomes by density-gradient centrifuging. For further explanation see text and legend to Fig. 3.

1967) shows that the enzyme is indeed confined to the external synaptosome membrane, but the resolution of the histochemical method is not sufficient to establish the functional location of the active centres of the enzyme.

A second fraction of bound acetylcholine (the 'stable-bound' fraction of Whittaker, 1959) survives hypo-osmotic treatment, and subfractionation of hypo-osmotically disrupted synaptosomes shows that this fraction of acetylcholine is present in synaptic vesicles (Whittaker et al., 1964). The subfractionation technique and the fractions obtained are summarized in Fig. 1. It will be seen that the particulate material is separated into six bands: a top hazy band (D) consists of almost pure synaptic vesicles (Fig. 2); beneath this there are three bands consisting of small (E, F) and larger (F, G) membrane fragments, a band (H) consisting of partially disrupted synaptosomes, and finally a pellet (I) containing small, intraterminal mitochondria. Studies with marker enzymes (Fig. 3) show that the plasma membrane marker Na,K-stimulated adenosine triphosphatase (NaK ATPase, bottom left diagram) is concentrated in fraction E–G (Hosie, 1965); acetylcholinesterase (Whittaker et al., 1964) and ganglioside (results of J. Eichberg quoted by Whittaker, 1966 and Mellanby and Whittaker, 1968) are also localized in these fractions and its seems likely that the membranes in them are mainly derived from the external synaptosome membrane. Many of the membranes, especially those in fraction G, are readily identified morphologically as 'synaptosome ghosts', i.e. synaptosomes with reasonably intact external membranes but lacking most of the typical organelles (synaptic vesicles, intraterminal mitochondria) of the synaptosome cytoplasm. By contrast, the mitochondrial marker succinate dehydrogenase (SDH) is localized sharply in fraction I, as would be expected from the morphology of the fraction.

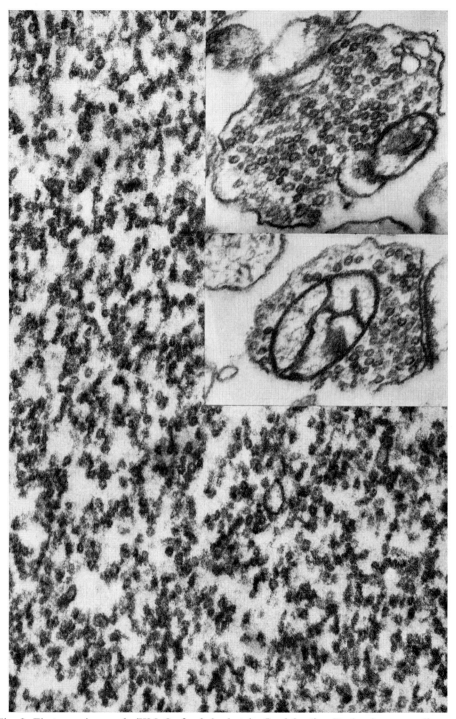

Fig. 2. Electron-micrograph (KMnO$_4$ fixed, lead stained) of fraction D showing mono-disperse synaptic vesicles identical in morphology to vesicles of intact synaptosomes (insert). Note that one of the latter has a portion of postsynaptic membrane still adhering to its periphery. Electron-micrograph prepared by Dr. M. N. Sheridan. Magnification × 70 000.

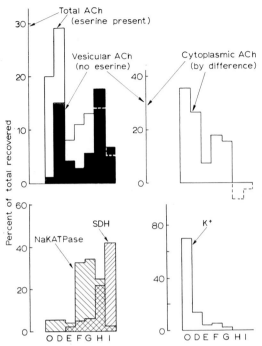

Fig. 3. Distribution of marker substances in subfractions of disrupted synaptosomes. Abbreviations: ACh, acetylcholine; SDH, succinate dehydrogenase, NaK ATPase, Na,K-stimulated adenosine triphosphatase. For nomenclature of fractions see text and Fig. 1.

The clear top layer (fraction O) contains about 70% of the potassium (Fig. 3, bottom right diagram), lactate dehydrogenase and other soluble cytoplasmic constituents of the synaptosome (Mangan and Whittaker, 1966; Whittaker *et al.*, 1964); and control experiments with bovine serum albumin have shown that soluble materials do not equilibrate throughout the gradient during dummy runs. Note that there is no second peak in fraction H, showing that the synaptosomes in this fraction are too severely damaged to retain soluble constituents.

The distribution of acetylcholine down the gradient (top-left diagram) is in striking contrast to the three markers already mentioned. In the absence of an anticholinesterase, when only the 'stable-bound' fraction (black blocks) survives, a characteristic bimodal distribution is seen, with a peak in the mono-disperse synaptic vesicle fraction (D) and a second peak in fraction H, which also contains synaptic vesicles. Note that fraction H, as we should expect from its content of damaged synaptosomes, contains three of the four markers, vesicular (acetylcholine), external membrane (NaK ATPase) and mitochondrial (SDH), and lacks only the soluble cytoplasmic (K⁺), whereas fraction D lacks NaK ATPase and SDH, showing its freedom from fragments of external membrane and mitochondria, and contains only a small amount of soluble cytoplasm by diffusion from fraction O.

If synaptosomes are disrupted in the presence of an anticholinesterase, the 'labile-bound' acetylcholine is preserved. The distribution of free acetylcholine down the

TABLE I

COMPARTMENTS OF BRAIN ACETYLCHOLINE (ACh)

	Type of ACh	Fraction	Presumed location
(I)	Free ACh	S_3 from eserinized homogenate	Cell sap from cell bodies or disrupted synaptosomes
(II)	Bound ACh:	P_2 or B from uneserinized homogenate	Synaptosomes
	(a) 'labile'	O from eserinized P_2 or B	Synaptosomal cytoplasm
	(b) 'stable'	(1) D from uneserinized P_2 or B	Synaptic vesicles
		(2) H from same	Synaptic vesicles in partially disrupted synaptosomes

gradient after separation of the disrupted synaptosomes into their subfractions can be estimated as the difference between the total and 'stable-bound' fractions. As seen in the top right-hand diagram of Fig. 3, the fraction containing most of the free acetylcholine is fraction O; however, the distribution is more spread out than would be expected for a soluble cytoplasmic constituent such as K^+; this discrepancy may be accounted for by continued leakage of acetylcholine from vesicles during their progress down the gradient; recent work with isolated vesicles has shown that their osmotic stability is relative rather than absolute.

The types of acetylcholine found in brain homogenates are thus three in number, free acetylcholine, labile-bound acetylcholine and stable-bound acetylcholine: their subcellular localization is summarized in Table I. The question now arises whether these various types of bound acetylcholine have any physiological significance or

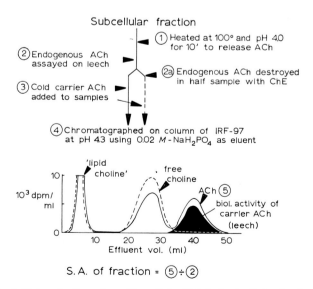

Fig. 4. Determination of specific activity (S.A.) of subcellular fractions.

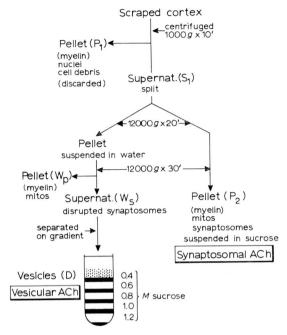

Fig. 5. Isolation of intact synaptosomes and synaptic vesicles for determination of the specific activities of synaptosomal cytoplasmic and vesicular acetylcholine. In some experiments (see Table II), synaptosomal acetylcholine was determined not in intact synaptosomes suspended in sucrose but in synaptosomes osmotically disrupted by suspension in water containing 50 μM eserine to inhibit loss of cytoplasmic fraction (*cf.* Fig. 3).

whether there is in reality only one pool of acetylcholine, *e.g.* vesicular, from which the others are formed by redistribution during homogenization.

An attempt has now been made to investigate this problem (Chakrin and Whittaker, 1968) by labelling the acetylcholine pools *in vivo* using [³H]choline as a precursor.

Since choline is a ubiquitous metabolite, it was necessary to separate acetylcholine from other choline derivatives in order to determine the amount of radioactivity which had been incorporated into acetylcholine. This was done (Fig. 4) by separating extracts on the weak acid ion-exchange resin IRF-97 (formerly XE-97) as described by Gardiner and Whittaker (1954). In view of the small amount of acetylcholine present, cold carrier acetylcholine was added after assaying the amount of endogenous acetylcholine using the leech micro-assay of Szerb (1961) as modified by Whittaker *et al.* (1964). The location of acetylcholine in the column effluent could then be readily determined by biological assay.

The identity of the radioactivity associated with carrier acetylcholine was routinely checked in a parallel run by incubating a sample of the extract with cholinesterase, adding cold carrier acetylcholine and chromatographing as before. Under these conditions (dashed line), no radioactivity was found to be associated with the carrier, but there was an augmentation of a peak having the same retention volume and reactions as free choline. A third peak of radioactivity with negligible affinity for the resin was eluted in the void volume and is described as lipid choline. No attempt was made to characterize the two peaks of low retention volume completely.

The complete procedure was as follows: [³H]choline (20 μC of specific radioactivity 150–200 mC/mmole in 100 μl of 0.9 % w/v sodium chloride solution) was injected into the exposed cortical tissue of anaesthetized guinea pigs or rabbits in 4–5 portions by means of a 50-μl Hamilton microsyringe. After 1 h the brain was removed; the cortical tissue was dissected, gently scraped free of myelin and homogenized in 0.32 M sucrose. Two identical crude synaptosome pellets were prepared from the homogenate essentially as shown in Fig. 5. One pellet was suspended in sucrose (or in water containing 50 μM eserine sulphate); this gave the amount x_s and specific activity r_s of total synaptosomal acetylcholine when analyzed according to the scheme given in Fig. 4. The other was suspended in water, and from the water suspension was prepared the synaptic vesicle fraction (D); this gave the amount x_v and specific activity r_v of vesicular acetylcholine. From these the amount $(x_s—x_v)$ and specific activity $[(x_s r_s—x_v r_v) / (x_s—x_v)]$ of the cytoplasmic ('labile-bound') fraction of acetylcholine could be calculated. In separate experiments cortical tissue was homogenized in sucrose containing 50 μM eserine and centrifuged at 100 000 g for 60 min: the supernatant so obtained was similarly analysed according to the scheme shown in Fig. 4.

Considerable amounts of radioactivity were found in the soluble cytoplasmic fraction O from uneserinized water suspensions of synaptosomes (fraction P₂), but as shown in Fig. 6 (upper diagram), none of the radioactivity was attributable to acetylcholine. In the synaptic vesicle fraction D (Fig. 6, lower diagram), there was less total radioactivity, but an appreciable amount was associated with cold carrier acetylcholine. In order to make certain that none of the radioactivity in the acetylcholine isolated from fraction D could represent soluble radioactive choline products (including free acetylcholine) diffusing from fraction O, use was made of gel filtration to eliminate non-vesicular components from fraction D. This technique is illustrated in Fig. 7. If samples of the synaptic vesicle fraction were passed through columns of Sephadex G-50 (bead form) pre-equilibrated with 0.4 M sucrose (*i.e.* sucrose iso-osmotic to the vesicle preparation) most of the radioactivity passed through in the void volume along with protein and other macromolecular constituents (including vesicles). However, when the vesicle preparation was passed through a column equilibrated with 0.005 M tris buffer pH 7.4 (strongly hypo-osmotic), the radioactivity emerging in the void volume was markedly reduced, and most of it now appeared in the non-occluded volume. This shows that most of the radioactivity is associated with a substance released from vesicles by hypo-osmotic stress. Fig. 8 shows that this substance is mainly acetylcholine. This chromatogram is that of the void volume effluent of a vesicle fraction passed through a column of G-50 equilibrated with 0.4 M sucrose before acid extraction and chromatography. It will be noted that most of the radioactivity is associated with acetylcholine, though there is apparently a small amount of choline (probably produced by hydrolysis of acetylcholine during manipulation) and some 'lipid–choline' which may represent [³H]choline incorporated into the vesicle wall. This last material may account for the osmotically-insensitive

References p. 222

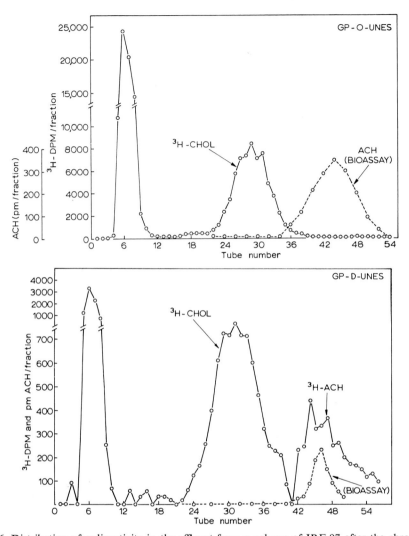

Fig. 6. Distribution of radioactivity in the effluent from a column of IRF-97 after the chromato-
graphic separation of an extract of fraction O (upper diagram) or fraction D (lower diagram) from
the guinea-pig brain. The preparation and chromatography of the extracts was essentially as shown
in Figs. 1, 4 and 5; the synaptosomes were suspended in uneserinized water to destroy the cytoplasmic
fraction of total synaptosomal acetylcholine.

^{3}H emerging in the void volume of the hypo-osmotic column in Fig. 7. After cholinesterase treatment (dotted lines) the radioactivity of the acetylcholine peak is
transferred, as one would expect, to the choline peak, but the lipid–choline peak is
unaffected.

Table II shows the specific activity of the three pools of acetylcholine in brain
tissue determined by the techniques summarized in Figs. 4–6 1 h after injection of
[^{3}H]choline. It will be seen that although vesicular acetylcholine is labelled, its
specific activity is only about two-thirds that of total synaptosomal acetylcholine.

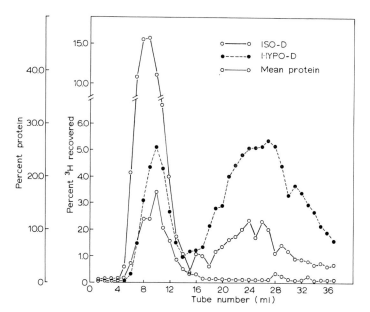

Fig. 7. Gel filtration of fraction D from an uneserinized water suspension of synaptosomes. The diagrams show the distribution of total radioactivity in the effluent from columns of Sephadex G-50 (bead form) equilibrated with 0.4 M sucrose (continuous thick lines) or 0.005 M tris buffer (pH 7.4) (dashed lines). The protein distribution (mean of both experiments, thin continuous lines) indicates that the initial peak of radioactivity is associated with the macromolecular phase.

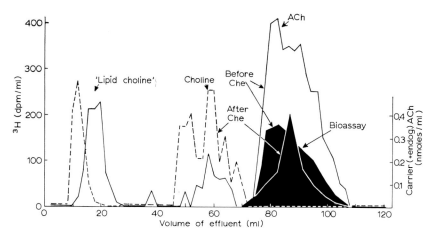

Fig. 8. Chromatogram similar to that of Fig. 6 but derived from the material from fraction D emerging in the void volume after gel-filtration. Continuous lines: radioactivity before cholinesterase treatment of extract. Dotted line: the same extract after cholinesterase treatment. Black blocks, bioassay of cold carrier acetylcholine and any endogenous acetylcholine also present.

Since there are about equal amounts of cytoplasmic and vesicular acetylcholine in synaptosomes (Whittaker, 1959) the cytoplasmic pool must have a specific activity about twice that of the vesicular at 1 h. The specific activity of the supernatant fraction is even lower — about one-third of the synaptosomal acetylcholine.

TABLE II

Units are disintegrations/min/pmole.

Expt.	Synaptosomal	Vesicular[d]	Supernatant[b]
1	7.2[a]	4.6 (63)	—
2	9.4[a]	5.1 (54)	—
3	6.3[a]	4.4 (69)	—
4	6.2	5.1 (83)	—
5	6.4	3.9 (61)	—
6	—	—	2.6
7	—	—	2.5
8	—	—	2.4
Mean $\pm$ S.D.	7.1 $\pm$ 1.8[c]	4.6 $\pm$ 0.3 (66 $\pm$ 5)[c]	2.5 $\pm$ 0.1

[a] Eserinized water suspension (see legend to Fig. 5).

[b] From eserinized homogenate

[c] Significantly different ($P < 0.01$) (paired t test).

[d] Figures in brackets: specific radioactivity as % of synaptosomal specific radioactivity.

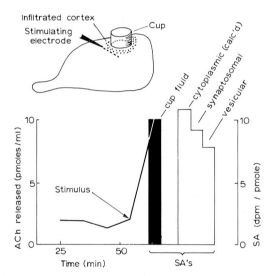

Fig. 9. Diagram summarizing (top) the technique for collection of acetylcholine released from the surface of the rabbit cortex at rest and after stimulating cholinergic afferents and (bottom) the release obtained and the specific activities of released (black block) and bound acetylcholine (white blocks).

The time course of labelling of the various pools has not yet been made but preliminary studies indicate that with fractions isolated half-an-hour after injection there is an even larger difference between the cytoplasmic and vesicular fractions, the former having over four times the specific activity of the latter.

It seems clear then, that newly formed acetylcholine appears earlier in the cytoplasmic compartment than in the vesicular; this is consistent with what has been deduced from the cytoplasmic localization of choline acetyltransferase (Fonnum,

TABLE III

COMPARISON OF SPECIFIC ACTIVITIES OF ACETYLCHOLINE (ACh) RELEASED FROM THE CORTEX OF RABBITS WITH THAT IN THE SUBCELLULAR POOLS

% Increase of ACh output on stimulation	Specific activity of ACh as dpm/pmole in:		
	Cup	Synaptosomes	Vesicles
+ 75	4.6	4.7	4.1
+430	10.0	9.1	7.8
+510	10.3	3.5	2.7

1967), namely that acetylcholine is synthesized in the cytoplasm of the synaptosome and transferred, by a mechanism that so far cannot be reproduced *in vitro* (Marchbanks, 1968), to the vesicles. It is, of course, possible that there is a population of osmotically labile and metabolically active vesicles that are capable of synthesizing acetylcholine more rapidly than the more stable vesicles that survive osmotic disruption: what has here been termed synaptosomal cytoplasmic acetylcholine would be the acetylcholine stored in these labile vesicles. However, there is no positive evidence for such a hypothesis at the present time.

In recent experiments with Dr. J. M. Mitchell, attempts have been made to determine the compartment(s) from which the acetylcholine released on stimulation is derived utilizing the 'Oborin cup' technique used extensively by him (Mitchell, 1965) to demonstrate the existence of cholinergic pathways to the cortex. The experimental arrangement and some of the results obtained are diagrammed in Fig. 9. A cup filled with eserinized saline is placed on the exposed occipital cortex of the rabbit and afferent cholinergic neurones stimulated by means of an electrode placed in the lateral geniculate body. The area of the cortex in the region of the cup is infiltrated with [³H]choline. The saline of the cup is replaced every 10 min and the acetylcholine content assayed to give the resting acetylcholine release. On applying a stimulus the acetylcholine content of the cup during the next collection period rises to a value up to five times that during rest. Immediately after stimulation and about 1 h after the initial infiltration of [³H]choline, the brain tissue in the vicinity of the cup is excised and the amounts and specific activities of the synaptosomal cytoplasmic and vesicular acetylcholine pools determined (white blocks, Fig. 9). As eserine had diffused into the brain tissue, cholinesterase was not fully active and a radiochemical assay (kindly performed by Dr. R. M. Marchbanks) using [¹⁴C]-acetylcholine in amounts equivalent to the endogenous concentration showed that free acetylcholine was not completely destroyed. This may account for the relatively small difference between the specific activities of the vesicular and total synaptosomal acetylcholine pools shown in Fig. 9. Nevertheless (Table III), the specific activity of the acetylcholine released into the cup was consistently *higher* than would be expected if it had arisen from the acetylcholine pool represented by the vesicles isolated in the D band. The result has been confirmed in experiments in which sampling of the tissue took place half-an-hour after infiltration of [³H]choline, when the specific activity of the vesicular acetylcholine is even lower relative to the cytoplasmic than at 1 h. This work shows that newly formed acetylcholine is preferentially released from the exposed cortex on stimulating afferent pathways and suggests that not all the released transmitter is derived from the 'stable-bound', vesicular pool, as defined by our subcellular fractionation procedures.

ACKNOWLEDGEMENTS

This work was supported by the U. K. Medical Research Council (Grant No. G 966/94/B) and by the U. S. Public Health Service (award of a Post-doctoral Fellowship and supply grant to Dr. L. W. Chakrin).

REFERENCES

CHAKRIN, L. W., AND WHITTAKER, V. P., (1968); The subcellular distribution of acetylcholine-methyl-³H synthesized by brain *in vivo*. In preparation.

FONNUM, F., (1967); The compartmentation of choline acetyltransferase within the synaptosome. *Biochem. J.*, **103**, 262–270.

GARDINER, J. E., AND WHITTAKER, V. P., (1954); The identification of propionylcholine as a constituent of ox spleen. *Biochem. J.*, **58**, 24–29.

GRAY, E. G., AND WHITTAKER, V. P., (1960); The isolation of synaptic vesicles from the central nervous system. *J. Physiol. (Lond.)*, **153**, 35–37 P.

GRAY, E. G., AND WHITTAKER, V. P., (1962); The isolation of nerve endings from brain: an electron-microscopic study of cell fragments derived by homogenization and centrifugation. *J. Anat. (Lond.)*, **96**, 79–88.

HEBB, C. O., AND WHITTAKER, V. P., (1958); Intracellular distributions of acetylcholine and choline acetylase. *J. Physiol. (Lond.)*, **142**, 187–196.

HOSIE, R. J. A., (1965); The localization of adenosine triphosphatases in morphologically characterized fractions of guinea-pig brain. *Biochem. J.*, **96**, 404–412.

LEWIS, P. R., AND SHUTE, C. D. D., (1966); The distribution of cholinesterase in cholinergic neurones demonstrated with the electron microscope. *J. Cell. Sci.*, **1**, 381–390.

MANGAN, J. L., AND WHITTAKER, V. P., (1966); The subcellular distribution of amino acids in guinea-pig brain. *Biochem. J.*, **98**, 128–137.

MARCHBANKS, R. M., (1968); Exchangeability of the bound acetylcholine of synaptosomes and synaptic vesicles. *Biochem. J.*, **106**, 87–95.

MELLANBY, J., AND WHITTAKER, V. P., (1968); The fixation of tetanus toxin by synaptic membranes. *J. Neurochem.*, **15**, 205–208.

MITCHELL, J. M., (1965); In: *Mechanisms of Release of Biogenic Amines*, U. S. VON EULER, S. ROSELL AND B. UVNÄS (Eds.), Wenner-Gren International Symposium Series, Vol. 5, Pergamon, Oxford.

SZERB, J. C., (1961); The estimation of acetylcholine, using leech muscle in a microbath. *J. Physiol. (Lond.)*, **158**, 8–9P.

WHITTAKER, V. P., (1959); The isolation and characterization of acetylcholine containing particles from brain. *Biochem. J.*, **72**, 694–706.

WHITTAKER, V. P., (1960); The binding of neurohormones by subcellular particles of brain tissue. Proc. IVth Int. Neurochem Symp.. Varenna, June 12–17, 1960. In: *Regional Neurochemistry: the Regional Chemistry, Physiology and Pharmacology of the Nervous System*, S. KETY AND J. ELKES (Eds.), Pergamon, Oxford, pp. 259–263.

WHITTAKER, V. P., (1966); Some properties of synaptic membranes isolated from the central nervous system. *Ann. N. Y. Acad. Sci.*, **137**, 982–998.

WHITTAKER, V. P., (1969); In: *Structure and Function of Nervous Tissue*, G. H. BOURNE (Ed.), Academic Press. New York, Vol. 2, chap. 1.

WHITTAKER, V. P., MICHAELSON, I. A., AND KIRKLAND, R. J. A., (1964); The separation of synaptic vesicles from nerve ending particles ('synaptosomes'). *Biochem. J.*, **90**, 293–305.

Contributions of New Impregnation Methods and Freeze Etching to the Problems of Synaptic Fine Structure *

KONRAD AKERT, HANS MOOR, KARL PFENNINGER AND CLARA SANDRI

Brain Research Institute, University of Zürich and Laboratory of Electron Microscopy, Department of General Botany, Swiss Federal Institute of Technology, Zürich (Switzerland)

INTRODUCTION

The present review is concerned with new information on synaptic fine structure that has been obtained recently in our laboratory by using iodide compounds of heavy metals for block staining as well as by examining synaptic areas in specimens prepared with the freeze-etching technique. The main interest revolves around synaptic vesicles, internal and external coats of nerve membranes and their specializations at the synaptic junction. It is hoped that the data might provide a basis for deeper understanding of the complex interplay of molecular mechanisms at the synapse, and that the methods involved may prove to be useful in monitoring experimental approaches to the problems of excitation, memory and individuality which remain great mysteries of living matter and especially the nervous tissue.

(1) Impregnation of synaptic vesicles

Various attempts have been made to obtain specific staining of synaptic vesicles. The most successful have been concerned with so-called granulated vesicles (see the contribution to this symposium by Tranzer *et al.*, 1969) which are known to store catecholamines and perhaps indolamines. The staining of so-called clear vesicles, especially at cholinergic sites, has recently been reported by Akert and Sandri (1968) and will be discussed here briefly.

The zinc-iodide–osmic acid (ZIO) method of Champy (1913) and Maillet (1962) was used for this purpose. It was for the first time clearly demonstrated that the black precipitation in nerve terminals and varicosities that are seen in ZIO-stained sections at the light microscopic level is based upon the specific impregnation of synaptic vesicles (Fig. 2). The problem of specificity of this method has been raised by several earlier investigators and seems far from being solved (the relevant literature was recently reviewed by Maillet, 1968).

---

* With the aid of the Swiss National Foundation for Scientific Research, Nos. 4356 and 4691.

References p. 239–240

(a) Specificity of vesicular impregnation

Consistent results were obtained when carefully dissected tissue blocks of peripheral and central nervous systems were impregnated according to the procedure
described by Akert and Sandri (1968). Within nerve terminals the reaction is limited
to synaptic vesicles. However, in other components of nerve tissue one may encounter reaction products in organelles such as the Golgi zone, lysosomes and even
in the glial and neuronal cytoplasm. While such observations clearly demonstrate
the limitations of the method, it is noteworthy that the ZIO stain of nerve terminals
can be considered the most specific of all "boutons techniques" that are presently
available. The reason for this statement is that other synaptic stains (Gray and Guillery,
1966) are based on the impregnation of neurofilaments or mitochondria both of
which are less specific components of nerve terminals than are synaptic vesicles.

(b) Specificity at cholinergic versus adrenergic sites

The positive correlation of vesicular impregnation at cholinergic sites and the
negative correlation at certain adrenergic sites (Akert et al., 1968) strongly suggest
a relationship with cholinergic transmitter mechanisms. The question is naturally
raised whether acetylcholine itself may provide the substrate for the reaction. At the
present time there is no direct evidence available in support of this hypothesis. Some
serious inconsistencies have been encountered in that vesicles at adrenergic sites
(e.g. the pineal gland) have undergone a clear-cut reaction with the ZIO mixture.
These controversial findings will be presented and discussed in detail elsewhere. At
the present time, a simple explanation of observed facts is not available.

It should be stressed, however, that the most indispensable element of the staining
compound seems to be the *iodide*. OsO_4 normally does not itself produce a positive
reaction within synaptic vesicles at known cholinergic sites (e.g. motor endplate,
sphincter iridis nerve terminals) with the exception of the electroplaque (Israel,
1969) whose vesicles contain a considerably higher concentration of acetylcholine.
An iodide compound of acetylcholine may be formed (Stanek, 1905), which is able
to reduce OsO_4. However, the positive reaction of certain non-cholinergic amine
storage granules may have a different explanation. The osmium component of the
ZIO mixture could react with the unsaturated bonds of catecholamines. This second

---

Fig. 1. Axo-dendritic synapse in the cat subfornical organ. Note the double synaptic plaque. The
presynaptic dense projections (dp) are faintly visible, while the postsynaptic appositional densities
(po) and the subsynaptic bodies (sb) are plainly seen. mv = multivesicular body; m = mitochondria;
sv = synaptic vesicles. Glutaraldehyde/OsO_4 fixation. Primary magnification 20 000 ×.
Fig. 2. Axo-dendritic synapse in the cat subfornical organ stained with zinc iodide–osmium (ZIO)
mixture (cf. Fig. 1). The clear synaptic vesicles (sv) are electronopaque. Dense-cored vesicles (dv),
mitochondria (m) and cytoplasmic membranes are unstained. Primary magnification 20 000 ×.
Fig. 3. Axo-dendritic synapse in the cat subfornical organ (cf. Fig. 1) stained with bismuth iodide
(BI) mixture. Appositional densities are clearly visible, especially the presynaptic dense projections
of Gray (dp). Although the synaptic vesicles (sv) failed to react to this stain, they stand out in the
negative because their contours are marked by a finely granular electronopaque coat. po = postsynaptic density; sb = subsynaptic bodies. Arrow = synaptic cleft with intracleft lines. Primary
magnification 20 000 ×.

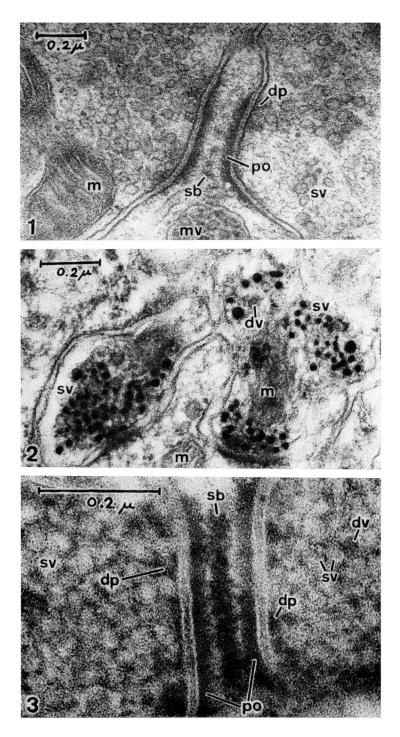

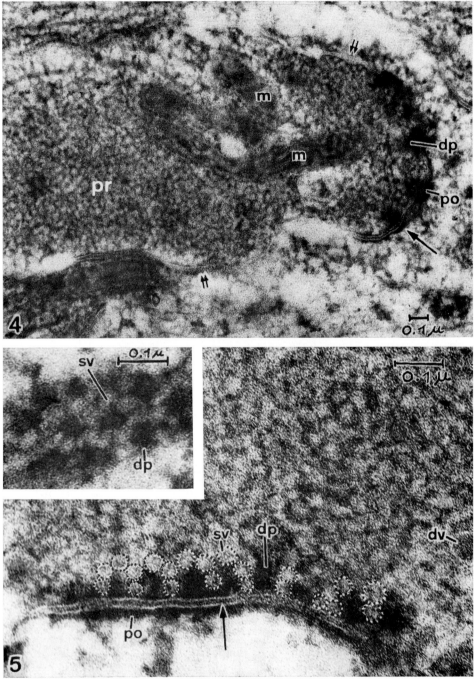

Fig. 4. The presynaptic dense projections (dp) of Gray in a cross-sectioned axon terminal (pr) stained with BI mixture. po = postsynaptic element (see also at arrow). m = mitochondria. Note the spiny contour of dense projections. Double arrows mark position of the plasmalemma. The unit membrane is spared, the inner and outer "fuzz" coats are stained. Primary magnification 20 000 ×.

Fig. 5. Presynaptic dense projections of Gray and the formation of a hexagonal *vesicular grid*. The spiny appearance of dense projections is due to "fuzz coat" surrounding the adjacent synaptic vesicles. dv = dense-cored vesicle; po = postsynaptic density; arrow = synaptic cleft with intracleft lines.

Inset: Tangential section through vesicular grid. Dark spots represent presynaptic dense projections (dp) in hexagonal arrangement with interconnecting filaments. Clear profiles between dense projections represent synaptic vesicles (sv), forming a rosette-like pattern. Note that each hole of the grid accommodates one single vesicle (*cf.* Fig. 6). Primary magnification 40 000 ×.

mechanism would seriously limit the specificity with respect to cholinergic binding capacity of the iodide component unless the catecholamines were eliminated experimentally before the reaction. Yet, so-called clear vesicles in nerve terminals of the cat dilator iris, vas deferens and spleen capsule yield positive ZIO staining reactions even after high doses of reserpine (15 mg/kg). Such vesicles, as well as their reaction product with ZIO, are morphologically not distinguishable from so-called cholinergic vesicles in the sphincter iridis terminals. They form a population within a given nerve terminal of only a few per cent, the whole of the remainder being non-reactive to ZIO (Akert *et al.*, 1968). This finding needs to be further investigated and discussed in the context of the Burn and Rand (1959) hypothesis.

(2) Impregnation of internal and external "fuzz" coats at the synaptic membranes

The term "fuzz" was recently used by F. O. Schmitt (cited by Lehninger, 1968) for the designation of an outer coat of the neuronal membrane. This coat is of low electron-density in pictures obtained with conventional ($KMnO_4$, OsO_4) fixation techniques and overlies the tramlines of the classical "unit membrane" of Robertson (1959). Application of the BI block impregnation of glutaraldehyde-fixed nerve tissue enables one to see both an external and an internal "fuzz" coat with local specializations in the region of synaptic contacts (Fig. 3). Such features can be readily detected at the post-synaptic membrane (*e.g.* the "postsynaptic web" of De Robertis, 1964), and previous studies in our laboratory (Fig. 1) have confirmed and extended the pioneering observations of Taxi (1965) and of Milhaud and Pappas (1966) with respect to postsynaptic bars and especially the subsynaptic bodies (Akert and Sandri, 1966; Akert *et al.*, 1967a, b). The following observations are primarily concerned with the "*presynaptic dense projections*" of Gray and with the *intracleft substance*.

(a) The presynaptic vesicular grid

Gray (1963, 1964) was the first to draw attention to small dense spots at the presynaptic membrane; these were particularly evident after phosphotungstic acid block staining. With the aid of the BI impregnation of non-osmicated material the densities are seen in abeyance of the membrane (Pfenninger *et al.*, 1969). In cross sections (Figs. 4, 5) one observes polyhedric bodies with spiny profiles which are spaced more or less regularly. These bodies are immediately surrounded by the contours of clear and dense-cored synaptic vesicles. Tangential sections reveal the regular hexagonal arrangement of the dense projections as well as the interconnecting filaments (Fig. 5, inset). Sections taken near the base of the grid, *i.e.* near the level of the presynaptic membrane, demonstrate that each of the free spaces between presynaptic dense projections contains one single synaptic vesicle (Fig. 5, inset). Based upon measured values of the diameters of dense projections and synaptic vesicles as well as their interdistances one may construct a three-dimensional model. It turns out that the dense projections form the nodal points of a grid and that each dense projection is surrounded by a monolayer of synaptic vesicles (Fig. 6). Thus, it seems appropriate to designate this structural complex "The presynaptic vesicular grid" (Fig. 7).

References p. 239–240

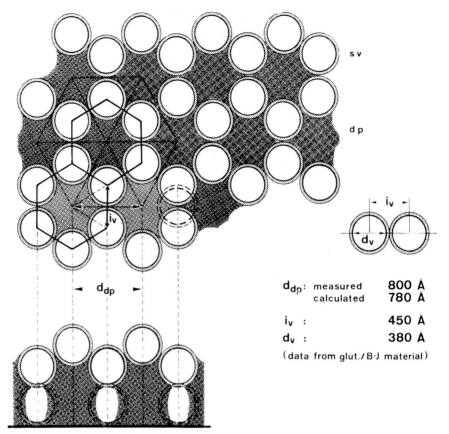

Fig. 6. The presynaptic vesicular grid. Reconstruction of geometrical relationships between pre-synaptic dense projections (dp) and synaptic vesicles (sv). *Upper diagram* represents tangential section of the grid, *lower diagram* represents cross-section. d = diameter; i = interval. The measured and calculated dimensions of grid and vesicles are within close range. The relationship between vesicles and dense projections as viewed in the cross-sectional reconstruction below can be detected in BI-stained cross-sections of synapses under optimal conditions (see Figs. 3 and 5).

Although not easily recognized in sample sections of synaptic areas, the vesicular grid pattern is suggestive in Figs. 3 and 5, and it was found to be present in a considerable number of electronmicrographs of our collection.

The plane of sectioning plays a decisive role for the demonstration of this unique and remarkable relationship between dense projections and vesicles. However, the basic configuration of the presynaptic grid may be truly unstable for reasons which will be discussed below, and this may provide an additional explanation for the fact that the arrangement of the vesicles as shown in the calculated reconstruction (Fig. 6) is not consistently seen in reality.

The significance of the vesicular grid at the presynaptic membrane is not yet clearly understood. The following two possibilities should be considered. (*1*) The grid arrangement "may play a role in guiding synaptic vesicles to special localities of the presynaptic membrane" (Gray, 1966). This suggestion is supported by the

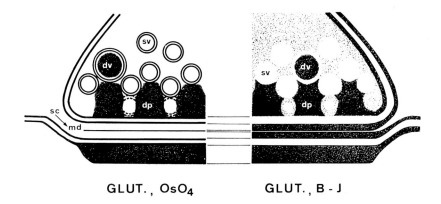

GLUT., OsO₄   GLUT., B-J

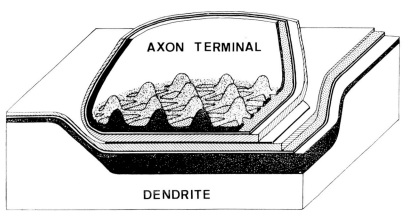

Fig. 7. Schematic reconstruction of synapse as viewed in BI-stained material. *Upper diagram*: Glutaral-dehyde–OsO₄ fixed synapse (left) is compared with one prepared with glutaraldehyde fixation and BI block staining (right). Note the spiny appearance of dense projections due to the indentation by adjacent vesicles. The intracleft lines seem to form thickenings of the *outer* "fuzz" coat of the cyto-plasmic neuronal membrane. The "true" synaptic cleft is minimal. *Lower diagram*: Three-dimensional reconstruction of the presynaptic grid of dense projections (without vesicles for sake of clarity) and the configuration of the synaptic cleft. Note that pre- and postsynaptic densities appear as specialized formations of the *inner* "fuzz" coat of the plasmalemma.

following morphological finding. The cytoplasmic surface of the synaptic terminal is covered by a thin "fuzz" coat (Pfenninger *et al.*, 1969) which is lacking in the holes of the presynaptic grid. Akert and Pfenninger (1969) have suggested that this situation would allow the synaptic vesicles to enter into an immediate contact with the electri-cally excitable membrane which is not present at other membrane sites of the terminal (Fig. 8). This constellation might favor the transmitter release from the presynaptic grid when the nerve impulse reaches the axon terminal, and may prevent it from occurring at other sites. (2) The dense projections may contain molecules which are of significance in the mechanisms of synthesis, release and repletion of transmitter

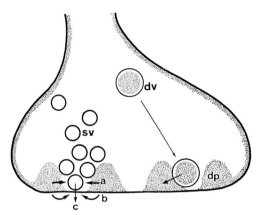

Fig. 8. Topographical relationships between vesicles and presynaptic grid. Arrows indicate functional pathways and interactions (hypothetical). *Clear vesicles* (sv) are randomly distributed in the terminal and regularly arranged within the grid. Only one single vesicle is accommodated within a grid hole and allowed to be in close contact with adjacent dense projections as well as with the excitable membrane. The internal "fuzz" coat seems to be lacking in the holes. a = postulated interaction between presynaptic dense projections (dp) and vesicles before transmitter is released. b = excitatory process involving the presynaptic membrane and triggering transmitter release (c). At least one fraction of the synaptic vesicles might be derived from the plasmalemma by micropinocytosis (see Fig. 10). *Dense-cored vesicles* (dv) may be transported by axoplasmic flow from the cell-body and deposit important molecular constituents at the dense projections.

substances. The intimate relationship between vesicles and grid seems ideally suited for processes of chemical interaction.

The presynaptic grid as a highly organized structure raises the question of its formation. Aghajanian and Bloom (1967) have recently studied the dense projections of Gray in young and adult animals and — although they have failed to recognize the geometrical finesse in the three-dimensional arrangement of dense projections in the mature state — they have reported a remarkable observation. It appears that the immature neuropil may exclusively contain junctions with *symmetrical* membrane appositions as in desmosomes or intermediate junctions. In more advanced maturational stages they encountered increasingly focalized densities at the presynaptic site which eventually attained the profiles of separated dense projections. Thus, the dense projections would not only appear as a criterion of *synaptic polarity* (Gray, 1966), but — in the view of these authors — it may well serve as an indicator of *synaptic viability*. The significance of this notion is easily appreciated. An extended version of this concept can be offered on the basis of our present findings which tend to emphasize the degree of orderliness of presynaptic organization and to correlate levels of its three-dimensional structural evolution with levels of functional differentiation. If this process parallels that of synaptic viability it seems inevitable that the formation of vesicles at the terminal might be among the dynamic factors which bring about the transformation of the solid plaque into the vesicular grid! On the other hand, it should not be overlooked that confirmational evidence of this attractive hypothesis is not available at the moment because direct observations on the transformation are difficult to obtain.

A second problem concerns the origin of appositional densities. As mentioned before, it has been demonstrated in BI-impregnated material that an internal "fuzz" coat exists throughout the axon terminal (Pfenninger *et al.*, 1969). The appositional densities at the pre- and postsynaptic membranes are continuous with, and may be considered to be specializations of, this internal "fuzz" coat. The chemical nature of the material is not known, and no information is available with respect to chemical differences between appositional densities at synapses and other forms of cell contact. Conceivably, the skeleton of these densities may be formed by similar macromolecular constituents. More specific compounds may be formed or deposited secondarily. Akert and Pfenninger (1969) suggest that dense-cored vesicles might be involved in the molecular transport from the neuronal Golgi zone to the presynaptic dense projections (Fig. 8), analogous to the transport of catecholamine-storage granules (Dahlström, 1969).

Finally, the question is raised whether the presynaptic grid is an obligatory synaptic structure or limited to certain types of junction. Our own material is at the moment limited to synapses of the cat subfornical organ. However, presynaptic dense projections have been observed by Gray (1966), Aghajanian and Bloom (1967) and others in the spinal cord and in the cerebral cortex. Thus, the vesicular grid may indeed constitute an important element of central synapses. Nevertheless, more comparative work on this problem seems highly desirable. To mention only the following possibility: Gray (1969) has recently made systematic studies on structural differences between excitatory and inhibitory synapses. Convincing evidence has been accumulated by this author with respect to the "flat vesicle story" of Uchizono (1965). Moreover, Gray's electronmicrographs seem to suggest that appositional densities differ in the two types of synapse. Those with round vesicles seem to be associated with more conspicuous appositional densities than those with flat vesicles. This observation raises the question whether the presynaptic grid formation may be typical for excitatory junctions and whether it might be absent or less developed in inhibitory synapses. The problem is now under investigation in our laboratory.

In the same context one wonders whether the presynaptic grid exists in peripheral junctions. Miledi (see Gray and Guillery, 1966) has found dense spots opposite the junctional folds at the membrane of nerve terminals of frog endplates. Recent studies in our laboratory on neuromuscular junctions in the rat diaphragm have confirmed this observation by clearly demonstrating the presence of dense projections (Fig. 9).

(b) The intracleft substance

Lehninger (1968) has recently discussed the problem of the outer "fuzz" coat of the neuronal membrane and the adjacent intercellular space. Glycoproteins and polysialogangliosides seem to play an important role. However, it was not until periodic acid–silver methenamine (Rambourg and Leblond, 1967), lanthanum (Doggenweiler and Frenk, 1965; Revel and Karnovsky, 1967) and ruthenium red (Bondareff, 1967) were allowed to penetrate the corresponding compartments that morphological evidence became available at the ultrastructural level. More recently, Pfenninger

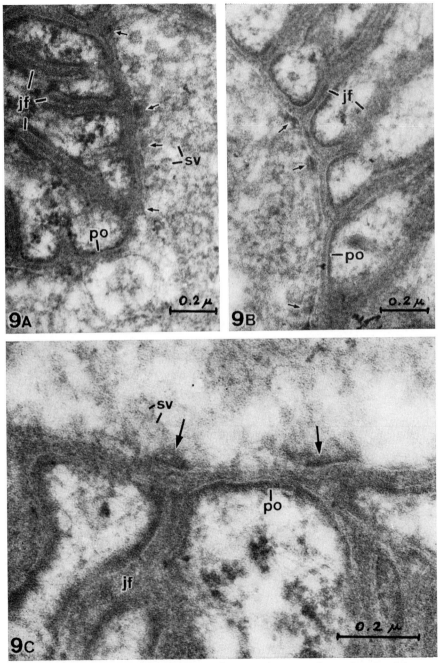

Fig. 9. Motor endplate of rat diaphragm after BI impregnation. Note that prejunctional dense spots (arrows) occur regularly opposite the junctional folds (jf). The postjunctional membrane apposition (po) is clearly seen. Synaptic vesicles (sv) are best seen in A; they seem to have a different appearance from those in presynaptic terminals (*cf.* Figs. 3, 4 and 5), and their relationship to the dense projections is less obvious. Primary magnification of A and B = 20 000 ×, of C = 40 000 ×.

et al. (1969) using the BI block stain, have obtained additional details on the outer coat of nerve membranes. *A double intracleft line* was demonstrated which can also be seen in material prepared with Westrum's combination (uranyl acetate and lead citrate) staining (Westrum, 1965a). This double line represents the outer coat of the plasmalemma which is somewhat thicker in the region of the synapse than elsewhere on the nerve terminal (Figs. 4 and 5). The findings are briefly summarized diagrammatically in Fig. 7. Further description of intracleft lines in synapses and other types of cell contact is to be found elsewhere (Akert and Pfenninger, 1969). The fact that the BI method fails to stain the basement membranes is in contrast with the specificity by which the capillary glycocalyx reacts with ruthenium red (Luft, 1966). Furthermore, the granular intracleft material demonstrated with the aid of ruthenium red (Bondareff, 1967) seems to be randomly arranged, while a clear-cut orientation of very fine electron-opaque granules in parallel with the plasmalemma is seen in BI-stained material. Thus, it seems that the outer membrane coat of neurons, especially at the synapse, may consist of a highly complex system of macromolecules (proteins, glycoproteins, glycolipids) which may be differentially affected by various histochemical reagents.

The functional significance of the intracleft substance at the synapse is at present mainly a matter for speculation. Recent results from our laboratory suggest that basic amino acids may be among the substrates of the BI reaction, and their presence in the junctional area may be critical for the "stickiness" to which the synapse owes its name.

(3) Freeze-etching of neuropil and synaptic junctions

The freeze-etching method (Moor and Mühlethaler, 1963) is known to provide high fidelity electronmicroscopic profiles of cells and tissues in the frozen state. In addition, it enables one to examine a surface view of plasmalemma and organelles. The subfornical organ (SFO) is ideally suited for such studies because it can be rapidly removed from the native brain without mechanical damage to the delicate texture of its neuropil. A further advantage is its relatively high synaptic density (Akert *et al.*, 1967b).

The investigations were based on 14 unfixed and 14 fixed cat SFOs. Fixation was performed with 3% buffered glutaraldehyde. Before the freeze-etching procedure began it was necessary to treat the fixed or unfixed specimens for 30 min in a Ringer solution containing 25–30% glycerol. Approximately 30% of the preparations turned out successfully; of these nearly 150 electronmicrographs were obtained. The majority of the pictures were derived from aldehyde-fixed material, although a sufficient number of unfixed control pictures was available for examination.

While details of this study will be reported in another communication (Moor *et al.*, 1969), we should like to present a brief summary of the principal findings with special emphasis on synaptic fine structure. Profiles of the *synaptic terminals* are readily identified on the basis of vesicles and mitochondria. *Synaptic sites* are characterized by the regularly apposed membranes, the slightly enlarged cleft and the accumulation of finely granulated material at the junctional membranes.

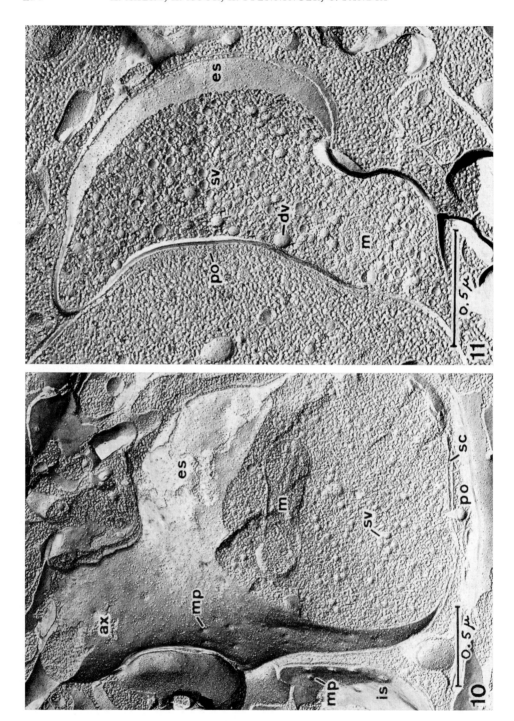

(a) Configuration and size of synaptic vesicles

All the vesicles observed in the SFO terminals (including those from aldehyde-fixed material) have *round* profiles (Figs. 10, 11, 12 and 13). This is in accord with the results of extensive studies on conventional glutaraldehyde–OsO_4-fixed sections of the same tissue. Thus, it appears that the SFO neuropil is not suitable for examining the problem of the so-called flat vesicles and their relationship with inhibitory synapses (see Gray, this volume, p.141).

Some vesicles are seen from the inside, others from the outside. By examining a large number of vesicles one gains the impression that the outer membrane surface is somewhat smoother and contains fewer and smaller granules than the inner surface. Size and shape of granules found at the inner surface of the vesicular membrane are similar to those found at the outer side of the plasmalemma.

The size of the synaptic vesicles is of particular interest from the point of view of maximal storage capacity for the transmitter molecules (Whittaker and Sheridan, 1965). For this reason, preliminary measurements of vesicular diameters were taken, and histograms of unfixed as well as prefixed freeze-etched material could be compared with that obtained from classical aldehyde-osmium fixed sections. The range and peaks of the histograms were surprisingly similar. In unfixed freeze-etched specimens the range of synaptic vesicles (including the large dark-cored) varied between 300 and 1000 Å and the peak distribution was at 500 Å (Moor *et al.*, 1969). Thus far, dark-cored and clear vesicles can be differentiated on the basis of size only. Comparison of freeze-etched and conventional material makes it possible to define the range for diameters of dark-cored vesicles between 600 and 1100 Å. Obviously, there is an intermodal overlap between the large profiles of clear vesicles and the small profiles of the dark-cored vesicles.

(b) Plasmalemma of presynaptic terminals. Micropinocytosis

Examination of freeze-etched neuropil reveals that plasmalemmal surfaces vary with respect to basic texture and granulations. These differences can be partly attributed to different cell types, to differences between inside and outside surfaces within cell types and possibly to regional differences of the latter. The present material is sufficiently large to make some statements concerning the difference between outside and inside surfaces of the plasmalemma near and at the axon terminal.

Fig. 10. Freeze-etched preparation of presynaptic nerve terminal. Cat subfornical organ. ax = preterminal axon. Note the external surface (es) covered with scattered granules giving a *rough* appearance. Micropinocytosis (mp) at the left side. is = inner surface of neuronal (?) plasmalemma. The cut surface of the bouton contains spherical profiles of synaptic vesicles (sv) and mitochondrion (m). Synaptic cleft = sc. Postsynaptic element = po. This specimen was fixed with 3% buffered glutaraldehyde. Primary magnification 20 000 ×.

Fig. 11. Freeze-etched presynaptic nerve terminal in the cat subfornical organ. It contains numerous convex and concave profiles of synaptic vesicles (sv) and one mitochondrion (m). The larger profiles represent dense-cored vesicles (dv). At the left is presumably a synaptic contact, blurred by an uncoated (white) zone. po = postsynaptic density (note the finely granulated material). The outer surface (es) of the plasmalemma is visible at the right. This specimen was fixed with 3% buffered glutaraldehyde. Primary magnification 20 000 ×.

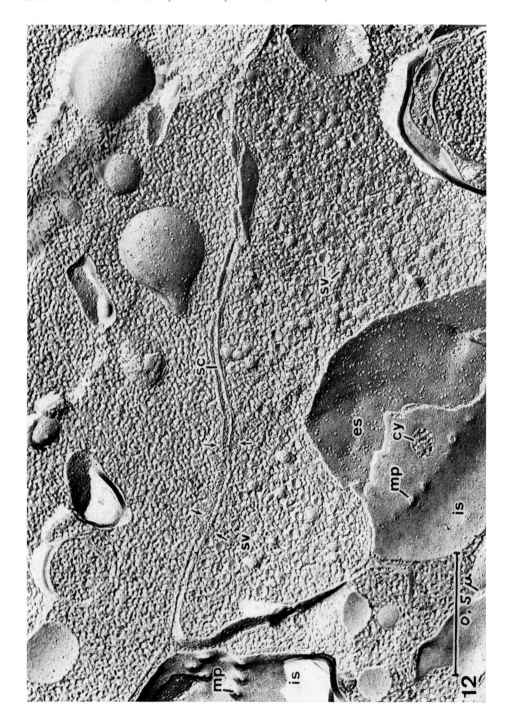

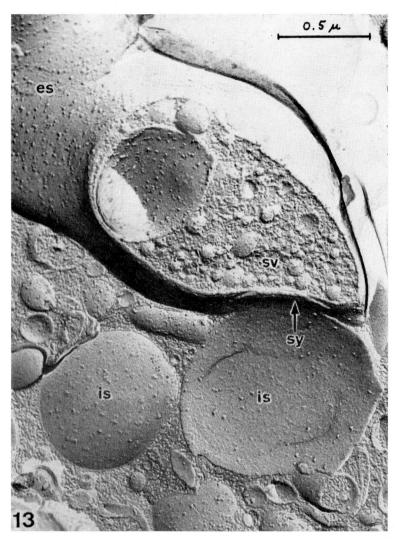

Fig. 13. Freeze-etched preparation of presynaptic nerve terminal. Cat subfornical organ. *This is an unfixed specimen*. Compare the outer rough surface of the plasmalemma (es) with that of fixed preparations in Figs. 8–10. The granules are larger and smoother. The profile of the bouton contains many large and small sized synaptic vesicles (sv). Arrow marks the site of a synaptic contact (sy). Note the *smooth* inner surface (is) of postsynaptic plasmalemma (dendrite?). Primary magnification 20 000 ×.

Fig. 12. Freeze-etched preparation of axosomatic synapse. Cat subfornical organ. The profile of the presynaptic terminal contains numerous spherical vesicles (sv). The synaptic cleft (sc) contains finely granulated material. The texture of the cytoplasm is particularly fine at the pre- and postsynaptic membranes, thus suggesting the site of appositional densities (arrows). Note the difference between the outer surface (es) of the bouton and the inner surface (is) of the plasmalemma of an adjacent element (neuron?). The latter is characterized by inward bulging pinocytotic vesicles (mp) and a small piece of adhering cytoplasm (cy). This specimen was fixed with 3% buffered glutaraldehyde. Primary magnification 20 000 ×.

Figs. 10, 11 and 12 illustrate the *outer surface* of three different boutons terminaux. The same type of surface granulation is seen in all instances. These pictures were taken from aldehyde-fixed material. The granules appear somewhat larger and more flat-topped in the unfixed state (Fig. 13) and resemble those described by Bischoff and Moor (1967a, b) and Branton (1967) on the "rough surface" of Schwann cell and oligodendroglial plasmalemma. The second feature of the outer surface of nerve terminals are the round holes approximately 600 Å in diameter which can be identified as micropinocytotic vesicles in the stage of formation (Fig. 10). They seem to correspond in form and size to those of the capillary endothelial cells, but the latter occur in more densely and regularly arranged populations. The observation of pinocytosis on the plasmalemma of axon terminals is not new. Brightman (1967) has shown this phenomenon in conventional electronmicroscopy. Using peroxidase molecules as tracer for the transport processes, the same author has convincingly demonstrated that substances may be transported by pinocytotic activity from the interstitial space into the nerve terminal. The present study confirms these observations and adds further support to the notion that at least part of the synaptic vesicle population receives its membrane from the plasmalemma. Thus far, the pinocytotic activity of the plasmalemma has been observed in the non-synaptic sites of the terminal. On the other hand, Westrum's (1965b) investigations by means of conventional electronmicroscopy have revealed occasional vesicles at the presynaptic membrane. Present studies with the freeze-etching method are not sufficient to decide whether pinocytosis into or from the synaptic cleft is an important process.

(c) Synaptic cleft and membrane appositions

The synaptic cleft is clearly pictured in Figs. 10 and 12. The presence of a finely granular material within the cleft (Fig. 12) confirms the findings reported earlier in this communication. The presence of synaptic densities is more difficult to ascertain with freeze-etched material. Close examination of the postsynaptic area in Fig. 12 shows that the cytoplasmic texture is extremely fine within an area roughly corresponding to the zone of the postsynaptic membrane apposition. Even more difficulty exists in verifying the presence of the "vesicular grid". Evidently, more detailed studies of the freeze-etched presynaptic area are necessary before comparison and correlation with conventional EM data can be successfully accomplished.

SUMMARY

(1) A brief survey is given on the results obtained with the zinc iodide–OsO_4 impregnation of presynaptic and prejunctional nerve terminals. Synaptic vesicles were stained selectively and a positive correlation with cholinergic sites was demonstrated. Negative as well as positive results were obtained at adrenergic sites. The nature of the histochemical reaction remains to be further clarified.

(2) Impregnation of synaptic junctions with bismuth iodide and subsequent contrasting with uranyl acetate and lead hydroxide gave significant details on the presynaptic membrane and its densities (Gray). In adult animals, the presynaptic

dense projections form a *grid structure* with the dense spots hexagonally arranged and interconnected with filamentous cross-bridges. The free spaces (holes) of the grid can accommodate one single synaptic vesicle. Thus, the formation is called the "*presynaptic vesicular grid*". Plasticity and functionally significant variations of this structure may possibly occur. The same method provided important details on the outer and inner coats of the plasmalemma of the presynaptic terminal. Within the synaptic cleft a double layered subunit is described.

(3) Freeze-etching preparations of synapses confirmed the "true" existence and spheric shape of synaptic vesicles. It revealed important differences between the outer and inner surfaces of the plasmalemma of presynaptic terminals. Furthermore, the presence of micropinocytosis at the surface of boutons terminaux was demonstrated.

ACKNOWLEDGEMENT

The authors wish to express their gratitude to Miss C. Berger for her skilful assistance in the freeze-etching preparation.

REFERENCES

AGHAJANIAN, G. K., AND BLOOM, F. E., (1967); The formation of synaptic junctions in developing rat brain: a quantitative electron microscopic study. *Brain Res.*, **6**, 716–727.
AKERT, K., AND PFENNINGER, K., (1969); Synaptic fine structure and neural dynamics. In: S. H. BARONDES (Ed.), *Cellular Dynamics of the Neuron*. I.S.C.B. Symposium, Paris, Academic Press, New York, in the press.
AKERT, K., AND SANDRI, C., (1966); A triple layered subsynaptic organelle in the subfornical organ of the cat. *Brain Res.*, **2**, 404–406.
AKERT, K., AND SANDRI, C., (1968); An electronmicroscopic study of zinc iodide–osmium impregnation of neurons. I. Staining of synaptic vesicles at cholinergic junctions. *Brain Res.*, **7**, 286–295.
AKERT, K., PFENNINGER, K., AND SANDRI, C., (1967a); Crest synapses with subjunctional bodies in the subfornical organ. *Brain Res.*, **5**, 118–121.
AKERT, K., PFENNINGER, K., AND SANDRI, C., (1967b); The fine structure of synapses in the subfornical organ of the cat. *Z. Zellforsch.*, **81**, 537–556.
AKERT, K., SANDRI, C., AND PFENNINGER, K., (1968); A new method for staining synaptic vesicles at peripheral and central synapses. In: D. S. BOCCIARELLI (Ed.), *Electronmicroscopy*, Vol. 2, Roma Tip. Pol. Vaticana, pp. 521–522.
BISCHOFF, A., AND MOOR, H., (1967a); Ultrastructural differences between the myelin sheath of peripheral nerve fibres and CNS white matter. *Z. Zellforsch.*, **81**, 303–310.
BISCHOFF, A., AND MOOR, H., (1967b); The ultrastructure of the "difference factor" in the myelin. *Z. Zellforsch.*, **81**, 571–580.
BONDAREFF, W., (1967); An intercellular substance in rat cerebral cortex: submicroscopic distribution of ruthenium red. *Anat. Rec.*, **157**, 527–536.
BRANTON, D., (1967); Fracture faces of frozen myelin. *Exp. Cell Res.*, **45**, 703–707.
BRIGHTMAN, M. W., (1967); The intracerebral movement of proteins injected into blood and cerebrospinal fluid of mice. In: A. LAJTHA AND D. H. FORD (Eds.), *Progress in Brain Research*, Vol. 29. *Brain Barrier Systems*. Elsevier, Amsterdam, pp. 20–37.
BURN, J. H., AND RAND, M. J., (1959); Sympathetic postganglionic mechanism. *Nature (Lond.)*, **184**, 163–165.
CHAMPY, C., (1913); Granules et substances réduisant l'iodure d'osmium. *J. Anat. (Paris)*, **49**, 323–343.

DAHLSTRÖM, A., (1969); Formation, transport and life span of amine storage granules in peripheral and central monoamine containing neurons. In: S. H. BARONDES (Ed.), *Cellular Dynamics of the Neuron*. I.S.C.B. Symposium, Paris, Academic Press, New York, in the press.

DE ROBERTIS, E. D. P., (1964); *Histophysiology of Synapses and Neurosecretion*. Pergamon, Oxford.

DOGGENWEILER, C. F., AND FRENK, S., (1965); Staining properties of lanthanum on cell membranes. *Proc. nat. Acad. Sci. (Wash.)*, **53**, 425–430.

GRAY, E. G., (1963); Electron microscopy of presynaptic organelles of the spinal cord. *J. Anat. (Lond.)*, **97**, 101–106.

GRAY, E. G., (1964); Tissue of the central nervous system. In: S. M. KURTZ (Ed.), *Electron Microscopic Anatomy*. Academic Press, New York, pp. 369–417.

GRAY, E. G., (1966); Problems of interpreting the fine structure of vertebrate and invertebrate synapses. *Int. Rev. Gen. & exp. Zool.*, **2**, 139–170.

GRAY, E. G., (1969); Electron microscopy of excitatory and inhibitory synapses: a brief review. In: K. AKERT AND P. G. WASER (Eds.), *Progress in Brain Research*, Vol. 31. *Mechanisms of Synaptic Transmission*, Elsevier, Amsterdam, pp. 141–155.

GRAY, E. G., AND GUILLERY, R. W., (1966); Synaptic morphology in the normal and degenerating nervous system. *Int. Rev. Cytol.*, **19**, 111–182.

ISRAEL, M., (1969); Cellular and subcellular localization of acetylcholine in electric organs with special reference to fractions derived from presynaptic part. In: S. H. BARONDES (Ed.), *Cellular Dynamics of the Neuron*. I.S.C.B. Symposium, Paris, Academic Press, New York, in the press.

LEHNINGER, A. L., (1968); The neuronal membrane. *Proc. nat. Acad. Sci. (Wash.)*, **60**, 1069–1080.

LUFT, J. H., (1966); Fine structure of capillary and endocapillary layer as revealed by ruthenium red. *Fed. Proc.*, **25**, 1773–1783.

MAILLET, M., (1962); La technique de Champy à l'osmium ioduré de potassium et la modification de Maillet à l'osmium–iodure de zinc. *Trab. Inst. Cajal Invest. biol.*, **54**, 1–36.

MAILLET, M., (1968); Étude critique des fixations au tétraoxyde d'osmium–iodure. *Bull. Ass. Anat. (Nancy)*, **53**, 233–394.

MILHAUD, M., AND PAPPAS, G., (1966); The fine structure of neurons and synapses of the habenula of the cat with special reference to subjunctional bodies. *Brain Res.*, **3**, 158–173.

MOOR, H., AND MÜHLETHALER, K., (1963); Fine structure in frozen-etched yeast cells. *J. Cell Biol.*, **17**, 609–628.

MOOR, H., PFENNINGER, K., SANDRI, C., AND AKERT, K., (1969); Freeze-etching of synapses. *Science*, in the press.

PFENNINGER, K., SANDRI, C., AKERT, K., AND EUGSTER, C. H., (1969); Contribution to the problem of structural organization of the presynaptic area. *Brain Res.*, **12**, 10–18.

RAMBOURG, A., AND LEBLOND, C. P., (1967); Electronmicroscope observations on the carbohydrate-rich cell coat present at the surface of cells in the rat. *J. Cell Biol.*, **32**, 27–53.

REVEL, J. P., AND KARNOVSKY, M. J., (1967); Hexagonal array of subunits in intercellular junctions of the mouse heart and liver. *J. Cell Biol.*, **33**, C7–C12.

ROBERTSON, J. D., (1959); The ultrastructure of cell membranes and their derivatives. *Biochem. Soc. Symp. (Cambridge, England)*, **16**, 3–43.

STANEK, J., (1905); Über das Cholinperjodid und die quantitative Fällung von Cholin durch Kaliumtrijodid. *Hoppe-Seylers Z. physiol. Chem.*, **46**, 280–285.

TAXI, J., (1965); Contribution à l'étude des connexions des neurones moteurs du système nerveux autonome. *Ann. Sci. nat. Zool. (Paris)*, **7**, 413–674.

TRANZER, J. P., THOENEN, H., SNIPES, R. L., AND RICHARDS, J. G., (1969); Recent developments on the ultrastructural aspect of adrenergic nerve endings in various experimental conditions. In: K. AKERT AND P. G. WASER (Eds.), *Progress in Brain Research*, Vol. 31. *Mechanisms of Synaptic Transmission*, Elsevier, Amsterdam, pp. 33–46.

UCHIZONO, K., (1965); Characteristics of excitatory and inhibitory synapses in the central nervous system of the cat. *Nature (Lond.)*, **207**, 642–643.

WESTRUM, L. E., (1965a); A combination staining technique for electron microscopy. 1. Nervous tissue. *J. Microscop.*, **4**, 275–278.

WESTRUM, L. E., (1965b); On the origin of synaptic vesicles in cerebral cortex. *J. Physiol. (London)*, **179**, 4–6P.

WHITTAKER, V. P., AND SHERIDAN, M. N., (1965); The morphology and acetylcholine content of isolated cerebral cortical synaptic vesicles. *J. Neurochem.*, **12**, 363–372.

Structure and Function of Acetylcholinesterase*

W. LEUZINGER

Departments of Biochemistry and Neurology, College of Physicians and Surgeons, Columbia University, New York, N.Y. (U.S.A.)

INTRODUCTION

During the last decade cellular membranes have been investigated intensively by electron microscopy combined with biochemical and biophysical methods. Although only 100 Å thick, membranes were found to be the site of a great diversity of proteins and enzymes, as illustrated *e.g.* by mitochondrial membranes.

In view of the central role of enzymes and proteins in cell mechanisms, it appears reasonable to assume that they also play an essential role in the elementary process of excitable membranes, *i.e.* in bioelectrogenesis. The following facts seem to be evidence for such an assumption (Nachmansohn, 1966, 1967):

(*1*) Acetylcholine (ACh) and the enzymes hydrolyzing and forming it: Acetylcholinesterase (ACh-ase) and choline *O*-acetyltransferase (choline acetylase), have been shown to be present in all types of conducting fibers of nerve and muscle throughout the animal kingdom. They are found in motor and sensory, "cholinergic" and "adrenergic", peripheral and central fibers, in invertebrates and in vertebrates, etc.

(*2*) ACh-ase, an enzyme relatively specific for ACh and distinctly different from other esterases, is localized in the excitable membranes of axons and muscle fibers as well as in those of junctions, *i.e.* in the membranes of nerve terminals and in the postsynaptic membranes.

(*3*) ACh-ase hydrolyzes ACh in a few micro-seconds, a prerequisite for attributing to the ester the role proposed by Nachmansohn of a trigger in the generation of bioelectric currents, since 1000 or more impulses may be propagated per second, so that the trigger must be removed with sufficient rapidity.

(*4*) An extraordinarily high concentration of the enzyme has been found in the electric organs of electric fish; these organs, the most powerful bioelectric generators developed by nature, are highly specialized in their function. Although formed by 3% of protein and 92% of water, 1 kg (fresh weight) of electric tissue of *Torpedo* and *Electrophorus* hydrolyzes 3–4 kg of ACh per hour. The tissue has been instrumental in the analysis of the proteins specifically associated with bioelectrogenesis.

(*5*) Specific and potent inhibitors of ACh-ase have been shown to block electrical

* Supported in part by the United States Public Health Service grants NB 03304 and NB 07743 and by the National Science Foundation grants GB 4844 and GB 7149.

References p. 245

activity in a great variety of nerve fibers, *e.g.* physostigmine reversibly, and diisopropylphosphofluoridate (DFP) irreversibly. Thus, electrical activity requires the activity of the enzyme present in the excitable membrane, supporting the assumption of its essential role in the permeability changes.

(6) In axons exposed to organophosphates under conditions leading to an irreversible block of electrical activity, powerful specific activator of the phosphorylated enzyme, pyridine-2-aldoxine methiodide, may, under appropriate conditions, restore electrical activity.

(7) The presence of a protein, the ACh-receptor, has been demonstrated in many axonal membranes. It has been shown that ACh and its congeners produce effects on the electrical parameters of axons similar to those previously observed on the junctional membranes, provided that the structural barriers for lipid-insoluble quaternary nitrogen derivatives are inadequate to prevent the compounds to reach the receptor or are reduced by chemical treatment.

(8) With the monocellular electroplax preparation of *Electrophorus*, the protein nature of the ACh-receptor has been established.

(9) Lipid-soluble inhibitors of the ACh-receptor, that are analogs of ACh, such as certain local anesthetics, block electrical activity in all excitable membranes, thus demonstrating the essential role of the ACh-receptor protein in bioelectrogenesis and supplementing the essential role of the enzyme.

Based on all these observations and data, Nachmansohn (1959) has postulated that ACh is released by excitation in the excitable membranes as a specific signal and causes a conformational change of the ACh-receptor, thereby possibly releasing Ca^{2+} ions, bound to carboxyl groups of the protein. Ca^{2+} ions have been known for a long time to be involved in the excitability of nerve and muscle fibers; the Ca^{2+} ions released may induce further conformational changes of phospholipids and other polyelectrolytes. The end result of this sequence of chemical reactions is the change of ion permeability permitting the movement of 20 000–40 000 ions, or more, across the membrane per molecule of ACh released. These reactions thus act as typical amplifiers of the signal given by ACh. ACh-ase, by hydrolyzing ACh, permits the receptor to return to its original conformation; the barrier of the ion movements is thereby reestablished.

ACETYLCHOLINESTERASE

As mentioned before, several proteins are associated with the function of ACh, among them the ACh-receptor, ACh-ase and choline *O*-acetyltransferase.

Based on indirect biochemical evidence, the localization of ACh-ase in excitable membranes had been postulated for more than two decades. Recently direct evidence has been obtained in many laboratories by histochemical techniques and electron microscopy. However, whereas it is easy to demonstrate the localization of the enzyme in the membrane of *non-myelinated* fibers, in *myelinated* fibers the presence of the enzyme in the membrane appeared to be irregular or absent. Since even in a slice of 1000 Å thickness or less, structural barriers may impair the reaction between the enzyme in the membrane and the added compounds, Brzin (1966) applied a detergent, Triton 100 X, to slices of an isolated sciatic nerve. After the treatment he found ACh-ase in the plasma membrane, located between the axoplasm and the myelin sheath.

The enzyme as well as the receptor have been shown, by using potent and specific inhibitors, to be essential for electrical activity in all excitable membranes.

The analyses of ACh-ase became feasible because of the availability of the electric organ of electric fish. Several hundred-fold purification of ACh-ase, extracted from electric tissue of *Electrophorus* was obtained in the early 1940's (Rothenberg and Nachmansohn, 1947). Partially purified preparations were adequate for kinetic studies which yielded information about the active sites of the enzymes. These analyses led to the understanding of the mode of action of many drugs which effect the nervous system, such as organophosphates (Nachmansohn and Wilson, 1951).

Meanwhile, there was very little information concerning the protein properties of ACh-ase. The main obstacle has been that sufficient amounts of pure enzyme protein have not been available. It thus appeared desirable to attempt a large-scale purification of ACh-ase for the study of protein structure and its properties. Last year, large-scale purification by 7 readily reproducible steps was accomplished. Subsequently, the crystallization of the enzyme became possible (Leuzinger and Baker, 1967a, b).

From 10 kg starting material about 70 mg of a homogeneous protein are obtained. The specific activity is 750 mmoles of ACh hydrolyzed per mg protein per hour.

The crystals are extremely well formed. The most common form of growth observed is a short, thick prism of regular cross-section, a form compatible with true hexagonal symmetry. The complex pyramidal termination shown by some crystals, however, may imply a crystal system of lower order. The crystals exhibit low birefringence so that it is impossible at present to determine whether they are uniaxial or biaxial.

The amino acid analysis did not reveal any special features except that amino sugars were present, namely: glucosamine, galactosamine and probably talosamine.

The isoelectric point has been found to be at pH 5.03. On the base of electrofocusing experiments, the molecular weight of the native enzyme has been determined by equilibrium centrifugation, together with Dr. Goldberg at the Pasteur Institute in Paris, in a condition where it is known to behave as a single species. From these experiments one can conclude that the molecular weight of the enzyme is 260 000. This result is in good agreement with previously reported values of 240 000 (Lawler, 1961) and 250 000 (Leuzinger and Baker, 1967a, b). The large value of the molecular weight of the enzyme indicated that ACh-ase contained several polypeptide chains. Hence, a protein solution containing 6 M guanidine hydrochloride and 0.02 M mercaptoethanol was centrifuged to ascertain whether denaturation and dissociation of the enzyme occurred. The data from these experiments analyzed by calculations similar to those of Ullmann (1968), show that the molecular weight of the protein subunit under these conditions is about one quarter of that of the intact enzyme. Under

the experimental conditions the subunits appear to be homogeneous, and even though
the behaviour in the ultracentrifuge is not a very good test for homogeneity one can
at least assume that the subunits do not differ significantly in molecular weight.
It thus can be concluded that the native molecule of ACh-ase consists of four subunits
of an average molecular weight of 64 000 $\pm$ 4 000. A close analysis of electron
micrographs indicates the same number.

The important question is now whether the subunits are identical or non-identical.
To answer that, a preliminary experiment of disc electrophoresis was performed in
the presence of 8 M urea. Two distinct bands were observed, indicating two different
chains. For the identification of the carboxyl-terminal amino acids, hydrazinolysis
was employed. A reaction time of 30 h provided maximum recovery of free amino
acids. Serine and glycine were recovered in equal amount, very close to 2 moles of
each per mole of ACh-ase and represent the carboxyl-terminal of two polypeptide
chains. Although leucine, alanine, aspartic acid and threonine are present at 0.5 mole/
mole ACh-ase, it is not significant, because some non-specific liberation of free
amino acids is known to occur from other positions than the carboxyl-terminal
when high molecular weight proteins are treated with hydrazine. To confirm these
results, enzymatic hydrolysis of ACh-ase by carboxypeptidase was undertaken as a
complementary method to the chemical hydrazinolysis. Only carboxypeptidase A
was used, because hydrazinolysis did not reveal any basic C-terminal amino acids.

The differences in velocity of the release of amino acids because of the two different
chains of ACh-ase make the results complex and difficult to interpret. Hence, no
conclusions can be made about the sequence, except for the terminal positions.
Only the values for serine and glycine, known to be the C-terminal residues based
on the previous experiments, should be evaluated critically. The rate of liberation
of serine confirms unequivocally the presence of two moles of C-terminal serine per
mole of enzyme. Glycine is generally released at a slower rate than serine. This is
also evident within the first half hour of the enzymatic hydrolysis. The explanation
for the rather high value of glycine after 20 h of digestion is probably due to its
occupation of a penultimate position in one type of chain, while alanine may occupy
the second position in the other type. Final conclusions about the sequence can be
drawn only after the separation of the chains (Leuzinger et al., 1969).

DISCUSSION

The analyses suggest that the enzyme is a dimer, each protomer consisting of two
non-identical chains. The non-identity of the two groups of polypeptide chains is
supported by the determination of the number of active sites of ACh-ase. Three
independent methods show that ACh-ase has only two active sites (unpublished).
Thus it seems reasonable to assume that the molecule may be a dimeric hybrid.
The α-chain of ACh-ase may be said to contain the active site, while the function
of the β-chains remains unknown at present; or α- and β-chains together may form
an active unit. If the first assumption should be true, the question may be raised,
whether the β-chains may be the receptor protomer. Our experimental data do not

exclude such a possibility. Should receptor and esterase be the same macromolecular component of the membrane, one could assume that this component exists in two conformational states, one representing the polarized state, and the other the depolarized state of the excitable membrane.

However, other information based on *in vitro* studies of the enzyme (Karlin, 1967) and on experiments conducted *in vivo* on the monocellular electroplax preparation (Karlin and Winnik, 1968), contradicts such an assumption. Eventually, a final answer must await the separation of the two chains.

Contemporary biochemistry has made it increasingly apparent that characterization of an enzyme requires studies not only in solution but also within the frame of the natural macromolecular assembly of the cell, in view of the many cooperative effects, regulatory and control mechanisms, on which the activity of an enzyme depends. The availability of crystals and of pure protein in adequate amounts in combination with the monocellular electroplax preparation (Schoffeniels, 1957), and the membrane-bound enzyme obtained by fractionation of cell fragments (Karlin, 1965), has thus opened the possibility of studying the characteristics of ACh-ase on a cellular, subcellular, and molecular level.

ACKNOWLEDGEMENT

The author is most grateful to Professor David Nachmansohn for his encouragement and his helpful discussions of the manuscript.

REFERENCES

BRZIN, M., (1966); The localization of acetylcholinesterase in axonal membranes of frog nerve fibers. *Proc. nat. Acad. Sci. (Wash.)*, **56**, 1560–1563.

KARLIN, A., (1965); The association of acetylcholinesterase and membrane in subcellular fractions of the electric tissue of electrophorus. *J. Cell Biol.*, **25**, 159–169.

KARLIN, A., (1967); Chemical distinctions between acetylcholinesterase and the acetylcholine receptor. *Biochim. Biophys. Acta (Amst.)*, **139**, 358–362.

KARLIN, A., AND WINNIK, M., (1968); Reduction and specific alkylation of the receptor for acetylcholine. *Proc. nat. Acad. Sci. (Wash.)*, **60**, 668–674.

LAWLER, H. C., (1961); Turnover time of acetylcholinesterase. *J. biol. Chem.*, **236**, 2296–2301.

LEUZINGER, W., AND BAKER, A. L., (1967a); Acetylcholinesterase I: Large scale purification, homogeneity, amino acid analysis. *Proc. nat. Acad. Sci. (Wash.)*, **57**, 446–451.

LEUZINGER, W., AND BAKER, A. L., (1967b); Crystallization of acetylcholinesterase. *Science*, **156**, 540.

LEUZINGER, W., GOLDBERG, M., AND CAUVIN, E., (1969); Molecular properties of acetylcholinesterase. *J. Mol. Biol.*, **40**, 365.

NACHMANSOHN, D., (1959); *Chemical and Molecular Basis of Nerve Activity*. Academic Press, New York.

NACHMANSOHN, D., (1966); Chemical control of the permeability cycle in excitable membranes during electrical activity. *Ann. N.Y. Acad. Sci.*, **137**, 877–900.

NACHMANSOHN, D., (1967); La membrane excitable. Macromolécules liées à la bioélectrogénèse. *Bull. Soc. Chim. biol., (Paris)*, **49**, 1177–1189.

NACHMANSOHN, D., AND WILSON, I. B., (1951); The enzymic hydrolysis and synthesis of acetylcholine. *Advanc. Enzymol.*, **12**, 259.

ROTHENBERG, M. A., AND NACHMANSOHN, D., (1947); Studies on cholinesterase III. Purification of the enzyme from electric tissue by fractional ammonium sulfate precipitation. *J. biol. Chem.*, **168**, 223–231.

SCHOFFENIELS, E., (1957); An isolated single electroplax preparation. *Biochim. biophys. Acta (Amst.)*, **26**, 585–596.

ULLMANN, A., (1968); Private communication.

Polyphasic Synaptic Activity

L. TAUC

Laboratory for Cellular Neurophysiology, Centre for Studies on Nervous Physiology, Centre National de la Recherche Scientifique, Paris (France)

In chemical synapses the transmitter released by the presynaptic neuron is believed to combine with specific receptor molecules in the postsynaptic neuronal membrane. This combination produces permeability changes for specific ions, and thus electric currents are created in the postsynaptic neuron which either depolarizes and excites it or hyperpolarizes and inhibits it. The measurable potential changes are so-called postsynaptic potentials. It had long been thought that a presynaptic neuron could exert only one type of action on all neurons with which it was in contact. This concept seemed to be a direct consequence of the principle of Dale (1935) postulating that the same transmitter substance is released from all the terminals of a given neuron. Furthermore, it was believed that the nature of the transmitter would determine the nature of its action, that is excitatory or inhibitory.

Experiments on the ganglion cells of Mollusca have shown (Tauc and Gerschenfeld, 1961, 1962) that a single transmitter substance, namely acetylcholine, is responsible for excitation on some cells and for inhibition in other cells in the same ganglion. It was clearly demonstrated that the polarity of the synaptic action is determined by differences in the properties of the postsynaptic neuron and not by the nature of the transmitter, which is the same for both receptors. Later it was found (Kandel *et al.*, 1967) that a single presynaptic neuron, using acetylcholine as the transmitter, was able to produce excitation in some of the neurons with which it is in contact and inhibition in others. It appears therefore that the type of response is determined by the postsynaptic neuron and that a presynaptic neuron cannot be designated, in general, as inhibitory or excitatory. It can only be considered excitatory or inhibitory with respect to the neuron with which it forms synaptic contact (Fig. 1).

But even this limited distinction between excitatory and inhibitory interneurons is to be questioned in instances when their activation produces, in the postsynaptic neuron, a complex response occurring in several phases. Such polyphasic responses have been observed in vertebrates on the cholinergic synapses of sympathetic postganglionic cells and of Renshaw cells. In the sympathetic ganglion (Eccles and Libet, 1961; Libet, 1964, 1965) stimulation of preganglionic fibres produces a complex response in the postsynaptic cells, which is recorded intracellularly (Libet and Tosaka, 1966; Tosaka *et al.*, 1968; Koketsu and Nishi, 1967; Nishi and Koketsu, 1968a)

References p. 256–257

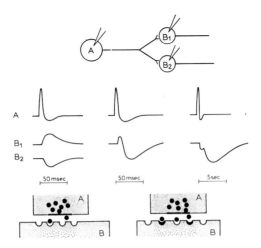

Fig. 1. Schematic representation of some possible modalities of synaptic interaction between three neurons (A, B1 and B2, see upper scheme). Discharge in cell A might produce respectively: excitatory postsynaptic potential in cell B1 and inhibitory postsynaptic potential in cell B2 (left middle column); biphasic potential in one of the cells B (central column); double inhibition in cells B (right column). The lower part of the figure represents a scheme of possible relationship between transmitter (represented by filled circles) liberated by presynaptic neuron A, and single receptor (left) or two re-ceptors (right) designated by different semicircles and situated on the postsynaptic neuron B.

as a fast depolarization reminiscent of a classical EPSP, followed by a much slower depolarization of several seconds duration — the so-called slow EPSP. The fast and slow EPSPs are separated in some cells by a hyperpolarizing slow wave called the slow IPSP. There is strong evidence that the fast and slow EPSP are produced by the action of the same transmitter, namely acetylcholine, on two different receptor sites in the postganglionic cells. The fast EPSP apparently results from the activation of nicotinic receptors, the slow EPSP from the activation of muscarinic receptors. The latter react more slowly and produce a prolonged polarization of the post-ganglionic cell (Eccles and Libet, 1961; Takeshige and Volle, 1964a, b, 1965; Volle, 1966a, b). The origin of the hyperpolarizing inhibitory PSP is still not clear (but see Eccles and Libet, 1961; Tosaka and Libet, 1965; Kobayashi and Libet, 1968; Nishi and Koketsu, 1968b). Nicotinic and muscarinic receptors are also involved in the response of Renshaw cells to the stimulation of cholinergic afferents (Curtis and Ryall, 1966a, b, c).

Polyphasic responses were demonstrated in *Aplysia* and related Mollusca with the description of a peculiar synaptic response called inhibition of long duration (Tauc, 1958, 1959, 1968). This inhibition consists of a short depolarizing phase followed by a long-duration hyperpolarizing inhibitory phase. Another type of inhibition of long duration has recently been described which consists of a fast hyperpolarizing phase followed by a slow hyperpolarizing phase (Kehoe, 1967). Two other types of biphasic response are known. One is found in the giant cells of the buccal ganglion of the mollusc *Navanax*, and is not treated here (Levitan and Tauc, unpublished), and the other appears between the two giant cells in *Aplysia* and has been called the

biphasic postsynaptic potential. In contrast with the other described forms of polyphasic response this BPSP seems to result from an electrical transmission process
(Hughes and Tauc, 1965, 1968; Biedebach *et al.*, 1968).

INHIBITION OF LONG DURATION (ILD)

Inhibition of long duration appears in cells which have been designated as HILDA
cells (Gerschenfeld and Tauc, 1964). The common property of these cells is the presence of a hyperpolarizing, inhibitory wave several seconds or minutes in duration;
in DILDA cells the inhibition of long duration is preceded by a fast depolarizing

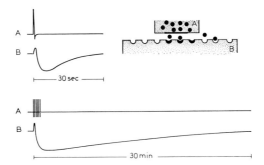

Fig. 2. Inhibition of long duration observed in the *Aplysia* R15 cell. Upper left drawing, unitary
response; lower drawing, prolongation of inhibition after repetitive discharge. Upper right, scheme
of possible interaction between single transmitter and two different receptors, each one being responsible for a part of the response. A, presynaptic neuron; B, postsynaptic neuron.

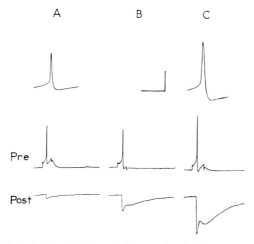

Fig. 3. Effects of intracellularly injected tetra-ethylammonium in the neuron presynaptic to a HILDA
cell. The size and the duration of the presynaptic spike represented in the first and second row at
different speeds (calibration: 20 mV, 100 msec and 1 sec respectively), progressively increases during
the injection and so does the amplitude of both phases of the postsynaptic response represented in the
lower row. A, before injection; B, 15 min of injection; C, 45 min of injection. (From Kehoe, 1968b.)

phase (Fig. 2), and in HILDA cells by a fast hyperpolarizing phase (Fig. 3). Acetylcholine depolarizes DILDA cells whereas it hyperpolarizes HILDA cells.

In an identifiable cell in the abdominal ganglion of *Aplysia* — cell R15 — (according
to the classification of Frazier *et al.*, 1967) previously called by us "OBERON",
a unitary ILD, resulting from the activity of a single interneuron, is represented by
a fast excitatory phase, about 300 msec in duration, followed by an inhibition usually
prolonged over 15–30 sec (Fig. 2). In other DILDA cells a unitary ILD is not observed. Moreover the first excitatory phase does not always appear clearly in these
cells, and the inhibition is usually shorter than that in R15.

By artificially changing the membrane potential the long-duration hyperpolarizing
phase can be reversed in polarity, and a study of this reversal potential has disclosed
the participation of potassium ions (Tauc, 1968). In addition it seems that the concomitant activation of a sodium–potassium pump plays an important role (Ascher,
1968, personal communication). It appears that ILD is due to the action of a chemical
transmission mechanism but the chemical nature of the transmitter is unknown.
There is suggestive evidence that dopamine might be the substance responsible,
for ILD can be imitated by the injection of dopamine on the axonal synaptic zone
of DILDA cells (Ascher *et al.*, 1967). However more detailed investigations (Ascher,
personal communication) suggest that even in DILDA-type cells there is more than
one type of ILD.

The inhibitory phase of ILD shows peculiar cumulative effects. When the interneuron responsible is repetitively activated, the hyperpolarization not only increases
in amplitude but also in duration, and the latter increase appears to be directly related
to the quantity of the initial input. In R15, after a short burst of activity, the inhibitory phase can be prolonged for over 30 min in spite of the fact that during all
this time the presynaptic neuron remains silent (Tauc, 1968). If one attempted to
produce such an effect using only classical inhibitory postsynaptic potentials it would
be necessary to maintain a high frequency discharge in the presynaptic neuron for
the entire period.

The character of the ILD appearing in HILDA cells is better known. Not only
have identifiable HILDA cells been found in the pleural ganglion of *Aplysia* but
also it has been possible to penetrate the presynaptic interneuron responsible for the
ILD (Kehoe, 1967, 1968a, b) (Fig. 3). Each of the two phases has been found to result
from different permeability changes. The initial fast inhibition phase is due to a
chloride permeability change whereas the second inhibitory phase results from a
change in potassium permeability.

What is remarkable is that injection of acetylcholine imitates both the fast and slow
phases of the physiological response and uses the same ionic mechanism (Fig. 5).
For both physiological and ACh responses, the changes in chloride and potassium
permeability appear nearly simultaneously but are of different duration; the difference
in duration explains the biphasic form of the phenomenon. The responses to natural
transmitter and to ACh injection are identically affected by blocking drugs. The
chloride permeability change can be blocked by *d*-tubocurarine, hexamethonium,
strychnine and several other cholinolytic drugs except atropine (Fig. 4). None of

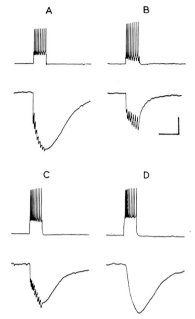

Fig. 4. Records from the presynaptic (upper traces showing spikes) and postsynaptic HILDA neuron (lower traces) showing double inhibition. A, test; B, in the presence of tetra-ethylammonium (10^{-4} M) which selectively blocks the slow inhibitory phase; C, test; D, in the presence of d-tubocurarine (10^{-3} g/ml) which selectively blocks the fast inhibitory phase. (Time basis, 2 sec; 20 mV for spikes, 5 mV for the synaptic response). (Courtesy of J. S. Kehoe, 1968.)

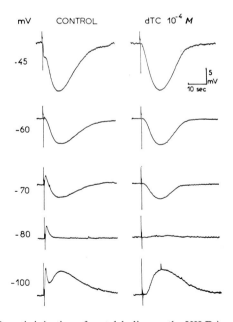

Fig. 5. Effects of electrophoretic injection of acetylcholine on the HILDA cell, at different membrane polarizations. Left column, control; right column, in the presence of d-tubocurarine (10^{-4} M) which selectively blocks the fast initial phase. (Courtesy of J. S. Kehoe, 1968.)

the classically known cholinolytic drugs had any effects on the second phase which, however, could be selectively blocked by tetra-ethylammonium (Fig. 4) (Kehoe, 1968a).

The concentration of tetra-ethylammonium necessary to block the receptors producing the change in potassium permeability was very low (Figs. 4 and 5), and it appears that at that concentration the potassium permeability is not directly affected by this drug. Indeed at this concentration tetra-ethylammonium has no effect on the potassium permeability change produced by the injection of dopamine. One has to admit that at this concentration the action of tetra-ethylammonium is exerted only on the level of the specific receptor to acetylcholine.

But the ability of tetra-ethylammonium at higher concentration to modify the potassium permeability, and thus the shape of the action potential, has been used to demonstrate that no interneuron is interposed between the penetrated presynaptic and postsynaptic cells (Kehoe, 1968b). Tetra-ethylammonium was injected electrophoretically into the presynaptic neuron through an intracellular micropipette, and as a consequence a prolongation of the spike was observed. At the same time both phases of the postsynaptic potential increased considerably in amplitude (Fig. 3). Since the distance from the soma to the presynaptic site is short (both neurons are situated in the same ganglion), the modification of the spike observed in the soma was no doubt also felt at the presynaptic site, and the increased spike duration produced increased the liberation of transmitter (cf. Hagiwara and Tasaki, 1958; Takeuchi and Takeuchi, 1962; Miledi and Slater, 1966). The fact that both fast and slow phases were affected excludes the possibility of an interneuron being placed between the penetrated cells.

There is consequently very strong evidence that acetylcholine liberated on HILDA cells by an interneuron combines with two different receptors, one acting on chloride and the other on potassium permeability mechanisms. Those receptors that are not affected by any of the classical cholinolytic drugs represent a peculiar cholinoceptive structure. Yet it does not represent a unique exception. In the giant cells of Navanax, inhibitory acetylcholine receptors were found that were not blocked by any of the classical cholinolytic agents, and tetra-ethylammonium was without effect (Tauc and Levitan, 1968, unpublished).

As in DILDA cells, the long inhibition in HILDA cells presents cumulative effects, although not so prolonged. This is interesting because it shows that once the transmitter combines with the receptor it appears to be protected from the destructive enzyme, acetylcholinesterase, which has been shown to be present in high concentrations in this Aplysia structure. This explains how long-lasting modifications in the postsynaptic structures can be maintained without repetitive presynaptic activity.

BIPHASIC POSTSYNAPTIC POTENTIAL (BPSP)

Two giant cells have been described in the Aplysia central nervous system; the left and the right giant cell (LGC and RGC). Although their cell bodies are located in the left pleural ganglion and visceral ganglion, respectively, they have a similar size, show identical membrane properties and distribute their axons quasisymmetrically. They seem to be homologous and functionally symmetrical (Hughes and Tauc, 1963).

When the RGC is selectively activated by direct intracellular stimulation, a biphasic postsynaptic potential is observed in the LGC (Hughes and Tauc, 1965, 1968). The BPSP consists of a fast depolarizing phase about 200 msec in duration followed by a slow hyperpolarizing phase about 3 sec duration (Fig. 6). The amplitude of each of these phases is about 500 μV, naturally opposite in polarity. Both phases differ from EPSPs and IPSPs observed in the same cell. Stimulation of the LGC also produces a BPSP in the RGC but such a BPSP can only be measured at the level of the right pleural ganglion and is undetectable in the soma of the RGC because of the long distance between the visceral and the pleural ganglion.

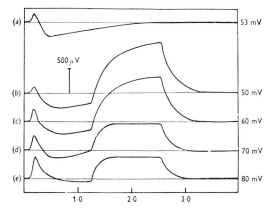

Fig. 6. Biphasic postsynaptic potential as recorded in the right giant cell at different membrane potentials. (a) At normal resting level; (b), (c), (d), (e) at different imposed polarization levels. The electrotonic potential superposed on the inhibitory phase is produced by a transmembrane constant square current pulse; the modification of its amplitude indicates the presence of anomalous rectification. (From Hughes and Tauc, 1968.)

With repetitive stimulation the amplitude of the inhibitory phase diminishes progressively if the interval between two presynaptic spikes is shorter than 2–3 sec. Concurrently, the depolarizing phase exhibits a small increase which can be interpreted as resulting from the diminution of the inhibitory phase. This diminution of the inhibitory phase at high repetition rates is responsible for the peculiar manner in which the BPSP summates upon repeated stimulation. At low frequencies, less than 3/sec, the net effect of the summed potentials is a hyperpolarization and inhibition. At higher frequencies the effect is a depolarization and excitation.

When the LGC is artificially hyperpolarized, the excitatory phase increases in size and the inhibitory phase diminishes (Fig. 6). The diminution in the inhibitory phase is more intense than one would deduce from the modifications of the membrane conductance which are concomitant with the polarization changes. These modifications of the excitatory and inhibitory phase seemed at first to indicate that a chemical mechanism was involved in the formation of the BPSP. This concept was strengthened by the fact that modifications of the potassium concentration in the

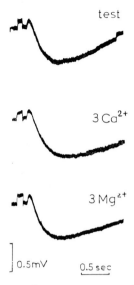

Fig. 7. Evolution of the biphasic postsynaptic potential in the presence of physiological solutions with increased Ca^{2+} and Mg^{2+} content. The absence of modifications points to a possible electrical mechanism. (Biedebach, Meunier and Tauc, unpublished.)

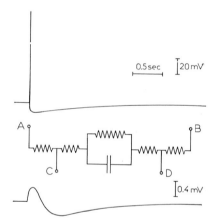

Fig. 8. Scheme showing equivalent RC circuitry which transforms the presynaptic spike with its exceptionally long after-potential (upper trace), into a response similar to the biphasic postsynaptic potential (lower trace). A and B, points of input; C and D, points of output. (Meunier and Tauc, 1968, unpublished.)

outside medium considerably affected the inhibitory phase in such a way as would be expected if a potassium permeability change were the basis of this inhibitory hyperpolarizing phase.

However, when the magnesium/calcium ratio was changed in the outside medium (Biedebach *et al.*, 1968), no effect was observed in the shape of the BPSP (Fig. 7). This was indeed strong evidence against a neuro-humoral mechanism. Finally it was found that the duration of the after-potential of the presynaptic spike could be 3 sec and thus comparable in duration to the inhibitory phase of the BPSP. Furthermore when such an action potential is passed through an adequate low pass RC filter, one can produce a potential change having exactly the form of a BPSP. Indeed the excitatory phase represents the spike, highly attenuated by the filter, whereas the slow after-potential passes the filter practically unaffected (Fig. 8). As a consequence the BPSP seems most likely to result from an electrical type of transmission.

The modifications of the two phases produced by hyperpolarization of the postsynaptic cell body can be explained by admitting that this polarization change could also affect the presynaptic neuron and modify the shape of the presynaptic spike. Similarly one can assume that it was the presynaptic spike which was mainly affected by modifications in the ionic composition of the outside medium. Owing to the considerable distance of the two giant cells, polarization of one of them cannot affect the membrane potential of the other. Only a conducted spike can reach the electrical synapse and affect the other cell.

The BPSP thus represents a rare case of electrically transmitted inhibition. The only other known inhibitory electrical synapse affects the Mauthner nerve cell; but there the mechanism is completely different and the duration of action is much shorter.

SUMMARY AND CONCLUSION

It appears that in many cases the neuronal interaction might produce a complex response in the postsynaptic neuron. With one exception, represented by the electrical synapse responsible for the BPSP, the mechanism so far demonstrated was based on the plurality of different postsynaptic receptors to the same transmitter substance. Each type of receptor had a different action on the postsynaptic membrane, which was manifested by differences in the duration or permeability changes effected. But the modifications might also be of another nature. For instance it seems now that activation of such receptors might act upon the sodium–potassium ionic pumps (Kobayashi and Libet, 1968; Libet and Tosaka, 1968; Nishi and Koketsu, 1968a; Ascher, personal communication; Kandel, personal communication). Another remarkable feature of this "additional" receptor seems to be the long duration of the effects which they can produce and which greatly surpasses that of classical synaptic action.

Although never demonstrated, another possible mechanism can be proposed to explain some other polyphasic synaptic effects. One cannot discard the possibility that a single presynaptic neuron can release more than one transmitter. Such a mechanism would be as effective as those mentioned above, but would in addition introduce new variables consisting in the separate control of presynaptic release through differences in timing, in the rate of metabolism of the two transmitters and in their inactivation mechanisms.

REFERENCES

ASCHER, P., KEHOE, J. S., AND TAUC, L., (1967); Effets d'injections électrophorétiques de dopamine sur les neurones d'Aplysie. *J. Physiol. (Paris)*, **59**, 331–332.

BIEDEBACH, M., MEUNIER, J. M., AND TAUC, L., (1968); Bases ioniques du potentiel postsynaptique biphasique chez l'Aplysie. *J. Physiol. (Paris)*, **60**, 220.

CURTIS, D. R., AND RYALL, R. W., (1966a); The excitation of Renshaw cells by cholinomimetics. *Exp. Brain Res.*, **2**, 49–65.

CURTIS, D. R., AND RYALL, R. W., (1966b); The acetylcholine receptors of Renshaw cells. *Exp. Brain Res.*, **2**, 66–80.

CURTIS, D. R., AND RYALL, R. W., (1966c); The synaptic excitation of Renshaw cells. *Exp. Brain Res.*, **2**, 81–96.

DALE, H. H., (1935); Pharmacology and nerve endings. *Proc. roy. Soc. Med.*, **28**, 319–332.

ECCLES, R. M., AND LIBET, B., (1961) Origin and blockade of the synaptic responses of curarized sympathetic ganglia. *J. Physiol. (Lond.)*, **157**, 484–503.

FRAZIER, W. T., KANDEL, E. R., KUFFERMAN, I., WAZIRI, R., AND COGGESHALL, R. E., (1967); Morphological and functional properties of identified neurons in the abdominal ganglion of *Aplysia californica*. *J. Neurophysiol.*, **30**, 1288–1351.

GERSCHENFELD, H. M., AND TAUC, L., (1964); Différents aspects de la pharmacologie des synapses dans le système nerveux central des Mollusques. *J. Physiol. (Paris)*, **56**, 360–361.

HAGIWARA, S., AND TASAKI, I., (1958); A study on the mechanism of impulse transmission across the giant synapse of the squid. *J. Physiol. (Lond.)*, **143**, 114–137.

HUGHES, G. M., AND TAUC, L., (1963); An electrophysiological study of the anatomical relations of two giant nerve cells in *Aplysia depilans*. *J. exp. Biol.*, **40**, 469–486.

HUGHES, G. M., AND TAUC, L., (1965); A unitary biphasic postsynaptic potential (BPSP) in *Aplysia* "brain". *J. Physiol. (Lond.)*, **179**, 27–28.

HUGHES, G. M., AND TAUC, L., (1968); A direct synaptic connexion between the left and right giant cells in *Aplysia*. *J. Physiol. (Lond.)*, **197**, 511–527.

KANDEL, E. R., FRAZIER, W. T., WAZIRI, R., AND COGGESHALL, R. E., (1967); Direct and common connections among identified neurons in *Aplysia*. *J. Neurophysiol.*, **30**, 1352–1376.

KEHOE, J. S., (1967); Pharmacological characteristics and ionic bases of two component postsynaptic inhibition. *Nature (Lond.)*, **215**, 1503–1505.

KEHOE, J. S., (1968a); Blocage sélectif par l'ion tétraéthylammonium d'une inhibition cholinergique résistant au curare. *C.R. Acad. Sci. (Paris)*, in the press.

KEHOE, J. S., (1968b); A single presynaptic neurone mediates a two component postsynaptique inhibition. *Nature (Lond.)*, in the press.

KOBAYASHI, H., AND LIBET, B., (1968); Electrogenesis of slow postsynaptic potentials in sympathetic ganglion cells. XXIV Int. Congr. Physiol. Sci., Washington. *Proc. Int. Union Physiol. Sci.*, **7**, No. 724, 242.

KOKETSU, K., AND NISHI, S., (1967); Characteristics of the slow inhibitory postsynaptic potential of bullfrog sympathetic ganglion. *Life Sci.*, **6**, 1827–1836.

LIBET, B., (1964); Slow synaptic responses and excitatory changes in sympathetic ganglia. *J. Physiol. (Lond.)*, **174**, 1–25.

LIBET, B., (1965); Slow synaptic responses in autonomic ganglia. In: D. R. CURTIS AND R. H. MCINTYRE (Eds.), *Studies in Physiology*, Springer, Berlin, pp. 160–165.

LIBET, B., AND TOSAKA, T., (1966); Slow potentials recorded intracellularly in sympathetic ganglia. *Fed. Proc.*, **25**, 270.

LIBET, B., AND TOSAKA, T., (1968); Slow inhibitory and excitatory postsynaptic responses recorded intracellularly in mammalian sympathetic ganglia. *Nature (Lond.)*, in the press.

LIBET, B., CHICHIBU, S., AND TOSAKA, T., (1968); Slow synaptic responses and excitability in sympathetic ganglia of the bullfrog. *J. Neurophysiol.*, **31**, 383–395.

MILEDI, R., AND SLATER, C. R., (1966); The action of calcium on neuronal synapses in the squid. *J. Physiol. (Lond.)*, **184**, 473–498.

NISHI, S., AND KOKETSU, K., (1968a); Early and late afterdischarges of amphibians sympathetic ganglion cells. *J. Neurophysiol.*, **31**, 109–121.

NISHI, S., AND KOKETSU, K., (1968b); Underlying mechanism of ganglionic slow IPSP and posttetanic hyperpolarization of pre- and postganglionic elements. XXIV Int. Congr. Physiol. Sci., Washington. *Proc. Int. Union Physiol. Sci.*, **7**, No. 961, 321.

TAKESHIGE, C., AND VOLLE, R. L., (1964a); Modification of ganglionic responses to cholinomimetic drugs following preganglionic stimulation, anticholinesterase agents and pilocarpine. *J. Pharmacol. exp. Ther.*, **146**, 335–343.

TAKESHIGE, C., AND VOLLE, R. L., (1964b); A comparison of the ganglion potentials and block produced by acetylcholine and tetraethylammonium. *Brit. J. Pharmacol.*, **23**, 80–89.

TAKEUCHI, A., AND TAKEUCHI, N., (1962); Electrical changes in pre- and postsynaptic axons of the giant synapse of *Loligo*. *J. gen. Physiol.*, **45**, 1181–1193.

TAUC, L., (1958); Processus post-synaptique d'excitation et d'inhibition dans le soma neuronique de l'Aplysie et de l'Escargot. *Arch. ital. Biol.*, **96**, 78–110.

TAUC, L., (1959); Sur la nature de l'onde de surpolarisation de longue durée observée parfois après l'excitation synaptique de certaines cellules ganglionnaires de Mollusques. *C.R. Acad. Sci. (Paris)*, **249**, 318–320.

TAUC, L., (1968); Some aspects of postsynaptic inhibition in *Aplysia*. In: *Structure and Function of Neuronal Inhibitory Mechanism*, Stockholm, 1966. Pergamon, Oxford, pp. 377–382.

TAUC, L., AND GERSCHENFELD, H. M., (1961); Cholinergic transmission mechanism for both excitation and inhibition in Molluscan central synapses. *Nature (Lond.)*, **192**, 366–367.

TAUC, L., AND GERSCHENFELD, H. M., (1962); A cholinergic mechanism of inhibition synaptic transmission in a molluscan system. *J. Neurophysiol.*, **25**, 236–262.

TOSAKA, T., AND LIBET, B., (1965); Slow postsynaptic potentials recorded intracellularly in sympathetic ganglia of frog. *Intern. Congr. Physiol. (Tokyo)*, p. 905.

TOSAKA, T., CHICHIBU, S., AND LIBET, B., (1968); Intracellular analysis of slow inhibitory and excitatory postsynaptic potentials in sympathetic ganglia of the frog. *J. Neurophysiol.*, **31**, 396–409.

VOLLE, R. L., (1966a); Modification by drugs of synaptic mechanisms in autonomic ganglia. *Pharmacol. Rev.*, **18**, 839–869.

VOLLE, R. L., (1966b); Muscarinic and nicotinic stimulant actions at autonomic ganglia. *Int. Encyclop. Pharmacol. Therap.*, section 12, vol. 1, Pergamon, Oxford, p. 110.

Synaptic Transmission in the Sensory Relay Neurons of the Thalamus*

K. MAEKAWA** AND ANNA ROSINA***

Department of Neurophysiology, Max-Planck Institute for Psychiatry, Munich (Germany)

INTRODUCTION

The elucidation of functional properties of dendrites has long been a central problem in the study of the electrophysiological activity of the brain.

The special synaptic morphology of the thalamo–cortical relay neurons (TCR) facilitates the neurophysiological study of dendritic function in these neurons. Synaptic organization of the sensory relay neurons of the thalamus has been extensively studied by means of electron microscopy as well as with the aid of various staining methods (Colonnier and Guillery, 1964; Glees, 1941; O'Leary *et al.*, 1965; Peters and Palay, 1966; Scheibel and Scheibel, 1966; Smith *et al.*, 1964; Szentágothai, 1963, 1967a, b; Szentágothai *et al.*, 1966; Tömböl, 1966–67), and the conclusions can be briefly summarized as follows. The axon terminals of the sensory input fibers make synaptic contact exclusively with the peripheral part of TCR neurons. Axo-dendritic synapses in the lateral geniculate body (LGB) show a peculiar complex organization which Szentágothai (1963) calls a "glomerular" synapse. The "glomerulus" consists of a "claw-shaped" presynaptic ending of optic fibers in close contact with spheroid protrusions of peripheral parts of the nerve cell dendrites. Non-optic terminals are also involved in the "glomerulus" which is surrounded by a glial sheath.

This synaptic morphology is present with minor differences in all TCR nuclei (Szentágothai, 1967a, b). In this paper the "glomerular" synapses are considered to play an important role in the high-safety synaptic transmission (Rose and Mountcastle, 1959) of TCR neurons.

METHODS

Experiments on the LGB were performed on nembutalized cats (10–20 mg/kg) which were immobilized by flaxedil and artificially ventilated. Glass microelectrodes

---

* This study was supported by the Deutsche Forschungsanstalt für Psychiatrie. Part of these results was reported at the Frühjahrstagung der Deutschen Physiologischen Gesellschaft, Mainz, 1968.
** Present address: Behavior Research Institute, Gunma University Medical School, Maebashi-shi, Gunma (Japan).
*** Present address: Istituto di Fisiologia Umana, Università di Milano, Milano (Italy).

References p. 264

filled with 2 M K-citrate (20–40 MΩ resistance) were inserted into the nucleus which had been exposed by aspiration of the overlying cortex. After enucleation of the optic bulb the exposed contralateral optic nerve (OT) was electrically stimulated with a bipolar silver electrode. Diffuse light pulses of short duration were used to stimulate the ipsilateral eye.

Experiments on the ventrobasal complex (VB) of the thalamus were also performed on cats lightly anesthetized with nembutal and immobilized with succinylcholine chloride. The method has been fully described in a previous paper (Maekawa and Purpura, 1967b). Polarizing currents were injected through the recording micro-electrode with the aid of a modified bridge circuit (Araki and Otani, 1955)*.

RESULTS

Intracellular recordings were obtained from about 200 LGB neurons identified through the monosynaptic response elicited by contralateral OT stimulation or through the response to diffuse light on the ipsilateral intact eye. The latter group (about 30 % of the total sample) was not influenced by the contralateral OT stimulus except for a few binocularly innervated neurons.

The latency of monosynaptic EPSP elicited by contralateral OT stimulation ranged between 1.5 and 2.5 msec. A typical example of OT-evoked monosynaptic EPSP is illustrated in Fig. 1A. The monosynaptic EPSP of 1.5 msec latency and 3.3 mV

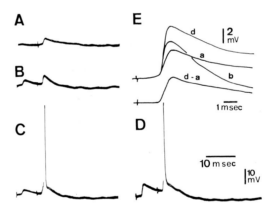

Fig. 1. Monosynaptic EPSP evoked in a LGB neuron by contralateral OT stimulation. (A) Sub-threshold OT stimulus elicits a monosynaptic EPSP of 3.3 mV amplitude. (B) A larger EPSP is elicited by the second stimulus of a double shock (7 msec interval) which secures a spike discharge in C. (D) OT stimulus intensity is increased and the fast-rising large EPSP (6.6 mV) is elicited by the first shock. (E) The photographically enlarged tracings labeled a, b and d correspond to the EPSP of A, the second of B and the first of D respectively. The time course of the potential difference between a and d was obtained by algebraic subtraction $(d - a)$. Note that this potential difference $(d - a)$ parallels the time course of the EPSP in A (a).

* Results on the VB neurons are part of a study (during 1965–1966) in collaboration with Dr. D. P. Purpura; Departments of Anatomy and Neurology, College of Physicians and Surgeons, Columbia University, New York, N.Y. (U.S.A.).

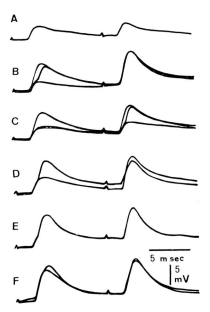

Fig. 2. Step-like augmentation of OT evoked monosynaptic EPSP. (A) Double OT stimuli (11 msec interval) produce 3 mV monosynaptic EPSPs. (B–D) OT stimulus intensity is increased. Each trace was formed by superimposition of 2–3 responses produced by consecutive stimuli at 0.8/sec frequency. Note various combinations of summation of two EPSP components and notches on the rising phase of EPSPs. (E–F) Stronger OT stimuli produce large EPSPs with less frequent decomposition.

amplitude was followed by a very small and long-lasting recurrent IPSP (Maekawa and Rosina, in preparation). The second of a pair of stimuli, separated by 7 msec, elicited a large fast-rising EPSP (B) which could trigger a spike discharge (C). When the stimulus intensity was increased (D), a fast-rising EPSP of 6.6 mV was produced by the first shock of the double stimuli.

Enlarged EPSP tracings are superimposed in E (upper trace): *a*, *b* and *d* correspond to the EPSP of A, the second of B and the first of D, respectively. The potential difference between *a* and *d*, obtained by subtraction, is shown in the lowermost trace (*d*—*a*), which parallels the time course and the amplitude of *a*. This observation strongly suggests that the large EPSP (*d*) is the synchronized summation of two smaller EPSPs (*a*). The smaller amplitude and fast decay of the EPSP (*b*) could be due to the change in membrane conductance during the IPSP produced by the first OT shock.

This kind of step augmentation of EPSP was not uncommon during OT activation in LGB neurons. In Fig. 2A, monosynaptic EPSPs of 3 mV were elicited by double OT stimuli (11 msec interval). The stimulus intensity of Fig. 2A was set at a threshold to produce the monosynaptic EPSP. The EPSPs appeared in an "all-or-none" fashion. The OT stimulus intensity was slightly increased from B to D, and stepwise summation of various pairs of EPSPs was observed. All records (B to D) are formed by superimposition of traces of consecutive responses elicited by OT stimuli at a frequency of 0.8/sec. The summation of two components was clearly demonstrated by the decomposition on the rising phase of EPSPs. The upper components also oc-

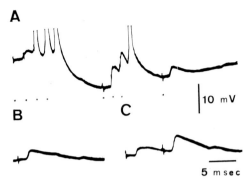

Fig. 3. Summation of EPSPs monosynaptically evoked by OT pulse train. Same LGB neuron as in Fig. 1. Top of spikes cut off for better illustration; spike amplitude as in Fig. 1. (A) Summated sub-threshold EPSPs, produced by OT pulse train (500/sec), secures high frequency spike discharges after second OT shock. Same OT pulse train delivered during IPSP produced by first train pulses: signifi-cantly augmented monosynaptic EPSPs summate and secure a spike discharge at a lower firing level. Note that last single OT stimulus produced a similar small EPSP to that in the control (B). (B–C) Control subthreshold EPSPs evoked by single and double stimuli.

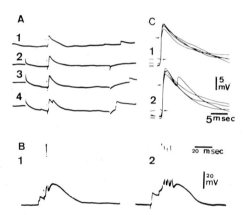

Fig. 4. Intracellular recording from a ventrobasal neuron. (A 1–4) Short latency monosynaptic EPSP evoked by medial lemniscal stimulation. A1 is a control response; in A2–4 hyperpolarizing current is injected through the recording microelectrode with increasing current intensity. Maximum current intensity at A4 about $1 \cdot 10^{-8}$ amp. Slight decomposition is observed on the rising phase of EPSPs. Note small component EPSP superimposed on falling phase of EPSP in A4. (C) Superimposed tra-cings of photographic enlargement of lemniscal-evoked EPSPs with (C2) and without (C1) hyperpolar-ization. Two horizontal arrows indicate decomposition on rising phase of EPSPs. Note that the fast rising component (between the two arrows) shows less fluctuation in amplitude than the slow rising components. (B) Spike discharges are secured when lemniscal evoked EPSPs summate with spontaneous EPSPs. Note decomposition in the spontaneous EPSPs (A4 and B1) and large after-depolarizing wave following spike potentials (B1, 2). (Maekawa and Purpura, unpublished results.)

casionally failed to be elicited and showed "all-or-none" behavior. Stronger OT stimulation (E, F) elicited larger EPSPs with less-frequent decomposition of the rising phase.

It is well known that the LGB neurons can respond to high frequency OT stimu-lation (Bishop *et al.*, 1962). Such high safety in synaptic transmission by LGB neurons was observed to be due to effective summation and marked augmentation of OT-evoked EPSP, an example of which is illustrated in Fig. 3. Subthreshold OT stimuli given at 500/sec produced a repetitive spike discharge after summation of the first two monosynaptic EPSPs. During the IPSP produced by the first pulse train, the same OT pulse train produced significantly augmented EPSPs which summated to secure a neuron discharge at a slightly lower firing level. This marked augmentation of EPSPs did not appear to be due to the membrane potential level difference, since a single OT stimulus delivered 10 msec after the second pulse train produced only a small EPSP similar to the control EPSP (the first EPSP of A and B).

Effective summation of EPSPs and high synaptic security were also observed in the ventrobasal (VB) neurons in the thalamus (Maekawa and Purpura, 1967b). An example of intracellular recording from a VB neuron is illustrated in Fig. 4. A monosynaptic EPSP was elicited by medial lemniscal stimulation at medullar level (A1). As already reported (Maekawa and Purpura, 1967b), a membrane hyperpolarization, induced by current injection through the recording microelectrode (A2–4), produced but a small increase in amplitude of the lemniscal-evoked EPSP in the majority of VB neurons. These minor effects were considered to result from the remote distribution of lemniscal axon terminals on the dendrites of VB neurons.

Small but clearly detectable decompositions were observed on the rising phase of the lemniscal-evoked EPSPs. Superimposed drawings of lemniscal-evoked EPSPs without (C1) and with hyperpolarization (C2) are shown. Two inflections (upper and lower arrows) appear on the rising phase of the EPSPs. The major fluctuating part of the EPSPs appears to be the slow-rising component whereas the fast-rising component (between the two arrows) is fairly constant in amplitude. These subthreshold lemniscal-evoked EPSPs summated with spontaneous EPSPs and triggered spike discharges as shown in B. Summated EPSPs showing decomposition also occurred spontaneously (right of A4 and B1).

CONCLUDING REMARKS

Emphasis has been placed on the characteristic stepwise summation of EPSPs observed during monosynaptic activation of TCR neurons by specific sensory input.

The OT-evoked monosynaptic EPSPs in LGB neurons were not infrequently observed to comprise several components, some of which behaved in an "all-or-none" manner and summated effectively to secure neuronal discharge (see also Bishop et al., 1958; Fuster et al., 1965; and Morlock et al., 1965).

This "all-or-none" behavior of EPSPs has already been reported for thalamic ventrobasal neurons (Maekawa and Purpura, 1967b), as well as in Purkinje cells (Eccles et al., 1966). A similar type of unitary EPSP has been described in thalamic ventrolateral neurons (Purpura et al., 1965, 1966).

It has been suggested that such EPSPs result from the activation of a large area of the postsynaptic membrane by terminals of a single presynaptic axon (Bishop et al., 1958; Eccles et al., 1966). In view of the recent morphological data which show that in TCR neurons each dendrite participates in the "glomerular" synapses it might be argued that a glomerular complex behaves as an elementary depolarizing component

References p. 264

of TCR cells. Clearly, the synchronized summation of elementary glomerular EPSPs originating in different dendrites might significantly contribute to preserving the high safety of sensory transmission in TCR neurons.

REFERENCES

ARAKI, T., AND OTANI, T., (1955); Response of single motoneurons to direct stimulation in toad's spinal cord. *J. Neurophysiol.*, **18**, 472–485.

BISHOP, P. O., BURKE, W., AND DAVIS, R., (1958); Synaptic discharge by single fibre in mammalian visual system. *Nature (Lond.)*, **182**, 728–730.

BISHOP, P. O., BURKE, W., AND DAVIS, R., (1962); The identification of single units in central visual pathways. *J. Physiol. (Lond.)*, **162**, 409–431.

COLONNIER, M., AND GUILLERY, R. W., (1964); Synaptic organization in the lateral geniculate nucleus of the monkey. *Z. Zellforsch.*, **62**, 333–355.

ECCLES, J. C., LLINAS, R., AND SASAKI, K., (1966); The excitatory synaptic action of climbing fibers on the Purkinje cells of the cerebellum. *J. Physiol. (Lond.)*, **182**, 268–296.

FUSTER, J. M., CREUTZFELDT, O. D., AND STRASCHILL, M., (1965); Intracellular recording of neuronal activity in the visual system. *Z. vergl. Physiol.*, **49**, 605–622.

GLEES, P., (1941); The termination of optic fibers in the lateral geniculate body of the cat. *J. Anat. (Lond.)*, **75**, 434–441.

MAEKAWA, K., AND PURPURA, D. P., (1967a); Intracellular study of lemniscal and non-specific synaptic interactions in thalamic ventrobasal neurons. *Brain Res.*, **4**, 308–323.

MAEKAWA, K., AND PURPURA, D. P., (1967b); Properties of spontaneous and evoked synaptic activities of thalamic ventrobasal neurons. *J. Neurophysiol.*, **30**, 360–381.

MAEKAWA, K., AND ROSINA, A., (1968); Postsynaptic potentials in lateral geniculate neurons induced by optic tract activation. XXXIV. Tagung der Deutschen Physiologischen Gesellschaft, Mainz. *Pflügers Arch. ges. Physiol.*, **300**, R 101–102.

MAEKAWA, K., AND ROSINA, A., (1969); Synaptic organization of the lateral geniculate neurons in cats. In preparation.

MORLOCK, N. L., PEARLMAN, A. L., AND MARSHALL, W. H., (1965); Single unit study of post-tetanic potentiation and second subnormality in the lateral geniculate body of cats. *Exp. Neurol.*, **11**, 38–47.

O'LEARY, J. L., SMITH, J. M., TIDWELL, M., AND HARRIS, A. B., (1965); Synapses in the lateral geniculate nucleus of the primate. *Neurology (Minneap.)*, **15**, 548–555.

PETERS, A., AND PALAY, S. L., (1966); The morphology of laminae A and A1 of the dorsal nucleus of the lateral geniculate body of the cat. *J. Anat. (Lond.)*, **100**, 451–486.

PURPURA, D. P., SCARFF, T., AND MCMURTRY, J. G., (1965); Intracellular study of internuclear inhibition in ventrolateral thalamic neurons. *J. Neurophysiol.*, **28**, 487–496.

PURPURA, D. P., MCMURTRY, J. G., AND MAEKAWA, K., (1966); Synaptic events in ventrolateral thalamic neurons during suppression of recruiting responses by brain stem reticular stimulation. *Brain Res.*, **1**, 63–76.

ROSE, J. E., AND MOUNTCASTLE, V. B., (1959); Touch and kinesthesis. *Handbook of Physiology*, Sect. 1, Vol. 1. Amer. Physiol. Soc., Washington, D.C., pp. 387–429.

SCHEIBEL, M. E., AND SCHEIBEL, A. B., (1966); Patterns of organization in specific and non-specific thalamic fields. In D. P. PURPURA AND M. D. YAHR (Eds.), *The Thalamus*, Columbia Univ. Press, New York, pp. 13–46.

SMITH, J. M., O'LEARY, J. L., HARRIS, A. B., AND GAY, A. J., (1964); Ultrastructural features of the lateral geniculate body of the cat. *J. comp. Neurol.*, **123**, 357–378.

SZENTÁGOTHAI, J., (1963); The structure of the synapse in the lateral geniculate body. *Acta anat. (Basel)*, **55**, 166–185.

SZENTÁGOTHAI, J., (1967a); Models of specific neuron arrays in thalamic relay nuclei. *Acta morph. Acad. Sci. hung.*, **15** (2), 113–124.

SZENTÁGOTHAI, J., (1967b); The anatomy of complex integrative units in the nervous system. In K. LISSÀK (Ed.), *Results in Neuroanatomy, Neurochemistry, Neuropharmacology and Neurophysiology*. Akadémia Kiadò, Budapest, pp. 9–45.

SZENTÁGOTHAI, J., HÁMORI, J., AND TÖMBÖL, T., (1966); Degeneration and electron microscope analysis of the synaptic glomeruli in the lateral geniculate body. *Exp. Brain Res.*, **2**, 283–301.

TÖMBÖL, T., (1966–67); Short neurons and their synaptic relations in the specific thalamic nuclei. *Brain Res.*, **3**, 307–326.

Forms of Spontaneous and Evoked Postsynaptic Potentials of Cortical Nerve Cells

O. CREUTZFELDT, K. MAEKAWA* AND L. HÖSLI**

Department of Neurophysiology, Max Planck Institute of Psychiatry, Munich (Germany)

INTRODUCTION

Several factors determine the shape and size of postsynaptic potentials of nerve cells: the amount of transmitter liberated by an impulse, the total synaptic area occupied by the axo-soma-dendritic contacts arising from one single afferent fibre, the membrane resistance and — as was recently pointed out again (Rall, 1967) — the location of the synapse relative to the soma. This situation is comparable to the situation of end-plate potentials and their spread along the muscle fibre (Fatt and Katz, 1951), but complicated by the geometry of cortical cells. Distantly located synapses will produce in the soma a relatively slowly rising flat PSP, and centrally located synapses a large and steeply rising PSP, even if the PSPs have the same size and form at the site of their origins. It was therefore proposed that the "shape index" of an EPSP might give an indication of its place of origin (Rall, 1967). This interpretation was supported by the observation that EPSPs whose shape index indicated a distant location (*i.e.* smooth and small EPSPs), were less influenced by intracellularly applied currents than the steeper, supposedly proximal EPSPs (Nelson and Frank, 1967). In cortical cells, it was observed that EPSPs elicited by electrical stimulation of non-specific thalamic nuclei were only little influenced by intracellular current injection, whereas VL-elicited EPSPs were increased by polarizing and decreased by depolarizing currents (Creutzfeldt and Lux, 1964). This may indicate a distant location of the "non-specific" synapses on the apical dendrites and a more proximal location of the "specific" synapses. On the other hand, it is generally assumed that inhibitory synapses are located on the soma although a definite proof of this statement has not yet been presented for neo-cortical neurons.

This presentation points to the variety of cortical PSPs. Examples of spontaneous EPSPs and IPSPs will be shown and differences between PSPs elicited by transcallosal volleys, by VL-afferents and by antidromic stimulation will be demonstrated.

---

* Present address: Behaviour Research Institute, Gunma University Medical School, Maebashi-shiʾ Gunma (Japan).
** Present address: Abteilung für Neurophysiologie, Neurologische Universitätsklinik, Basel (Schweiz).

References p. 273

METHODS

The experiments were performed on nembutalized and curarized cats with the usual precautions for sufficient artificial respiration and temperature control. Intracellular recordings were made from the motor cortex (posterior lip of the precruciate gyrus) using essentially the same methods as those described earlier (Creutzfeldt *et al.*, 1964). Concentric stimulation electrodes were stereotactically placed into the nucleus ventralis lateralis (VL) of the thalamus, and bipolar electrodes into the pontine pyramidal tract. Three pairs of concentric electrodes were located on the contralateral motor cortex with one electrode corresponding to the homologous point of the ipsilateral recording site, and the two other electrodes about 2 mm from this point.

The responses were recorded on magnetic tape during the experiment and analysed later.

RESULTS

(a) Spontaneous post-synaptic potentials

Different spontaneous EPSPs are shown in Fig. 1. They are from the same cell and selected from a 2-h recording. Each type appeared repeatedly during all periods of the recording so that possible injury of the cell could not account for the differences.

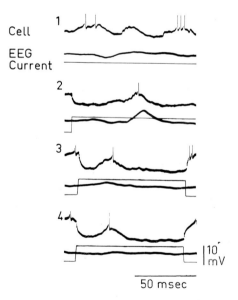

Fig. 1. Spontaneous EPSPs of a cortical nerve cell. Motor cortex, cat, nembutal anaesthesia. Selected examples from a 2-h recording. Action potential (about 30 mV) not fully shown. In 2–4 long polarizing current pulses are given in order to increase the firing threshold. (Recording of the current pulse: lower trace.) Middle trace, EEG. The records are selected with emphasis on the grouped EPSPs shown at about the middle of each trace. Note the clusters of fast "unitary" EPSPs in 1 and 2, the slow components in 3 and the smooth depolarization in 4.

Polarizing pulses of intracellularly applied current are given at 2-sec intervals in order to avoid too much firing. The EPSPs thus appeared less distorted by spikes. In this figure, the typical EPSPs are shown in order of increasingly smooth rising phases. In 1 and 2, the depolarizations in the middle of the traces are composed of a series of individual EPSPs which are well separated from each other. The individual EPSPs are steeper in 1 than in 2, but in both a considerable variability of rise times can be noted. It is reasonable to assume that both clusters of EPSPs are due to a discharge group of a single afferent fibre, and that each single step represents "unitary EPSPs" (Watanabe and Creutzfeldt, 1966; Burke, 1967) due to a single discharge of one fibre. If this be so, the variability of rise times within one cluster is worth noting. In Fig. 1, traces 3 and 4, smooth EPSPs are shown, in which smaller wavelets may be more or less clearly distinguished. Such smooth depolarizations can be of large or small amplitude. The shortest rise times of unitary EPSPs were only 1.5 msec, the longest could be 5–10 msec. Decay times of summed EPSPs did not depend on the rise times of the single unitary EPSPs or of the total rise time of compound EPSPs. As shown earlier, the rise time could not reliably be correlated with the amplitude (Watanabe and Creutzfeldt, 1966).

Spontaneous IPSPs showed a smaller variety of their rising slope but a considerable variability of their amplitude and duration. Fig. 2 shows some examples which are taken from the same cell as that in Fig. 1. In A, large rhythmical IPSPs are shown which follow clusters of rhythmical spike activity. The downward slopes show some

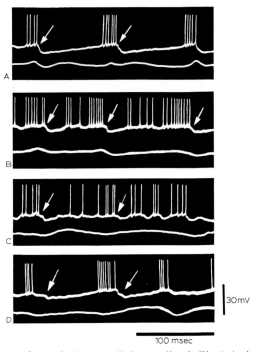

Fig. 2. Spontaneous IPSPs of a cortical nerve cell. Same cell as in Fig. 1. Action potentials retouched. The traces are selected in order to show IPSPs (arrows) of different duration (see text).

steps which indicate summation of several smaller IPSPs, although a superimposition of EPSPs belonging to the preceding excitatory burst cannot be ruled out completely. The return of the membrane potential is slow, the total duration of the IPSP about 70 msec. The IPSPs in B–C are smaller and shorter (20–30 msec in B, around 20 msec in C, and as short as 10–15 msec in D). The rise times did not differ considerably and were about 2 msec except in A. This also suggests that in A several IPSPs were superimposed resulting in a large compound IPSP.

(b) Evoked post-synaptic potentials

Post-synaptic potentials were evoked by electrical stimulation of the ventrolateral nucleus of the thalamus, the bulbar pyramid and the contralateral cortex (transcallosal stimulation). It was found that the EPSPs elicited by contralateral cortical stimulation (via the corpus callosum) had slower rise times than those elicited by VL stimulation or by stimulation of the bulbar pyramid. Examples from one cell are shown in Fig. 3. Weak single electrical stimuli applied to the homologous field of the contalateral hemisphere produced, after a latency of 8–10 msec, a slowly rising depolarization which reached the threshold after about 5 msec (Fig. 3A). When the cell was hyperpolarized so that the post-synaptic depolarization did not always reach the threshold (Fig. 3B), several irregular steps could be recognized on the rising slope. The peak was reached after 15–20 msec. If the stimulus intensity was increased, a short latency EPSP appeared which had a shorter rise time (1.5 msec) than that

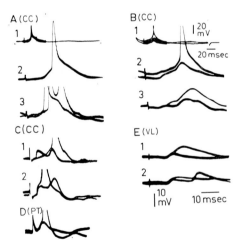

Fig. 3. EPSPs elicited by electrical stimulation of different afferents. Motor cortex, cat, nembutal anaesthesia. A and B, Weak, single electrical shocks to the homologous area of the contralateral cortex (transcallosal stimulation). Trace 1, slow record (time and calibration upper right corner); 2 and 3, different records with faster sweep speed (calibration and time below E). In B a weak polarizing pulse was given in order to show full development of callosal EPSP. C, Strong stimulation of the contralateral cortex provokes a short latency, sharp EPSP. In C1 a weak and strong stimulus are superimposed in order to show the difference in the responses. D, Stimulation of the bulbar pyramid (recurrent EPSP). E, EPSPs after weak VL stimulation without IPSP.

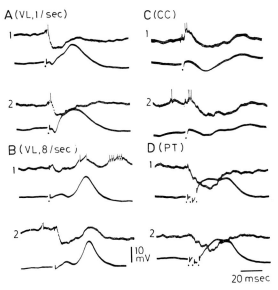

Fig. 4. Postsynaptic reactions after stimulation of different afferents. Cat, nembutal, motor cortex. Action potential (35 mV) not fully shown. Lower trace EEG. A, VL stimulation 1/sec. Short excitation cut off by early large IPSP. B, VL stimulation 8/sec. Note enhancement of secondary smooth EPSP ("augmenting EPSP") which was sometimes noted during 1/sec stimulation (A1). The initial EPSP is very small and does not lead to firing during 8/sec stimulus series. C, EPSP–IPSP sequence after callosal stimulation. Note the slow initial rise of the IPSP. D, IPSPs after repetitive stimulation of bulbar pyramids (dots below EEG record). Note the similarity of this composed IPSP to the transcallosal IPSP (in C).

evoked by weak stimulation (Fig. 3C; in C_1 a weak and a strong stimulus are superimposed). Pyramidal stimulation evoked in this cell a collateral EPSP whose rise time was 2 msec (Fig. 3D), and weak VL stimulation evoked an EPSP with a rise time of 3–3.5 msec, which may be followed by a second depolarizing potential of slower or slightly faster rise time (Fig. 3E, 1 and 2).

It is thus possible to demonstrate in this cell EPSPs of somewhat variable rise times and slope by stimulation of different inputs and intensity. Besides the rise times of the individual EPSPs which were probably of unitary nature, the summating behaviour was also different. The weak contralateral cortical stimulation led to a series of slowly summating EPSPs, the weak ventrolateral thalamic stimulus to one or two discrete EPSPs, and strong contralateral cortical as well as the antidromic pyramidal stimulus to one or two discrete EPSPs.

By ventrolateral thalamic stimulation two types of EPSPs could be elicited, especially if repetitive stimuli of the augmenting type were used (Klee and Offenloch, 1964; Nacimiento et al., 1964). An example is shown in Fig. 4. Single VL-stimuli (Fig. 4A) produced a short primary EPSP followed by an IPSP on which a slow depolarization may have been superimposed concomitant with a large negative wave in the EEG record. This secondary broad EPSP was enhanced at 8/sec stimulation (Fig. 4B), which also resulted in a typical augmenting response. The IPSP may be reduced during this rhythmic stimulation (Fig. $4B_1$; see also Nacimiento et al., 1964).

The difference between the primary and secondary EPSPs is clearly seen: the primary EPSP is small and has a rise time of 1.5 msec, which is best seen in Fig. 4B$_1$ where it is not cut off by the large IPSP; the secondary EPSP is larger and has a slow total rise time. Irregular bumps may sometimes suggest a compound potential composed of several unitary EPSPs (A$_2$, B$_2$), but the main depolarization consists mostly of a smooth depolarization.

IPSPs may have a steep or a flat initial slope. IPSPs with total rise times of 3–5 msec or less are easily elicited by strong thalamic (VL) or antidromic pyramidal stimulation (Albe-Fessard and Buser, 1953; Phillips, 1959; Nacimiento *et al.*, 1964). An example is shown in Fig. 4A. Contralateral stimulation as a rule evoked slowly starting IPSPs (Fig. 4C). Single steps on the falling slope could mostly be recognized. Similar "slow" IPSPs could also be produced by weak repetitive antidromic stimulation (Fig. 4D) although here the single steps were more pronounced. This suggests that the trans-callosal IPSP is composed of several single IPSPs summating over some time (15–20 msec).

DISCUSSION

(a) *Excitatory postsynaptic potentials*

Before EPSP shapes of cortical nerve cells can be interpreted with relation to elec-trotonic distortion, the question must be answered whether the recorded potentials are indeed due to discharges of single afferent or intracortical fibres. No one would, of course, expect that one single synapse on a dendritic spine would lead to a potential which might be discovered as a discrete potential change by an electrode situated in the soma. But it must be appreciated that afferent fibres as well as some intra-cortical fibres, establish a large number of contacts during their course parallel to the apical dendrite (Ramón y Cajal, 1952; Colonnier, 1966; Szentágothai, 1967). A discharge of one single fibre may therefore well lead to a discrete "unitary" po-tential as in motoneurons (Burke, 1967). Analysis of EPSPs of cells of the motor and visual cortex strongly supports the view that at least most of the discrete in-dividual EPSPs are due to the discharge of single afferent fibres (Watanabe and Creutzfeldt, 1966; Creutzfeldt and Ito, 1968). The grouped EPSPs in Fig. 1, records 1 and 2 of this paper may then be interpreted as being caused by discharge groups of single afferent fibres. But since the unitary EPSPs are composed of several local EPSPs with different distances from the soma (according to the multiple contacts of single afferents), a rigorous interpretation of these EPSPs on the basis of their shape index is not possible. All one can say is that they originated not far from the soma.

EPSPs like those shown in Fig. 1, records 3 and 4, pose similar problems of inter-pretation. They may either be due to the slightly asynchronous activity of many small EPSPs so that single steps cannot be discriminated, or they may also be due to the ac-tivity of individual fibres with multiple contacts far from the soma. An attempt was made to discriminate between these two possibilities by comparing the amplitude histo-grams during different degrees of polarization of the membrane potentials, but no clear conclusion was reached because of the large variability of amplitudes of such EPSPs. We are therefore only able to guess that these slow potentials are due to the grouped and temporally dispersed activity of many fibres each having possibly only a few contacts distant from the soma.

The interpretation of EPSPs evoked by stimulation of different fibre groups would be more promising if we knew the exact location of these afferents. Here the neurophysiologist needs the help of the neuroanatomist. In the motor cortex extensive studies in this direction have not been done to our knowledge. In the visual cortex, Globus and Scheibel (see Scheibel and Scheibel, 1968) assume that the specific afferents terminate on the central parts of the apical dendritic shafts, callosal afferents on the oblique branches of the apical dendrites and recurrent collaterals possibly on the basal dendrites. Should such an organization also exist in the motor cortex, one would expect sharp and distinct EPSPs after VL stimulation, flatter ones from the callosal afferents and steep EPSPs from recurrent collaterals. The results of our study indeed point in this direction but are not yet sufficient fully to prove this hypothesis Here again the question arises whether the clope of an individual EPSP is due to the degree of synchrony of several afferent EPSPs or to the location of fibre terminals responsible for one "unitary" EPSP. The collateral EPSPs after pyramidal tract stimulation showed an all-or-nothing behaviour and are thus probably due to the discharges of individual fibres. A location of their synapses close to the soma is therefore highly suggestive. Callosal EPSPs after weak contralateral cortical stimulation are mostly of composite nature. It is known from earlier extracellular studies (Creutzfeldt *et al.*, 1956) that single stimulation of the motor cortex with short shocks mostly evokes single, only sometimes double and rarely multiple, discharges. It is therefore probable that the broad composite EPSPs originate from several fibres converging on the same cell. However, the individual EPSPs are mostly flat and therefore may arise somewhat more distant from the soma. The short latency EPSP sometimes observed after strong contralateral cortex stimulation may be explained by the shortened latency of the cellular response under the stimulation electrode. But since this is not always seen with short pulses (Creutzfeldt *et al.*, 1956) it seems more probable that these short latency EPSPs after strong contralateral stimulation are due to antidromic excitation of transcallosal fibres, which invade the corresponding recurrent collaterals. Unfortunately, this was not further tested in our present experiments. In any case, the similarity of these short latency callosal EPSPs to the recurrent pyramidal EPSPs is obvious.

EPSPs after VL stimulation are mostly cut off by the subsequent IPSP. Only with weak stimulation, it is possible to obtain isolated single EPSPs. These are as a rule slightly steeper than callosal and flatter than antidromic EPSPs. This does not necessarily point to a more distant location of the VL synapses, but may be due to the slight temporal dispersion of the single synaptic potentials originating at each contact of the specific afferent thalamo-cortical fibre during its parallel course along the apical dendrite.

It is clear from these preliminary findings that a straightforward interpretation of cortical EPSPs in terms of the cable theory is not yet possible. It is altogether questionable whether a satisfactory theoretical analysis of cortical EPSPs in terms of the dendritic cable theory may be possible at all, because of the variable and complex geometry of nerve cells and of their synaptic contacts. This makes it impossible to expect a complete conformity between experimental results and theoretical treatment as could be demonstrated so elegantly for the end-plate potential in the muscle fibre by Fatt and Katz (1951). The "shape index" (Rall, 1967) of EPSPs therefore cannot be more than a qualitative suggestion. As such it may be helpful.

(b) Inhibitory postsynaptic potentials

Cortical IPSPs are known for their long duration (Creutzfeldt et al., 1966). The observations were made during experiments using electrical stimulation of cortical afferents or efferents. In the visual cortex it was shown recently that individual IPSPs may be as short as 15–20 msec (Creutzfeldt and Ito, 1968). Such short IPSPs can also be seen in motor cortex neurons during spontaneous activity and after weak electrical stimulation of afferents. This suggests that the "unitary" IPSP is much shorter than the large IPSP after stimulation of a great number of afferents (or recurrent collaterals). The graded changes in its amplitude and duration with stimulus strength of afferent pathways (Watanabe et al., 1966) also strongly suggest the composite nature of the large cortical IPSPs after strong stimulation. In our experiments the slope of the initial falling phase of IPSPs was different after stimulation of different afferents: it was steep after thalamic and strong antidromic pyramidal, but slow after contralateral stimulation. A slowly starting IPSP can also be produced by appropriate timing of weak pyramidal tract stimuli. The slow course of callosal IPSPs is therefore most easily explained by the temporal dispersion of the summating "unitary" IPSPs, which are caused by the poorly synchronized firing of the cortical cells after callosal stimulation. This would also imply a recurrent inhibitory mechanism for transcallosally evoked IPSPs, a hypothesis which is further supported by other characteristics of these IPSPs (publication in preparation). At present, there is no indication that the different slope of IPSPs may be due to a variable location of inhibitory synapses.

SUMMARY

In the anaesthetized cat, the post-synaptic activity of motor cortex cells was investigated intracellularly. Spontaneous EPSP's with different rise times and slopes were demonstrated and their possible origins at different sites of the dendritic membrane is discussed. EPSPs after electrical stimulation of the bulbar pyramid (antidromic stimulation), the nucleus VL of the thalamus and the contralateral cortex (transcallosal stimulation) were recorded. The rise time and slope of the single components of the composed EPSPs (unitary EPSPs) differed, recurrent PT–EPSPs being mostly shorter than VL–EPSPs. The "unitary" components of transcallosal EPSPs were longer than the VL– and PT–EPSPs, but with strong stimulation short latency steep EPSPs could be elicited which were interpreted as recurrent EPSPs due to antidromic stimulation of callosal fibres. The limitation of an interpretation of cortical EPSPs in terms of shape indices is discussed. Individual IPSPs can be of short duration (15–20 msec). The long-lasting IPSPs usually observed are composite in nature. Contralateral stimulation leads to slowly summating IPSPs. The different forms and shapes of cortical IPSPs can be satisfactorily explained by their summating behaviour. There is at present no reason to assume different sites of inhibitory synapses.

REFERENCES

ALBE-FESSARD, D., AND BUSER, P., (1953); Exploration de certaines activités du cortex moteur chez le chat par microélectrodes: dérivations endo-somatiques. *J. Physiol. (Paris)*, **45**, 14–16.

BURKE, R. E., (1967); Composite nature of the monosynaptic excitatory postsynaptic potential. *J. Neurophysiol.*, **30**, 1114–1137.

COLONNIER, M., (1966); The structural design of the neo-cortex. In: J. C. ECCLES (Ed.), *Brain and Conscious Experience*, Springer, Berlin, pp. 1–23.

CREUTZFELDT, O. D., AND ITO, M., (1968); Functional synaptic organization of primary visual cortex neurones in the cat. *Exp. Brain Res.*, **6**, 324–352.

CREUTZFELDT, O., AND LUX, H. D., (1964); Zur Unterscheidung von "spezifischen" und "unspezifischen" Synapsen an corticalen Nervenzellen. *Naturwissenschaften*, **51**, 89–90.

CREUTZFELDT, O., BAUMGARTNER, G., AND SCHOEN, C., (1956); Reaktionen einzelner Neurone des senso-motorischen Cortex nach elektrischen Reizen. *Arch. Psychiat. Nervenkr.*, **194**, 597–614.

CREUTZFELDT, O. D., LUX, H. D., AND NACIMIENTO, A. C., (1964); Intracelluläre Reizung corticaler Nervenzellen. *Pflügers Arch. ges. Physiol.*, **281**, 129–151.

CREUTZFELDT, O. D., LUX, H. D., AND WATANABE, S., (1966); Electrophysiology of cortical nerve cells. In: D. P. PURPURA AND M. D. YAHR (Eds.), *The Thalamus*, Columbia University Press, New York, pp. 209–235.

FATT, P., AND KATZ, B., (1951); An analysis of the end-plate potential recorded with an intracellular electrode. *J. Physiol. (Lond.)*, **115**, 320–270.

KLEE, M. R., AND OFFENLOCH, K., (1964); Post-synaptic potentials and spike patterns during augmenting responses in cat's motor cortex. *Science*, **143**, 488–489.

NACIMIENTO, A. C., LUX, H. D., AND CREUTZFELDT, O. D., (1964); Postsynaptische Potentiale von Nervenzellen des motorischen Cortex nach elektrischer Reizung spezifischer und unspezifischer Thalamuskerne. *Pflügers Arch. ges. Physiol.*, **281**, 152–169.

NELSON, P. G., AND FRANK, K., (1967); Anomalous rectification in cat spinal motoneurones and effect of polarizing currents on excitatory postsynaptic potential. *J. Neurophysiol.*, **30**, 1097–1113.

PHILLIPS, C. G., (1959); Actions of antidromic pyramidal volleys on single Betz cells in the cat. *Quart. J. exp. Physiol.*, **44**, 1–25.

RALL, W., (1967); Distinguishing theoretical synaptic potentials computed for different soma-dendritic distributions of synaptic input. *J. Neurophysiol.*, **30**, 1138–1169.

RAMÓN Y CAJAL, S., (1952); *Histologie du Système Nerveux de l'Homme et des Vertébrés.* Vol. II. Reedited by CSIC, Instituto Ramón y Cajal, Madrid.

SCHEIBEL, M. E., AND SCHEIBEL, A. B., (1968); On the nature of dendritic spines — Report of a work shop. *Commun. Behav. Biol., Part A*, **1**, 231–265.

SZENTÁGOTHAI, J., (1967); The anatomy of complex integrative units in the nervous system. In: K. LISSADE (Ed.), *Results in Neuroanatomy, Neurochemistry, Neuropharmacology and Neurophysiology*, Akademiai Kiado, Budapest, pp. 9–45.

WATANABE, S., AND CREUTZFELDT, O. D., (1966); Spontane post-synaptische Potentiale von Nervenzellen des motorischen Cortex der Katze. *Exp. Brain Res.*, **1**, 48–64.

WATANABE. S., KONISHI, M., AND CREUTZFELDT, O. D., (1966); Postsynaptic potentials in the cat's visual cortex following electrical stimulation of afferent pathways. *Exp. Brain Res.*, **1**, 272–283.

Electrical Coupling Between Myocardial Cells

S. WEIDMANN*

Department of Physiology, University of Berne (Switzerland)

The feeling may arise that the problems of cell-to-cell contact between cardiac cells, and between visual cells, are rather remote from the main topic of the present symposium. Nevertheless, the next three contributors hope to show that there are enough parallels to justify their presence at Einsiedeln.

In the days of light microscopy, morphologists had diverging views on the structure of the contacts between nerve cells. Held, as late as 1929, described protoplasmic continuity between nerve cells at the synaptic junctions (reticular theory). Cajal and many others (for references see Eccles, 1959), on the other hand, maintained that the nerve cell was an independent entity and that there was no structural continuity between cells. It was not until the advent of high resolution electron microscopy (Palade and Palay, 1954) that this controversy was finally settled in favour of Cajal. The divergence of views is hardly surprising since the two rival theories were based (as many theories are) on the interpretation of structures just beyond the resolving power of the scientific instruments then available (cit. from Katz, 1966).

For heart muscle the concept of a morphological syncytium was universally accepted, mainly on the ground of functional evidence. The law of "all-or-nothing excitability" as well as conduction without decrement made heart muscle comparable, from a functional point of view, to a single fibre of skeletal muscle or nerve. To the cardiac electrophysiologists, therefore, the demonstration by Sjöstrand and Andersson (1954) of *cytoplasmic discontinuity* at the level of the intercalated disks came as a somewhat unpleasant surprise. Either we would have to revise our concepts of propagation by local circuit currents; or alternatively, we would have to postulate that the two membranes in close contact have a much lower electrical resistance than a corresponding area of outside cell membrane.

ARGUMENTS IN FAVOUR OF HIGH-RESISTANCE JUNCTIONS

In a number of publications that appeared between 1960 and 1964 the Cleveland group (Hoshiko, Sperelakis, Berne, Tarr and Keller) have presented evidence in favour of the concept of functionally independent cells. The specific location of acetylcholinesterase near the disks (Joó and Csillik, 1962) added confidence to the

* Financial support was provided by grant 3535 of the Swiss National Science Foundation.

References p. 280–281

assumption that transmission from cell to cell was chemical in nature. The arguments by the Cleveland group will now be stated one at a time, together with the alternative explanations that can be provided for the Group's experimental findings. It is not expected that the evidence can be fully weighed by the reader without studying the original literature.

(1) Current is made to flow between the tips of two microelectrodes. Potential difference is recorded by the same microelectrodes. When one cell is impaled the polarization resistance is about 12 MΩ, when two cells are impaled it rises to 24 MΩ, suggesting that all current has to leave and re-enter the tissue (Sperelakis et al., 1960a).

The electrodes were inserted at a *minimal* distance of 500 μ into a three-dimensional network. Under these conditions most of the current would indeed flow out and in again through surface membranes rather than take the pathway from cell to cell, even if the junctional resistance were low.

(2) After ion depletion of the interspace (2 h in isotonic sucrose) the longitudinal resistance of cat ventricular strips is high, suggesting a high cell-to-cell resistance (Sperelakis and Hoshiko, 1961).

In smooth muscle it has been demonstrated that prolonged exposure to purified sucrose solution results in a gradual rise of the longitudinal resistance, suggesting electrical uncoupling of cellular junctions (Tomita, 1968); and in the salivary gland of the midge, cells become electrically isolated from one another when Ca ions are withdrawn from the extracellular medium (Loewenstein et al., 1967). It thus seems possible that at the end of 2 h in Ca-free solution cardiac cells actually become electrically isolated from each other.

(3) Hypertonic solutions deprive the frog ventricle of all-or-nothing conduction, suggesting a failure of (chemical ?) cell-to-cell transmission (Sperelakis et al., 1960b).

In frog auricle that has been treated by hypertonic solutions the electron microscope reveals that the cell-to-cell junctions are disrupted. These structural changes are reversible and conduction can be re-established in normotonic solutions (Barr et al., 1965).

(4) When cat papillary muscle is stimulated by an electric field of longitudinally flowing current, all the cells are excited simultaneously (Sperelakis, 1963).

When this experiment is repeated with strands of parallel fibres from sheep ventricle, excitation does not occur simultaneously if currents of moderate strength are used (1–10 times threshold). These produce depolarization only at the end near the cathode, the excitation starting near the cathode and reaching the other end of the muscle strand by propagation. On the other hand, currents of more than 10 times threshold will initiate action potentials in other parts of the preparation (Weidmann, unpublished). This is theoretically possible if the bundle does not consist of ideally parallel fibres.

(5) If strips of frog ventricle are kept in Ca-free and Mg-free Ringer solution and strong electric fields (2–5 V/cm) are applied in a longitudinal direction, intracellular action potentials may be broken up into two components: spikes and slow waves. The possibility of splitting up the action potential suggests that the spike is generated at the "outside membrane", the slow wave or plateau at the junctional

membrane (Hoshiko and Sperelakis, 1962). However, Ca-free solution breaks up cell-to-cell contacts in varying degrees (Barr et al., 1965), and may produce leak currents. This may produce repolarization since a relatively small amount of additional outward current is required to cut short an action potential immediately after its peak (cf. discussion by Pillat, 1964), even in a preparation under seemingly normal conditions.

(6) Frog ventricular strips in Ca-free, Mg-rich (6–30 mM) solution, when treated with a longitudinal flow of direct current for several minutes, propagate action potentials in one direction only, from the former cathode to the former anode (Hoshiko and Sperelakis, 1961). It is assumed that current entry through the junctional membrane into the cell causes less damage to the mechanism of transmitter release than current exit at the other end of the individual cell.

An alternative explanation for these findings is that the longitudinal current transforms the membranes at the cell junctions into rectifying membranes. Admittedly, neither of these explanations is readily acceptable.

(7) Cardiac cells in tissue cultures may show slow diastolic potentials (pacemaker potentials) and spontaneous firing. The size of the pacemaker potentials can be influenced by current introduced into one cell by means of a microelectrode. This result is taken to signify that pacemaker potentials are post-synaptic potentials (Sperelakis and Lehmkuhl, 1964).

If it be assumed that the cluster of cells is the electrical unit rather than the single cell these results can equally well be accounted for. There will be electrical interaction between the part of the preparation near the current electrode and other parts which also have a tendency for generating pacemaker potentials.

(8) In cat papillary muscle, when current is injected by an intracellular electrode and potential is recorded by this and a second intracellular electrode, the amplitudes of the electrotonic potentials are either comparable (tips in same cell?) or the second electrode practically picks up no voltage change (tips in different cells?). While this result would seem to provide rather direct evidence in favour of high-resistance cell-to-cell contacts (Tarr and Sperelakis, 1964), several authors describing similar experiments find electrotonic potentials of well-measurable amplitude at distances from the polarizing intracellular electrode corresponding to several cell lengths (Woodbury and Crill, 1961; Tille, 1966; Tanaka and Sasaki, 1966). Here we are up against a difference in results rather than a divergence of possible explanations.

ARGUMENTS IN FAVOUR OF LOW-RESISTANCE JUNCTIONS

If two electrodes lead off from the surface of a heart, and if the tissue under one of them is damaged, a potential difference (injury potential) is recorded (Engelmann, 1877). In a few minutes this potential difference disappears. Engelmann assumes a process of "healing over" of the damaged fibres.

An alternative explanation to Engelmann's results is provided by Rothschuh (1951). Having performed essentially the same experiment, he proposes high-resistance

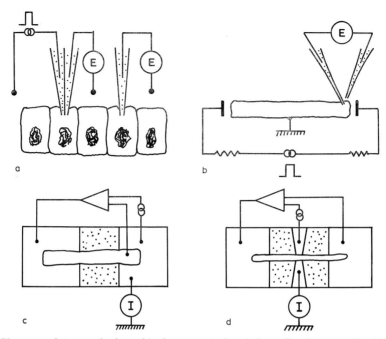

Fig. 1. Upper panel: two methods used to demonstrate electrical coupling between cells. (a) Epithelial gland; measurement of amplitude of electrotonic potential at various distances (Loewenstein *et al.*, 1967). (b) Bundle of cardiac fibres in a longitudinal electric field; measurement of decay of electrotonic potential from a healed-over end of the bundle (Weidmann, 1969). Lower panel: two methods used to displace the membrane potential to a new steady value (voltage clamp) and measure the corresponding current. Isotonic sucrose solution is used to minimize current flow through an extracellular pathway. (c) single gap and intracellular voltage control (Giebisch and Weidmann, 1967). (d) Double gap and extracellular voltage control (Rougier *et al.*, 1968).

intercalated disks and assumes that the damaged cells alone generate the injury current which disappears as soon as the cells are discharged.

(*2*) Ventricular "Purkinje fibres" or "Purkinje strands" of ungulates contain several Purkinje cells on their cross section. From cable analysis it is concluded that the inside longitudinal resistance of a "fibre" is so low (2–3 times that of Tyrode solution) that cell-to-cell contacts must be of the low-resistance type (Weidmann, 1952, 1969).

No doubts seem to exist as far as Purkinje fibres are concerned; but the question remains whether the situation is the same in ordinary myocardial fibres.

(*3*) When current is made to flow through bundles of mammalian *ventricular* fibres (Fig. 1b) the space constant (λ), *i.e.* the distance over which the electrotonic potential falls by a factor of e, is of the order of 1 mm. With a cell length of about 125 μ this result is possible only if the cell-to-cell resistance is low (Kavaler, 1959; Kamiyama and Matsuda, 1966; Weidmann, 1969).

(*4*) The method of "voltage-clamp" has successfully been applied to bundles of fibres of the frog auricle (Rougier *et al.*, 1968; Fig. 1c) and of the mammalian ventricle (Giebisch and Weidmann, 1967; Morad and Trautwein, 1968; Fig. 1d). The "clamped" part of the bundle has a length several times that of a single cell. The spatial distribution of the imposed potential change is almost uniform which is only possible if cells are electrically connected by a low-resistance pathway.

(5) When one half of a bundle of ventricular fibres is exposed to ^{42}K-Tyrode and the other half is continuously washed by radio-inactive Tyrode, a steady-state with respect to tissue ^{42}K is reached in about 6 h (Weidmann, 1966). The "washed" half of the bundle contains a considerable amount of radio-potassium. The results are explained on the assumption that ^{42}K is taken up into the fibres from the radio-active solution and diffuses to the other half of the bundle within the myoplasm and across low-resistance intercalated disks. A quantitative treatment of the data suggests that the permeability of the disk is about 5000 times greater than the permeability of the surface membrane to outward movement of ^{42}K.

The diffusion experiments (Weidmann, 1966) are open to the criticism that ^{42}K might have moved in the extracellular space, whence it might have been taken up into the myoplasm (Sperelakis, personal communication).

(6) When a mid-portion of a frog auricular bundle is in sucrose, its two ends being kept in Ringer, conduction fails (Barr *et al.*, 1965). Transmission can be re-established by connecting the two Ringer pools by a low ohmic resistance. This is the classical experiment to demonstrate propagation by local circuit currents (Osterhout and Hill, 1930).

A PERSONAL OPINION

By 1954 morphologists had demonstrated beyond all doubt that heart muscle is not a syncytium. It was then quite natural to ask whether our concept of impulse conduction was still tenable, or whether long-standing ideas had to be revised.

Weighing all the evidence for and against low cell-to-cell resistance, it seems permissible to conclude that cells are connected by low-resistance junctions, and that we may once more safely think about heart muscle *as if it were* a syncytium.

OTHER INSTANCES OF LOW-RESISTANCE CELL-TO-CELL CONTACTS

Up to 1959 the humoral mechanism was the universally accepted answer to the problem of synaptic transmission. Then Furshpan and Potter described a particular synapse (giant motor synapse of the crayfish) in which the electrical resistance between the pre- and the postsynaptic cells is low. Other examples soon followed. Bennett (1968) in a recent review lists no less than 12 examples in which electrical coupling has been demonstrated in vertebrate synapses.

In a variety of other tissues it has been shown that cells are connected by low-resistance junctions (Table I). The evidence for this rests either on electrical techniques (*e.g.* Loewenstein *et al.*, 1967; Fig. 1a) or on the micro-injection of a dye into a single cell, and the observation of its diffusion into neighbouring cells (Potter *et al.*, 1966).

The functional significance of a low-resistance pathway in cardiac and smooth muscle, or at a synapse, is evident, for it allows electrical transmission. In epithelia and epithelial glands the close contact between cells of a whole layer will effectively

TABEL I

EXAMPLES OF LOW-RESISTANCE CELL-TO-CELL CONTACTS

Selected references excluding heart muscle and electrical synapses

Tissue	Authors
Whole embryo of the squid	Potter et al., 1966
Glia cells	Kuffler, 1967
Liver cells	Loewenstein and Kanno, 1967
Intestinal smooth muscle	Nagai and Prosser, 1963
Somatic smooth muscle	DeBell et al., 1963
Skin epithelium	Loewenstein and Penn, 1967
Salivary gland cells	Loewenstein et al., 1967
Kidney tubular epithelial cells	Giebisch, 1968
Urinary bladder epithelial cells	Loewenstein et al., 1965
Ampullary canal of Lorenzini	Waltman, 1966
Visual cells	Smith and Bauman, 1969 (this symposium, p. 313)

increase the resistance to diffusion through the intercellular space, thus preventing the back-diffusion of the ions or molecules that have been transported by a "pump" mechanism. The significance of low-resistance pathways between glia cells and between liver cells remains, at present, somewhat less obvious.

REFERENCES

BARR, L., DEWEY, M. M., AND BERGER, W., (1965); Propagation of action potentials and the structure of the nexus in cardiac muscle. J. gen. Physiol., 48, 797–823.

BENNETT, M. V. L., (1968); Similarities between chemically and electrically mediated transmission. In F. D. CARLSON (Ed.), Physiological and Biochemical Aspects of Nerve Interaction, Prentice-Hall, Englewood Cliffs, N.J.

DEBELL, J. T., DEL CASTILLO, J., AND SANCHEZ, V., (1963); Electrophysiology of the somatic muscle cells of Ascaris lumbricoides. J. cell. comp. Physiol., 62, 159–177.

ECCLES, J. C., (1959); The development of ideas on the synapse. In: C. McC. BROOKS AND P. F. CRANEFIELD (Eds.), The Historical Development of Physiological Thought, Hafner, New York.

ENGELMANN, T. W., (1877); Vergleichende Untersuchungen zur Lehre von der Muskel- und Nerven elektricität. Pflügers Arch. ges. Physiol., 15, 116–148.

FURSHPAN, E. J., AND POTTER, D. D., (1959); Transmission at the giant motor synapses of the cray-fish, J. Physiol. (Lond.), 145, 289–325.

GIEBISCH, G., (1968); Some electrical properties of single renal tubule cells. J. gen. Physiol., 51, 315s–325s.

GIEBISCH, G., AND WEIDMANN, S., (1967); Membrane currents in mammalian ventricular heart muscle fibres using a "voltage clamp" technique. Helv. physiol. pharmacol. Acta, 25, CR 189–CR 190.

HOSHIKO, T., AND SPERELAKIS, N., (1961); Prepotentials and unidirectional propagation in myo-cardium. Am. J. Physiol., 201, 873–880.

HOSHIKO, T., AND SPERELAKIS, N., (1962); Components of the cardiac action potential. Am. J. Physiol., 203, 258–260.

JOÓ, F., AND CSILLIK, B., (1962); Cholinesterase activity of intercalated disks in mammalian heart muscle. Nature (Lond.), 193, 1192–1193.

KAMIYAMA, A., AND MATSUDA, K., (1966); Electrophysiological properties of the canine ventricular fiber, Jap. J. Physiol., 16, 407–420.

KATZ, B., (1966); Nerve, Muscle and Synapse. McGraw-Hill, New York.

KAVALER, F., (1959); Membrane depolarization as a cause of tension development in mammalian ventricular muscle. *Am. J. Physiol.*, **197**, 968–970.

KUFFLER, S. W., (1967); Neuroglial cells: physiological properties and a potassium mediated effect of neuronal activity on the glial membrane potential. *Proc. Roy. Soc. B*, **13**, 168, 1–21.

LOEWENSTEIN, W. R., AND KANNO, Y., (1967); Intercellular communication and tissue growth. I. Cancerous growth. *J. Cell Biol.*, **33**, 225–234.

LOEWENSTEIN, W. R., AND PENN, R. D., (1967); Intercellular communication and tissue growth. II. Tissue regeneration. *J. Cell Biol.*, **33**, 235–242.

LOEWENSTEIN, W. R., SOCOLAR, S. J., HIGASHINO, S., KANNO, Y., AND DAVIDSON, N., (1965); Intercellular communication: renal, urinary bladder, sensory and salivary gland cells, *Science*, **149**, 295–298.

LOEWENSTEIN, W. R., NAKAS, M., AND SOCOLAR, S. J., (1967); Junctional membrane uncoupling. Permeability transformations at a cell membrane junction. *J. gen. Physiol.*, **50**, 1865–1891.

MORAD, M., AND TRAUTWEIN, W., (1968); The effect of the duration of the action potential on contraction in the mammalian heart muscle. *Pflügers Arch. ges. Physiol.*, **299**, 66–82.

NAGAI, T., AND PROSSER, C. L., (1963); Electrical parameters of smooth muscle cells. *Am. J. Physiol.*, **204**, 915–924.

OSTERHOUT, W. J. V., AND HILL, S. E., (1930); Salt bridges and negative variations. *J. gen. Physiol.*, **13**, 547–552.

PALADE, G. E., AND PALAY, S. L., (1954); Electron microscope observations of interneuronal and neuromuscular synapses. *Anat. Rec.*, **118**, 335–336.

PILLAT, B., (1964); Über eine abnormale Verkürzung des Aktionspotentials in der relativen Refraktärphase des Herzmuskels, *Pflügers Arch. ges. Physiol.*, **280**, 326–332.

POTTER, D. D., FURSHPAN, E. J., AND LENNOX, E. S., (1966); Connections between cells of the developing squid as revealed by electrophysiological methods. *Proc. Natl. Acad. Sci. (U.S.)*, **55**, 328–336.

ROTHSCHUH, K. E., (1951); Über den funktionellen Aufbau des Herzens aus elektrophysiologischen Elementen und über den Mechanismus der Erregungsleitung im Herzen. *Pflügers Arch. ges. Physiol.*, **253**, 238–251.

ROUGIER, O., VASSORT, G., AND STÄMPFLI, R., (1968); Voltage clamp experiments of frog atrial heart muscle fibres with the sucrose gap technique. *Pflügers Arch. ges. Physiol.*, **301**, 91–108.

SJÖSTRAND, F. S., AND ANDERSSON, E., (1954); Electron microscopy of the intercalated discs of cardiac muscle tissue. *Experientia (Basel)*, **10**, 369–370.

SPERELAKIS, N., (1963); Additional evidence for high-resistance intercalated discs in the myocardium. *Circulat. Res.*, **12**, 676–683.

SPERELAKIS, N., AND HOSHIKO, T., (1961); Electrical impedance of cardiac muscle. *Circulat. Res.*, **9**, 1280–1283.

SPERELAKIS, N., AND LEHMKUHL, D., (1964); Effect of current on transmembrane potentials in cultured chick heart cells. *J. gen. Physiol.*, **47**, 895–927.

SPERELAKIS, N., HOSHIKO, T., AND BERNE, R. M., (1960a); Nonsyncytial nature of cardiac muscle: membrane resistance of single cells. *Am. J. Physiol.*, **198**, 531–536.

SPERELAKIS, N., HOSHIKO, T., KELLER, R. F., AND BERNE, R. M., (1960b); Intracellular and external recording from frog ventricular fibers during hypertonic perfusion. *Am. J. Physiol.*, **198**, 135–140.

TANAKA, I., AND SASAKI, Y., (1966); On the electrotonic spread in cardiac muscle of the mouse, *J. gen. Physiol.*, **49**, 1089–1110.

TARR, M., AND SPERELAKIS, N., (1964); Weak electrotonic interaction between contiguous cardiac cells. *Am. J. Physiol.*, **207**, 691–700.

TILLE, J. (1966); Electrotonic interaction between muscle fibres in rabbit ventricle. *J. gen. Physiol.*, **50**, 189–202.

TOMITA, T., (1969); The longitudinal tissue impedance of smooth muscle of guinea pig taenia coli. *J. Physiol. (Lond.)*, in the press.

WALTMAN, B., (1966); Electrical properties and fine structure of the ampullary canals of Lorenzini. *Acta physiol. scand., Suppl.*, **264**, 1–60.

WEIDMANN, S., (1952); The electrical constants of Purkinje fibres, *J. Physiol. (Lond.)*, **118**, 348–360.

WEIDMANN, S., (1966); The diffusion of radiopotassium across intercalated disks of mammalian cardiac muscle. *J. Physiol. (Lond.)*, **187**, 323–342.

WEIDMANN, S., (1969); Electrical constants of trabecular muscle from mammalian heart. In preparation.

WOODBURY, J. W., AND CRILL, W. E., (1961); On the problem of impulse conduction in the atrium. In: *Nervous Inhibition*, Pergamon, Oxford, pp. 124–135.

Homo- and Heterocellular Junctions in Cell Cultures:
An Electrophysiological and Morphological Study*

A. HYDE, B. BLONDEL, A. MATTER, J. P. CHENEVAL, B. FILLOUX
AND L. GIRARDIER

Departments of Physiology and Histology, University of Geneva (Switzerland)

INTRODUCTION

In the preceding contribution to this symposium, Weidmann has extensively discussed the problem of electrotonic coupling between cells of the cardiac Purkinje fibres and between cells of the myocardium proper. For both these tissues, there seems to remain little doubt that low-resistance intercellular junctions subserve the function of cell-to-cell propagation of excitation. Weidmann also gave some examples of other tissues in which evidence of electrotonic junctions has been found, and in which the role of electrotonic coupling does not seem to lie in the conduction of electrical signals. One can reasonably assume that, if electrotonic coupling is due to the presence of low-resistance connections between cells, then it will probably be associated with some degree of metabolic interaction between the interconnected cells, since the latters' ionic and micromolecular concentrations will tend to equalize across the junction. It seems fairly well established that the intracellular concentrations and movements of cations are fundamental to organic metabolism and cell permeability control, at least in certain tissues (Mosinger and Kujalova, 1966; Ho and Jeanrenaud, 1967; Letarte and Renold, 1967; Clausen *et al.*, 1968). In this context, it would seem highly interesting to study the properties of heterocellular junctions exhibiting electrotonic coupling.

Preparations containing such junctions can easily be obtained by culturing trypsin-dispersed heart cells. The cultures contain a mixture of cardiac myoblasts and fibroblasts in various proportions. Electrotonic coupling is regularly found between myoblast and myoblast, as was to be expected, and also, although to a lesser degree, between myoblast and fibroblast, and between fibroblast and fibroblast. Thus, cultures of cardiac cells offer the opportunity of investigating the properties of three functionally distinct types of junction.

A purely morphological comparison of myoblast–myoblast (M–M) junctions on the one hand, and of myoblast–fibroblast (M–F) and fibroblast–fibroblast (F–F) junctions on the other hand, suggested that the tighter electrotonic coupling found in the former was merely due to the lower resistance of the junctions between myo-

* This work was financially supported by the Swiss National Foundation for Scientific Research.

blasts. Indeed, large areas of tight apposition of membranes (nexuses) are readily found at M–M junctions, whilst at M–F and F–F junctions, only locally restricted contacts of the membranes are seen. However, a detailed analysis of the electro-physiological data showed that the situation was not quite so simple, and that the greater effectiveness of the M–M coupling was to a considerable extent due to the higher specific resistance of non-junctional membrane in these cells.

Furthermore, cultures containing a mixture of fibro- and myoblasts suggest that the metabolism of a cell can effectively be modified by the presence of low-resistance junctions connecting it to a neighbouring cell of a different type, since the membrane potential of fibroblasts is no less than 3 times higher in a culture containing myoblasts than in a pure fibroblast culture.

MATERIALS AND METHODS

(a) Cultures

(1) Culturing technique

The culturing technique was adapted from those described by earlier investigators (Fänge *et al.*, 1957; Crill *et al.*, 1959; Harary and Farley, 1963; Lehmkuhl and Spere-lakis, 1963; Mark and Strasser, 1966). The hearts of approximately a dozen 2- to 7-day-old Charles River rats of both sexes were excised as aseptically as possible, and minced together down to fragments 0.5–1 mm in diameter. The fragments were washed for two consecutive periods of 5 min in sterile phosphate buffer solution (PBS) (Dulbecco and Vogt, 1954) with gentle magnetic stirring. The PBS was then sucked off and discarded, and the fragments were resuspended in 10 ml of pre-warmed trypsin solution (0.25% trypsin in Ca^{2+}- and Mg^{2+}-free buffered saline). The vessel was placed in an incubator at 37° over a magnetic stirrer and left there for 10 min, during which time dissociation of cells took place. After 10 min the vessel was taken out of the incubator, the fragments were allowed to settle on the bottom, and the cloudy supernatant, containing a mixture of isolated fibro- and myoblasts, was gently sucked off, and either placed in a centrifuge tube with 5 ml cold culture medium, or discarded. The fragments of heart tissue were subjected to 8 such periods of trypsin digestion, and the resulting fractions were numbered in chronological order. The fractions retained for culturing were then centrifuged at approximately 1300 g for 5 min. The supernatant was discarded, and the pellets were resuspended in culture medium by gently sucking them up and down a large-bore pipette, pooled, and distributed in 6-ml aliquots into sterile polystyrene Petri dishes.

12 hearts usually provided an adequate inoculum for 6 dishes. The cultures were incubated at 37° with automatic pH control (pH maintained at 7.4 ± 0.05 by CO_2 in air against 7.1 mM HCO_3^-). 24 h later, the cultures were washed with warm PBS, in order to remove cells which had not become attached to the dish, and given 6 ml of fresh medium. Thereafter, medium renewals took place regularly at 48-h intervals.

The culture medium used in these experiments was Eagle's minimum essential medium (M.E.M. Powder Medium, Gibco) supplemented with 0.3 w/v lactalbumin hydrolysate + yeast extract (Difco Laboratories) and 10% v/v calf serum. As mentioned above, the pH was buffered by 7.1 mM NaHCO$_3$ against CO$_2$ in air. The osmolality of the complete medium, as determined by the freezing point method, was 270 mOsm/kg, and its ionic composition was as follows.

Cations (mequiv./l)		Anions (mequiv./l)	
Na$^+$	148	Cl$^-$	127.21
K$^+$	5.36	HPO$_4^{2-}$	0.95
Ca^{2+}	0.90	HCO$_3^-$	7.1
Mg^{2+}	0.48	Organic (amino acids etc.)	19.48

(2) Purification technique

Selection of the trypsinization fractions which were to be cultured or discarded was determined by the cell type desired. Fraction 1 was always discarded, since it mostly contained cellular debris.

Mixed cultures. When mixed cultures, containing at the outset approximately equal proportions of fibro- and myoblasts, were desired, all fractions except the first were retained for culturing.

Myoblast-enriched cultures. Predominantly myoblastic cultures were obtained by taking the hearts of 2-day-old rats, and by discarding the first 3 trypsinization fractions, which mostly contained fibroblasts. In addition, advantage was taken of the fact that fibroblasts became attached to the plastic dishes within 2–3 h after being placed in the incubator, while myoblasts required a longer period. The highest degree of myoblast enrichment was reached by decanting the cell suspension into fresh dishes after about 3 h in the incubator, since by that time most of the fibroblasts had firmly adhered to the initial dish, whereas the myoblasts were still floating free in the medium. In the most successful experiments, the degree of purity of myoblast cultures exceeded 95% for the first 3 days. However, mitotic activity is much higher in fibroblasts than in myoblasts (Mark and Strasser, 1966), so that after 5–6 days of incubation the degree of purity fell to about 50%. Hence the need for very large inocula, if one wishes a myoblast culture to attain confluence before the inevitable fibroblast contaminants have pervaded the culture to an intolerable degree. A more detailed account of the purification technique will appear elsewhere (Blondel *et al.*, 1969).

Fibroblast-enriched cultures. When predominantly fibroblastic cultures were desired, 6–7-day-old rats were selected, and only fractions 2 and 3 were cultured. After 3 h in the incubator, the medium, together with the unattached myoblasts, was discarded, and replaced by fresh medium.

(b) Intracellular recordings

The recording system consisted of 2 conventional micropipettes filled with 3 M KCl (15–30 MΩ resistance) mounted on 2 separate micromanipulators. Each microelectrode was connected *via* an Ag–AgCl wire to the central terminal of an independently mounted 3-terminal mercury switch, of which the 2 remaining terminals were connected respectively to a stimulus isolation unit, and to the input of a preamplifier with input capacity neutralization, an input resistance greater than $10^{12}\,\Omega$, and a grid current smaller than 10^{-13} A (M. J. Richez, Electronics Laboratory of the Faculty of Medicine, Geneva). With this arrangement, each microelectrode could be used alternatively to record transmembrane potential or to deliver current pulses, while at all times remaining intracellular. It was often possible to leave one of the microelectrodes in the same cell for over an hour without depolarizing it. The extracellular fluid was earthed through the 50 Ω output resistance of a calibration unit.

Square current pulses were delivered to the preparation through a stimulus isolation unit, a $10^8\,\Omega$ series resistance to ensure current constancy, and the input of a current monitor. The absence of interelectrode coupling was ascertained by routine checking.

The cells were observed through a phase-contrast microscope, with a total magnification of 500 $\times$. This proved sufficient to exclude confusion between fibroblasts and myoblasts, even when the latter happened to be quiescent.

(c) Experimental procedure

All impalements were carried out on confluent cultures in culture medium, at 30–32°.

At the outset, the mercury switches were in the "record" position, and remained so until both electrodes recorded almost identical resting and action potential amplitudes. One of the switches was then flipped into the "current" position, and hyper- or depolarizing pulses of current (5–20 nA, 120 msec duration) were passed through the corresponding microelectrode, while the other recorded the potential change across the membrane of the other impaled cell, some distance away. After a photograph of the electrotonic potential had been taken, the situation was reversed, and another record was taken. Finally, both microelectrodes were switched to the "record" position, and a control photograph was taken, in order to ascertain that neither cell had depolarized during the procedure. Records of impalements during which one or both cells depolarized by more than 5 mV were discarded. The distance between the two microelectrode tips was estimated with an eyepiece graticule. One of the microelectrodes was then withdrawn and inserted into another cell, and the whole procedure was repeated as many times as necessary to explore the field under observation. The interelectrode distances ranged from 3 to 400 μ. Only photographs on which the current pulse terminated just before the upstroke of an action potential were analyzed. When enough points had been obtained, the culture was fixed, dehydrated, and embedded according to the technique described by Matter *et al.* (1969). Semi-thin sections were cut perpendicular to the plane of the culture, and photographed through a phase-contrast microscope, in order to estimate the average thickness of the culture, which was based on at least 30 measurements at randomly selected points on the culture.

THEORY

A model had to be developed to permit interpretation of the measured input resistance in terms of the specific membrane resistance and of the lumped specific resistance of the intracellular medium. A sheet of cultured cells should be reasonably well described by a two-dimensional model, and the external medium can be made of negligible resistance by leaving a 3-mm layer of liquid over the cells, thus fulfilling two simplifying assumptions often made in describing electrotonic spread in heart muscle. The major difficulty arises in defining the geometry of the connections between cells, since identification of low-resistance junctions is impossible to ascertain morphologically as well as topographically without the help of the electron microscope.

Fortunately, the geometrical factor turns out to be of secondary importance. Four geometrically different models have been described (Woodbury and Crill, 1961; George, 1961; Tanaka and Sasaki, 1966), and all four lead to equations of the same form for the distribution of electrotonic potential as a function of the distance between the current electrode and the recording electrode.

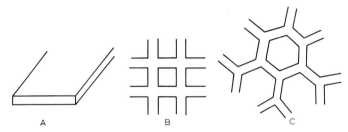

Scheme 1. A, 'Sandwich' model, Woodbury and Crill (1961). B, Rectangular lattice model, Tanaka and Sasaki (1966). C, Bifurcating lattice model, George (1961).

In steady state conditions, each of these models can be described by the differential equation

$$\frac{\mathrm{d}^2 V_{(r)}}{\mathrm{d}r^2} + \frac{1}{r} \cdot \frac{\mathrm{d}V_{(r)}}{\mathrm{d}r} - \frac{1}{\lambda^2} \cdot V_{(r)} = 0 \tag{1}$$

where r is the distance between the current electrode (at $r = 0$) and the recording electrode, $V_{(r)}$ is the potential at distance r, and λ the attenuation length, a constant which has to be defined for each model. The derivation of eqn. (1) for the "sandwich" model is given in the appendix (p. 306). The definition of λ in this case is

$$\lambda^2 = \frac{R_l \cdot d}{R_i}$$

where R_l = leakage resistance of a cm² of culture (Ωcm²)

$\quad R_i$ = specific resistance of intracellular medium, lumped for myoplasm and intercellular connections (Ωcm)

$\quad d$ = thickness of the sheet of cells (cm)

The suitable solution of eqn. (1) is a modified Bessel function (eqn. 11 in the Appendix). By a simple curve-fitting procedure described in the Appendix, the values of R_l and R_i can be estimated from the measured electrotonic spread of potential.

RESULTS

(a) Contractile behaviour

In mixed and myoblast-enriched cultures, spontaneous, rhythmic beating was always observed 24 h after culturing. At first, as reported by others (Harary and Farley, 1963; Lehmkuhl and Sperelakis, 1963; Mark and Strasser, 1966), individual cells or cell clusters beat at independent frequencies, but within 2–3 days in our conditions, as the cultures tended towards complete confluence, contractions became synchronous throughout. Complete confluence was achieved between 3 and 6 days after culturing, depending upon the density of viable cells in the initial inoculum. By the time mixed cultures had attained complete confluence, they contained approximately equal proportions of both cell types. The myoblasts tended to assemble in roughly circular clusters, whereas the fibroblasts filled in the empty spaces between the myoblast communities. In general each cluster of myoblasts was in contact with neighbouring clusters through one or more strands of myoblasts, and the whole myoblast population of the culture contracted simultaneously. Occasionally a cluster was found completely surrounded by fibroblasts. These isolated clusters also contracted synchronously with the remainder of the myoblast population. It was observed in young, mixed cultures, which had not yet reached complete confluence, that a pair of myoblasts which did not appear to touch each other, and which did not make contact with other myoblasts, beat synchronously provided a fibroblast was interposed between them. This finding is similar to the observations of Mark and Strasser (1966). At all temperatures between 37 and 30°, the frequency of spontaneous contractions was lower in mixed cultures than in "pure" myoblast cultures. This may be because mixed cultures were usually obtained from slightly older rats than "pure" myoblast cultures.

Occasionally, a solitary group of 2–3 myoblasts was found in a fibroblast-enriched culture. In that event, the myoblasts were either completely quiescent, or showed weak, sluggish contractions.

(b) Electrophysiology

(1) Myoblasts in "pure" cultures

A series of records obtained from a successful impalement of 2 myoblasts belonging to an almost pure myoblast culture (fibroblast contaminants estimated at less than 5%) is shown in Fig. 1. As can be seen on the first and last photographs of the series, the resting potentials of both cells were practically identical throughout the impalement. Resting potential values ranged from —55 to —75 mV (mean 63 $\pm$ 9.5 mV S.D.). The membrane potential during "diastole" was usually flat, but occasionally showed slow diastolic depolarization, as well as the rounded upstrokes of action

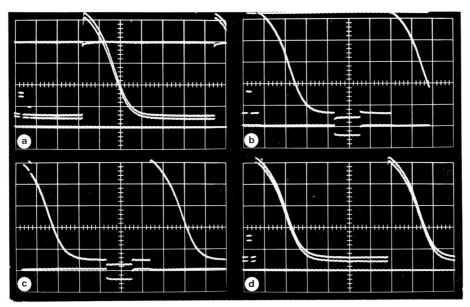

Fig. 1. Example of a set of transmembrane potential records obtained from a pair of cultured myo-blasts in a pure culture. The interelectrode distance was 50 μ. Frames a and d show the quasi-equality of the membrane potentials of both cells, before and after current had been passed respectively. Frames b and c show the electrotonic potentials when a square pulse of hyperpolarizing current (9 nA, 120 msec, bottom trace) was passed in succession through the two microelectrodes. Potential calibration pulse in all frames: 20 mV, 20 msec. O potential was one major division below the upper border of the graticule.

potentials typically associated with pacemaker activity. Pacemaker activity in cultured heart cells has already been reported by several authors (Lehmkuhl and Sperelakis, 1963; Crill *et al.*, 1959; Fänge *et al.*, 1957). In any given experiment, no more than 2–3 different cell clusters could be explored. Under these conditions it was observed that if one myoblast in a cluster displayed pacemaker activity, then the whole cluster showed the same behaviour. On the other hand, in most cultures it was difficult to locate the pacemaker even when as many as 50 impalements were made. Slow diastolic depolarization without rounded upstrokes of action potentials, indicative of driven cells with latent pacemaker potentiality, were also occasionally observed. The average resting potential of non-pacemaker cells was 62 mV ($n = 20$), that of pacemaker cells was 59 mV ($n = 38$), and that of latent pacemaker cells 59 mV ($n = 20$). The presence of a short plateau after the peak of the action potential was regularly observed in cultures derived from the hearts of very young rats (2–3 days old), whilst no plateau was noted in cultures of older hearts (6–8 days post natum). This finding is in broad agreement with the data of Bernard and Gargouïl (1963) and Bernard *et al.* (1968), who reported the presence of a plateau preceding repolarization in foetal rat heart and its disappearance after birth. As illustrated by Fig. 1, the amplitude of the membrane potential deflection due to the current pulse was usually identical to within a few tenths of a millivolt, whether the current was delivered through electrode 1 or electrode 2. Several voltage–current plots (Fig. 2) have shown

References p. 310–311

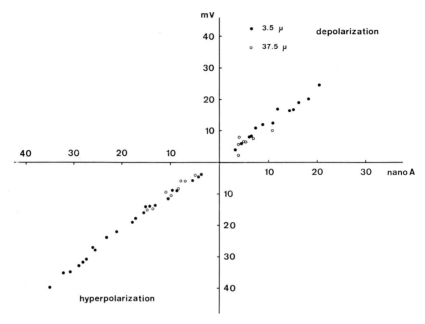

Fig. 2. Superimposed current–voltage plots obtained from two pairs of cultured myoblasts. Black circles, interelectrode distance 3.5 μ; both microelectrodes appeared to be in the same cell; pure culture. Open circles, interelectrode distance 37.5 μ; at least one cell junction was interposed between the electrodes; mixed culture.

that the junctions between cardiac myoblasts do not rectify to any appreciable degree within a considerable range of membrane potentials.

In all experiments, the transmembrane potential of one impaled cell was electronically subtracted from that of the other cell, and the subtraction trace displayed on the oscilloscope screen, enabling the observer to determine which of the two cells fired first. In this connection, it is of interest to point out that in "pure" myoblast cultures, as well as in mixed cultures, the firing sequence of a pair of impaled myoblasts was usually fixed throughout the entire observation period. Occasionally, however, an impalement of a pair of myoblasts showed variation of the firing sequence. Sometimes the switch of priority took place abruptly from one action potential to the next, as illustrated in Fig. 3, whilst in others it took place gradually, over several beats.

(2) Myoblasts in mixed cultures

The frequency with which pacemaker cells were impaled was not significantly different in mixed cultures from that encountered in "pure" myoblast cultures. The average resting potential of myoblasts in a mixed culture tended to be somewhat lower (mean 50 $\pm$ 10.3 mV S.D.) than in "pure" cultures.

Impalements in which one electrode was inserted into a myoblast, and the other into a fibroblast, showed that there was no fixed rule as to the sequence of firing: sometimes the myoblast fired first, at other times the action potential appeared first in the fibroblast.

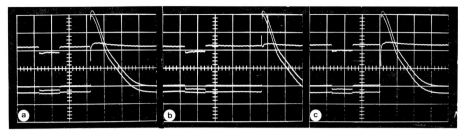

Fig. 3. Example of an abrupt switchover of the firing sequence of two myoblasts in a mixed culture. Three consecutive action potentials. The two bottom traces are the membrane-potential recordings, and the upper trace is the subtraction of one membrane potential from the other. The sharp spikes on the subtraction trace provide an indirect measurement of the delay between the upstrokes of the action potentials of both cells. Note the variation in the amplitude of these deflections from one action potential to the next, indicative of a variation in the firing delay, and the reversal of the firing sequence in the middle frame. Sweep speed 0.1 sec/division. Voltage calibration 20 mV per major graticule division.

(3) Myoblasts in fibroblast-enriched cultures

Impalements of solitary myoblast contaminants, occasionally found in fibroblast-enriched cultures, yielded resting potentials of the same magnitude as those of the surrounding fibroblasts. Low-amplitude (5–10 mV) upward deflections, synchronous with the sluggish contractions mentioned above, when these were present, were also observed. These deflections were also displayed by the fibroblasts in the immediate vicinity of the myoblast islets.

(4) Fibroblasts in "pure" cultures

Fibroblasts in "pure" cultures (less than 1% myoblasts) proved much more difficult to impale successfully than myoblasts. The membrane of fibroblasts seemed to tear with much greater ease than that of myoblasts. As a rule the membrane potential of fibroblasts in "pure" cultures showed a sharp transient, 35–40 mV in amplitude, at the moment of penetration, after which it stabilized at a value between —10 and —20 mV.

(5) Fibroblasts in mixed cultures

A striking difference was found between the membrane potential of fibroblasts in mixed cultures, as compared with "pure" fibroblast cultures. As stated above, the membrane potential of fibroblasts in "pure" fibroblast cultures usually stabilized at values between —10 and —20 mV. In contrast, fibroblasts belonging to a mixed culture exhibited resting potentials identical in amplitude to those of the surrounding myoblasts, i.e. —40 to —60 mV, as well as barely attenuated action potentials. Provided the criterion of a satisfactory double impalement was satisfied, i.e. quasi-equality of resting potentials of both cells, the total amplitude of the action potentials of a given fibroblast was roughly equal to that of the myoblast impaled in its neighbourhood.

A feature common to all double impalements, regardless of the nature of the cells impaled, was that the membrane potential of the first cell to be successfully penetrated

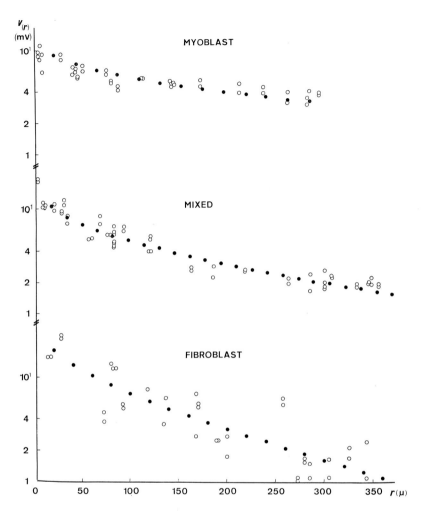

Fig. 4. From top to bottom: three semilogarithmic plots of the electrotonic potential against the interelectrode distance, obtained respectively from a pure myoblast, a mixed, and a pure fibroblast culture. The potential values were linearly normalized for $I_0 = 10^{-8}$ A. Open circles, experimental points. Black circles, best-fitting Bessel function, from which the attenuation lengths were obtained. The values of the latter were 1100 μ for the myoblast culture, 400 μ for the mixed culture, and 200 μ for the fibroblast culture.

regularly fell by a few millivolts at the moment the second cell was punctured. As sealing in of the second microelectrode proceeded, both membrane potentials gradually rose to their stabilization level. This phenomenon was also observed when one of the impaled cells was a myoblast and the other a fibroblast. The amplitude of the transient depolarization of the first-impaled cell was more markedly dependent on the interelectrode distance in fibroblast cultures than in myoblast cultures. This is in accord with the shorter attenuation length found in fibroblast cultures.

Typical examples of potential *versus* distance plots for a "pure" myoblast, a "pure" fibroblast, and a mixed culture, are shown in Fig. 4, in which the logarithmic ordinate

TABLE I

SUMMARIZED ELECTROPHYSIOLOGICAL RESULTS

λ = attenuation length, nV_0 = constant determined by the boundary conditions, r_i = effective resistance of intracellular phase, d = thickness of culture, Age = age of culture, R_i = lumped specific resistance of intracellular phase, R_l = leakage resistance of a cm² of culture. R_{l1} and R_{l1} were computed on the assumption that leakage of current occurred through the upper membranes only, $i.e.$ by halving the leakage current given by eqn. 12 (Appendix).

Predominant cell type	λ (μ)	$nV_0 \cdot 10^3$ (mV)	r_i (MΩ)	d (μ)	Age (days)	R_{i1} (Ωcm)	R_{l1} (Ωcm^2)	R_{i2} (Ωcm)	R_{l2} (Ωcm^2)
Myoblast	1100	2.19	1.39	2.06	4	286	16820	350	20691
Myoblast	1100	2.04	1.39	1.19	2	165	16820	202	20570
Myoblast	1100	1.59	0.98	3.92	3	384	11860	415	12826
Myoblast	1000	1.60	0.90	4.00	4	360	9000	388	9700
Myoblast	1000	1.60	0.90	3.95	3	356	9000	383	9700
Mixed	850	1.59	1.01	4.62	6	467	7297	517	8092
Myoblast	800	3.82	2.35	2.25	2	529	15000	574	16320
Myoblast	780	2.55	1.62	3.55	2	575	9856	621	10464
Mixed	700	1.66	1.02	–	4	–	5000	–	5439
Mixed	400	3.18	2.03	3.03	4	615	3250	691	3648
Fibroblast	250	12.10	7.31	–	6	–	4563	–	5968
Fibroblast	200	7.64	4.61	2.87	3	1325	1844	1556	2168
Fibroblast	180	11.46	7.06	6.78	4	4790	2287	6712	3208
Fibroblast	80	25.48	16.00	–	5	–	1021	–	3560

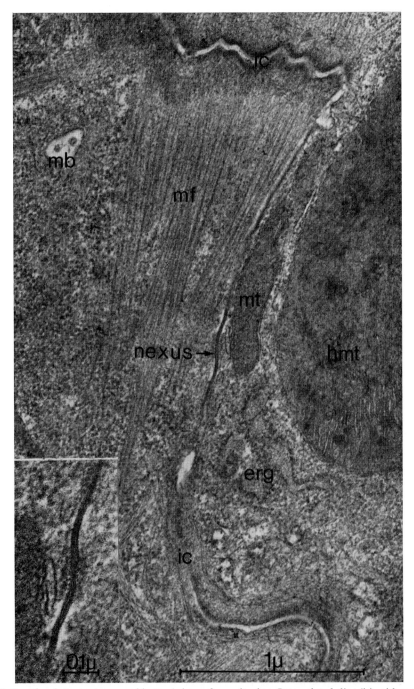

Fig. 5. Junction between two myoblasts, 4 days after culturing. Intercalated disc (ic) with a nexus showing the characteristic quintuple layered structure (see inset) with a thickness of 180 Å. A myofibril in the making (mf) is visible in the upper part of the disc, with dense Z band material adjoining the still denser material of the desmosome; mb, multivesicular body; mt, normal mitochondrion; hmt, hypertrophied mitochondrion; erg, ergastogplasm, magnification 50 000 ×. Inset: Magnification 100 000×.

represents $V_{(r)}$ linearly normalized for $I_0 = 10^{-8}$ A. Superimposed on the plots of the experimental points are the theoretical Bessel functions computed for the best-fitting values of λ and nV_0.

The results pertaining to electrotonic coupling in each case are presented in Table I. The data concerning mixed cultures were obtained from impalements of pairs of myoblasts only. However, impalements of myoblast–fibroblast pairs also showed a considerable degree of electrotonic coupling.

(c) Morphology

(1) M–M junctions

Marked ultrastructural differences exist between M–M junctions on the hand, and M–F and F–F junctions on the other hand. The regions of contact between cultured cardiac myoblasts (Fig. 5) closely resemble the intercalated discs of adult heart tissue. Two distinct specialized junctional structures, *i.e.* desmosomes and nexuses, are readily recognizable. The nexuses exhibit the characteristic five-layered structure, and their minimal overall thickness is consistently less than 180 Å with our fixation technique. These observations suggest that, structurally, the nexuses connecting cultured cardiac myoblasts are essentially the same as those of heart muscle *in situ*. In the latter tissue, after block-staining with uranyl acetate, and provided the section is adequately oriented with respect to the electron beam, the minimal overall thickness of nexuses is also consistently below 280 Å, and a 20-Å wide gap can regularly be resolved between the outer leaflets of the apposed unit membranes. Using a technique involving impregnation of blocks of myocardial tissue with colloidal lanthanum nitrate, Revel and Karnovsky (1967) were able to demonstrate that the nexal gap possesses a substructure which shows up as a periodic cross-striation in transverse sections and as an hexagonal lattice in tangential sections. The electrical implications of this observation are obvious, since an empty gap, even only 20-Å wide, would act as a shunt for current flowing through the nexus, whilst a closed honeycomb structure would not, or at least not to the same extent.

(2) M–F and F–F junctions

M–F junctions (Fig. 6) exhibit desmosomes, with their characteristic 100-Å wide intercellular cleft and their appositions of electron-dense material on either side of the cleft. However, in contrast to M–M junctions, they are apparently completely devoid of nexuses. They do present points of close contact, at which no intercellular gap is seen. The overall thickness of the merging membranes never falls below the value of twice the thickness of a unit membrane.

In our preparations, no desmosomes were seen at F–F junctions (Figs. 7 and 8). The only specialization encountered at these junctions consisted of focal contacts of the type described above for M–F junctions.

Examination of 10 such points of focal contact, at F–F junctions, was carried out with the aid of a goniometer. Tilting the sections through the appropriate angle showed a definite intercellular cleft in all of them, revealing that the 10 points of

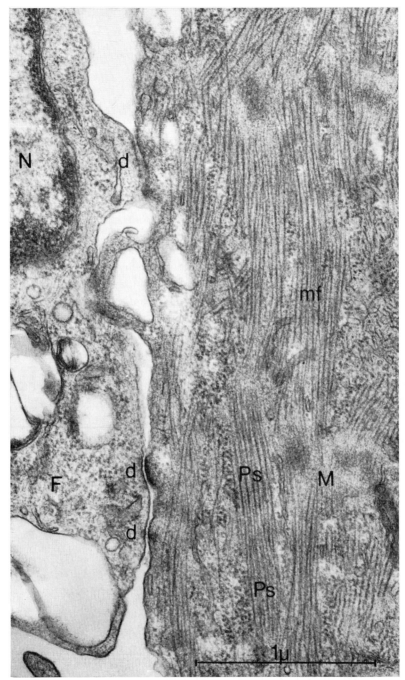

Fig. 6. Myoblast–fibroblast (M–F) junction in a 4-day-old culture, exhibiting a desmosome (d), but no nexus. N, nucleus; Ps, polysomes; mf, myofibrils. Magnification 49 000 ×.

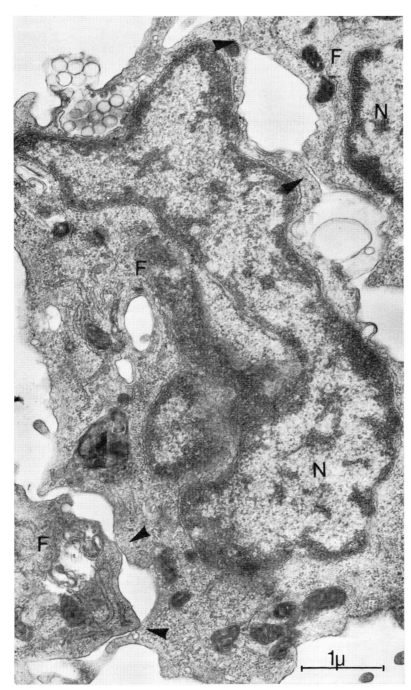

Fig. 7. Three fibroblasts (F) in contact with each other, in a 4-day-old culture. The arrows indicate the points of closest proximity. N, nucleus. Magnification 23 000 ×.

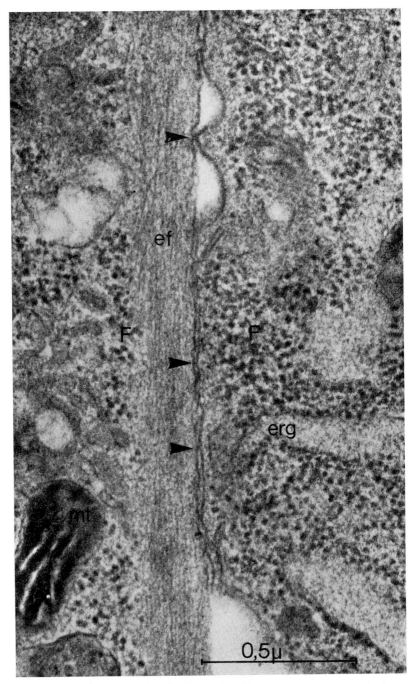

Fig. 8. Fibroblast–fibroblast (F–F) junction in a 4-day-old culture. There are small regions at which the outer leaflets of the apposed membranes apparently touch each other (arrows) but no nexuses; mt, mitochondrion in condensed form (due to hyperosmotic fixative); erg, ergastoplasm; ef, elementary fibrils. Magnification 85 000 ×.

contact subjected to goniometric analysis were, in reality, merely superposition artifacts. Sometimes the cleft material was almost electron-transparent, whereas in others it was markedly electron-dense. In Fig. 9, a point of apparent contact is visible at tilt angles between —30 and —6°; however, tilting the preparation through 0° to +24° reveals a cleft between the two apposed unit membranes. The cleft material is of very low electron-density. Fig. 10 shows apparent fusion of the membranes at tilt angles from —24 to —18°, then increasing separation of the membranes from —12 to +24°, followed again by apparent fusion at +30°. Even at tilt angles revealing definite separation, the cleft is filled with markedly electron-dense material. Thus the morphological substrate of electrotonic coupling through junctions of this type remains an open question.

DISCUSSION

A survey of recent literature shows that a wide variety of tissues exhibit electrotonic coupling of cells (for references, see Loewenstein, 1966; Bennett, 1968), and one is entitled to ask whether electrical interaction between cells of the same type is not the rule rather than the exception. The purpose of this investigation was to compare the electrotonic properties of two distinct kinds of intercellular junction, formed under identical culturing conditions, and to examine the possibility of metabolic interaction between cells of different types connected with each other through low-resistance junctions.

The results obtained with "pure" cultures of cardiac myoblasts and fibroblasts show that marked differences in the properties of the junctional membranes and plasma membranes existed between these two cell types, as well as differences in their resting potentials. These differences tended to disappear when cells of both types were intimately associated in mixed cultures.

(a) Intercellular junctions

Fig. 4 shows that in "pure" myoblast cultures the plot of the electrotonic potential against the interelectrode distance is remarkably smooth, and that the scatter is small. If the cultures were made of strings of cells in single file, and if high-resistance intercellular junctions be assumed, one might theoretically expect each displacement of the recording electrode from one cell to the next to show up as a definite step in the potential *versus* distance plot. However, this is not so in our preparation because, firstly, a culture is a relatively vast, continuous sheet of cells, and secondly because the curves are statistical. Therefore, instead of showing up as sharp discontinuities in the curves, high-resistance junctions would be reflected in the scatter (background noise) of the points. The experiments reported here show that the scatter was small in "pure" myoblast cultures, slightly larger in mixed cultures, and largest in "pure" fibroblast cultures, indicating that the resistance of F–F junctions is much larger than that of M–M junctions. This suggestion is further supported by a comparison of the calculated values of the overall specific resistance of the intracellular phase

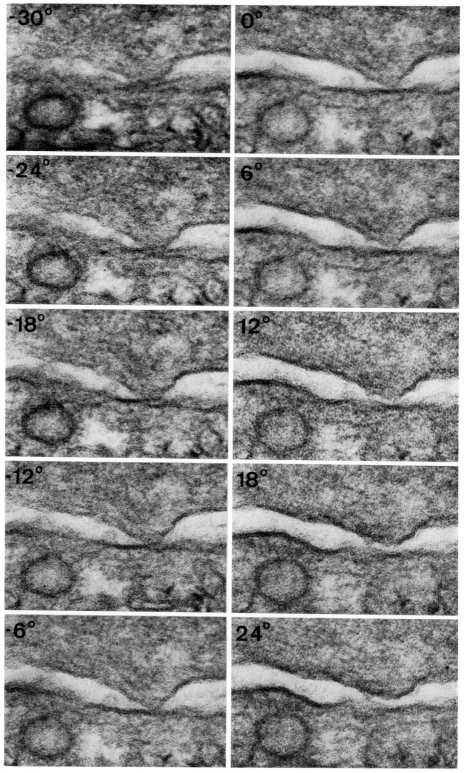

Fig. 9. Goniometric analysis of a junction between two cultured fibroblasts. The numbers refer to tilt angles. All micrographs were selected from a through-focus series. A point of apparent contact is visible at tilt angles between −30 and −6°. Tilting the section to + 24° reveals a cleft between the apposed unit membranes. Magnification 150 000 ×.

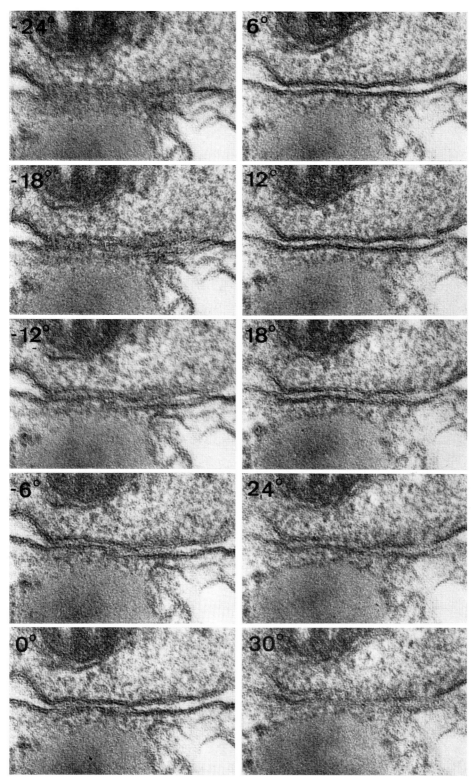

Fig. 10. Same as Fig. 9, except for high electron-density of cleft-material. Magnification 150 000 ×.

References p. 310–311

(R_{i2}, Table I) for both types of pure culture, and for mixed cultures. The mean value of R_{i2} was 419 Ωcm in "pure" myoblast cultures, 604 Ωcm in mixed cultures, and 4134 Ωcm in "pure" fibroblast cultures. It seems highly probable that most, if not all, of the difference between myoblast and fibroblast cultures in this respect is due to the lower effective resistance of the junctional structures between myoblasts.

The mean value of the overall specific resistance of the intracellular medium for cultured myoblasts (419 Ωcm) is 4 times greater than that reported for kid Purkinje fibres (Weidmann, 1952) and 3 times greater than that of calf and sheep Purkinje fibres (Coraboeuf and Weidmann, 1954). Since precise measurements of the nexal area have not been made so far for any of these cell systems, it is impossible to decide whether the specific junctional resistance is higher in cultured myoblasts than in Purkinje fibres, or whether the latter simply provide a larger area of nexus for the flow of current. However, examination of a large number of junctions between Purkinje cells and between cultured myoblasts in the electron microscope leads to a marked preference for the second hypothesis.

The absence of rectification by the intercellular junctions in "pure" cultures of both types, and in mixed cultures, has frequently been checked, since in each double impalement the current was passed alternately through both electrodes. No significant difference in the amplitude of the electrotonic potential was found. The absence of rectification is further illustrated by Fig. 2. Concerning this figure, it may be of interest to mention that a cell could often be depolarized by 30 mV or more without producing an action potential. Anodal break responses, on the other hand, were easily obtained.

Experiments involving injection of minute amounts of tracer substances into a cell and the observation of diffusion of the tracer into neighbouring cells have shown that even quite large molecules, such as fluorescein-labelled serum albumin, could cross at least some types of homocellular junction (Loewenstein, 1966). Diffusion of ions and molecules from one cell to another may be thought to play a part in cell-to-cell transmission of information, as for example in ensuring equivalent differentiation of cells of a given tissue subserving a given set of functions (Dulbecco, 1963). It may reasonably be expected that tight junctions between cells of different types (heterocellular junctions), no matter how tight they might be electrically, would show greater discrimination in the selection of molecules and ions that would be allowed to diffuse through the junctions. The experiments reported in this paper have shown that the resting potential of fibroblasts in mixed cultures is about 3 times higher than that of fibroblasts in pure cultures, suggesting that at least K^+ ions, and presumably also other small ions, must be able to diffuse freely across heterocellular junctions, and that the pumping of ions must be shared. In view of the considerable importance of the intracellular K^+ concentration in the control of many cellular enzymes, in particular those involved in phosphorylation (Kernan, 1965), one can easily imagine that the metabolism of fibroblasts might be profoundly altered by their association with myoblasts.

Another interesting fact concerning M–F junctions, as opposed to M–M junctions, is that in the former we have never seen the characteristic morphology of the nexus.

This observation suggests that formation of a nexus requires that the cells in contact be of the same kind, and may provide some information as to the mechanisms underlying cell-to-cell adhesion. The problem of the precise chemical nature of cell adhesion is still unsolved. However, various hypotheses have been put forward, and can be divided into two major categories: (*a*) hypotheses involving strictly physico-chemical phenomena, and (*b*) hypotheses invoking specific cellular functions. Hypotheses of the first category include: stabilization of an intercellular cement by divalent cations (Ringer, 1890; Chambers and Chambers, 1961); calcium-bridge bonding of cell surfaces (Steinberg, 1958; Ambrose, 1967); cell-to-cell adsorption due to the interplay of attractive and repulsive physical forces involving the zeta potentials of the cells; and the London–Van der Waals forces (for detailed discussion of this point, see Beumer *et al.*, 1957). Among the hypotheses of the second category, one can cite bonding between sterically complementary surface groups (Tyler, 1947; Weiss, 1947) and specific cell products acting on the cell surface (Moscona, 1962). The fact that nexuses do not occur at M–F and F–F junctions suggests that their formation requires some kind of specific affinity between the cells involved in the junction, and that the factors governing the formation of nexuses belong to the second category. On the other hand, tight junctions consisting of focal contacts of the outer leaflets of both unit membranes do not seem to require any kind of specific affinity, since they occur both at heterocellular (M–F) and homocellular (F–F) junctions. Further investigations in this field should include a comparative study of the behaviour of both types of junction under various chemical and physico-chemical conditions. Close contacts between cultured fibroblasts, obtained from adult guinea-pigs, have been described by Devis and James (1964). Some of the electron micrographs published by these authors show five-layered junctional structures which most probably represent nexuses.

(b) Plasma membrane

There is a significant negative correlation between the calculated values of R_l and the measured thicknesses of the cultures. This correlation is reasonably well described by a regression line within the limits of the observed range of thicknesses, *i.e.* from 1 to 6 μ, and the equation of the regression line for myoblast cultures is $R_l = 16788 - 2376\,d$, where R_l has the dimensions of $\Omega\,cm^2$ and d is expressed in μ. The explanation of this correlation is found in the geometry of the cell system. Consider Fig. 11, which shows 3 transverse sections through three different myoblast cultures. It can be seen that thickening of the cultures is due to an increase in the number of cell layers, rather than to thickening of the cells. The same holds for fibroblast cultures. If it be remembered that R_l is the leakage resistance of a cm^2 of culture, it becomes obvious that, all other factors being equal, R_l must decrease as the culture becomes more stratified, *i.e.* as the area of cell membrane per cm^2 of culture increases. It is equally obvious that R_l will tend to equal the specific membrane resistance in a strictly monolayer culture. Table I shows that for the thinnest cultures the value of R_l is between 15 000 and 20 000 $\Omega\,cm^2$ for myoblasts, and approximately 3000 $\Omega\,cm^2$ for

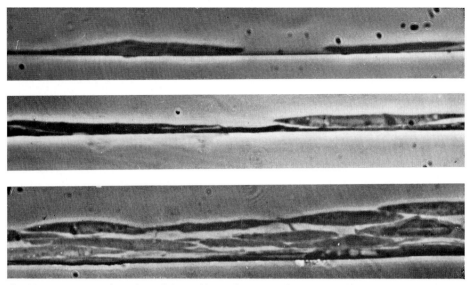

Fig. 11. Transverse sections through 3 myoblast cultures. The increase in thickness is due to stratification of the culture rather than to thickening of the cells.

fibroblasts. These values provide a fairly likely estimate of the specific membrane resistance of both cell types, and show that the ionic membrane permeabilities of myoblasts and fibroblasts are markedly different. That other differences, of a qualitative as well as quantitative nature, also exist between the membranes of the two cell types is suggested by the observation that, under identical culturing conditions, the fibroblasts became attached to the Petri dishes within less than 3 h, whereas the myoblasts required a much longer period.

In a preliminary investigation (Girardier *et al.*, 1967), an attempt was made to determine the specific membrane resistance of cultured myoblasts with a direct method. Completely isolated myoblasts belonging to very young, non-confluent cultures (24–48 h after trypsin dispersion), were impaled with a microelectrode mounted in a Wheatstone bridge, and their effective resistance was measured. The cells were then photographed, and their surface area was estimated with a planimeter. This method yielded a value of the specific membrane resistance of approximately 60 Ωcm². Two possible explanations can be put forward for the discrepancy between this result and the results of more recent work. In the first place trypsinization of the cells may cause the membrane resistance to collapse and the latter may take more than 48 h to recover. Secondly, the resting potential of completely isolated myoblasts is regularly low, around 30–40 mV, and it has not been possible to determine whether this is due to a completely isolated cell normally possessing a resting potential of this order, or if it is simply due to damage inflicted by the microelectrode. The second hypothesis seems the more likely, since the resting potential of isolated myoblasts never remained stable for more than a few minutes. If damage to the cell membrane were the cause of the low resting potential, then one would expect a considerable leakage of current to occur around the electrode tip, and the consequence of this state of affairs would naturally be a low effective resistance.

(c) Myoblast–fibroblast interactions

The ionic permeability of the fibroblast plasma membrane is much higher than that of the myoblast plasma membrane. The resting potential of fibroblasts in pure cultures is markedly smaller than that of myoblasts in pure cultures. Further investigation is needed to determine whether the difference in resting potential is due solely to the membrane-permeability factor, or to a difference in the mechanisms of ionic transport through the membranes as well.

The most striking finding is that the difference in magnitude of the resting potential between myoblasts and fibroblasts disappears when both cells are cultured together (mixed cultures). This seems to indicate that intimate association of heterotypic cells causes profound modifications in their membrane properties and/or metabolism, which have not as yet been analyzed experimentally. However, a purely qualitative observation, which may be of interest in this connection, is that satisfactory impalements of fibroblasts were much easier to obtain in mixed cultures than in pure cultures.

Electrotonic coupling between heterotypic cells may be a purely artificial phenomenon, due to the culturing procedure itself, and the pooling of solutes, which it entails, may play a part in the de-differentiation of cells in culture.

(d) Electrotonic spread

The results presented in this paper show that the average attenuation length, λ, is approximately 5 times larger in myoblast cultures than in fibroblast cultures. This would seem to indicate that electrical coupling through M–M junctions, whose function is to provide optimal conditions for cell-to-cell flow of current, is from the outset more efficient than through M–F and F–F junctions. Furthermore, it is tempting to speculate that the electrical connections between myocardial cells and cells of the Purkinje fibres are merely remnants of the electrotonic junctions which are known to exist between embryonic cells (Potter et al., 1966). However, this does not seem to be the case, and the impression prevails that tight electrical coupling of myocardial cells is an intrinsic property of these cells, resulting from early specialization of their regions of contact, and of their plasma membrane as a whole.

A further interesting finding was that the greater efficiency of electrical coupling between myoblasts, as compared with that of M–F and F–F junctions, is for a sizeable proportion due to the greater leakage resistance (R_l) of the myoblasts, and not simply to a lower junctional resistance, as might have been assumed on the basis of morphological findings alone. The mean value of the effective resistance of the intracellular medium (r_i) is approximately 7 times as great in fibroblast cultures as in myoblast cultures. Were the leakage resistances (R_l) of myoblast and fibroblast cultures equal, this would account for the space constant of myoblast cultures being only $\sqrt{7}$, or 2.45 times greater than that of fibroblast cultures. On the other hand, the mean leakage resistance of myoblast cultures is between 3.5 and 5.7 times greater than that of fibroblasts. Division of this factor by the ratio of myoblast effective internal resistance to fibroblast effective internal resistance reasonably accounts for the observed ratio of space constants.

A high specific membrane resistance would seem to be a most useful and economical property for a cardiac myoblast, since it would enable the cell to maintain a sufficiently high resting potential to keep its sodium system in readiness for repetitive action at a relatively low energy cost, and at the same time ensure favourable conditions for the electrotonic spread of excitation.

APPENDIX

(a) Derivation of the basic equations

The model can be schematically represented as in Fig. 12. Let d be the thickness of the sheet of cells, R_i the overall specific resistance of the intracellular medium (myoplasm and intercellular junctions in series), and I_0 the current delivered by one of the intracellular microelectrodes. I_0 divides into I_i, the internal current flowing radially

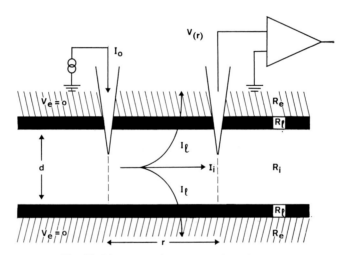

Fig. 12. Diagrammatic representation of the model.

within the myoplasm of the cells, and I_l, the current which escapes through the leakage resistance R_l. If we assume that there is no angular variation of I_i and I_l around the tip of the current electrode, at any finite distance r from the point of application of I_0 the internal current I_i produces a voltage drop $-\Delta V$ across a length Δr of internal medium:

$$-\Delta V = \frac{I}{2\pi r d} \cdot R_i \cdot \Delta r \tag{1}$$

Let

$$\frac{R_i}{d} = r_i \tag{2}$$

then

$$-\Delta V = \frac{I}{2\pi r} \cdot r_i \cdot \Delta r \tag{3}$$

In the differential form, (3) can be written:

$$-\frac{dV}{dr} = \frac{I}{2\pi r} \cdot r_i \tag{4}$$

Differentiating (4):

$$\frac{dI}{dr} = -\frac{2\pi}{r_i} \cdot (r \frac{d^2V}{dr^2} + \frac{dV}{dr}) \tag{5}$$

Furthermore, the density of current leaking outwards through the upper and lower rings of membrane of width Δr is related to the membrane potential V by the equation

$$-V = \frac{\Delta I}{4\pi r \Delta r} \cdot R_l \tag{6}$$

Photomicrographs of transverse sections through the cultures (Fig. 11) show that the lower aspect of the cells is entirely in contact with the bottom of the Petri dish, but nothing is known about the precise nature of the contact nor of its electrical resistance. Hence some uncertainty exists as to the leakage area of the bottom layer of cells. In the differential form, (6) becomes

$$\frac{dI}{dr} = -\frac{4\pi}{R_l} \cdot r \cdot V \tag{7}$$

If we assume the specific resistance of the extracellular fluid to be negligible and combine eqns. (5) and (7):

$$-\frac{4\pi}{R_l} \cdot r \cdot V = -\frac{2\pi}{r_i} (r \cdot \frac{d^2V}{dr^2} + \frac{dV}{dr}) \tag{8}$$

Let

$$\frac{R_l}{r_i} = \lambda^2 \tag{9}$$

References p. 310–311

then

$$\frac{d^2V}{dr^2} + \frac{1}{r} \cdot \frac{dV}{dr} - \frac{2}{\lambda^2} \cdot V = 0 \tag{10}$$

A particular solution of eqn. (10) meeting our boundary conditions for steady state is

$$V_{(r)} = nV_0 \, K_0 \, (x) \tag{11}$$

where $V_{(r)}$ = deflection of membrane potential due to current pulse I_0 at distance r from the current electrode

$\quad\quad n$ = constant depending on the boundary conditions

$\quad\quad V_0$ = V at finite distance r_0 from point source of current

$\quad\quad K_0(x)$ = $(\pi/2) \, i \, H_0^{(1)}(ix)$, *i.e.* modified zero order Bessel function of second kind with imaginary argument

$$x = \frac{r}{\lambda}$$

If one turns back to eqn. (7), one can see that the total amount of current which leaks out of the cells between the tips of both electrodes is

$$I_{l(r)} = -\frac{4\pi}{R_l} \cdot \int_{r_0}^{r} \cdot V_{(r)} \cdot dr \tag{12}$$

Replacing $V_{(r)}$ by its value in (10)

$$I_{l(r)} = -\frac{4\pi}{R_l} \cdot nV_0 \cdot \int_{r_0}^{r} rK_0 \, (x) \, dr \tag{13}$$

The internal current at distance r is

$$I_{i(r)} = I_0 - I_{l(r)}$$

Eqn. (4) can now be re-written

$$-\frac{dV}{dr} = \frac{r_i}{2\pi r} (I_0 - I_{l(r)}) \tag{14}$$

Since

$$\frac{r_i}{R_l} = \frac{1}{\lambda^2}$$

and letting

$$\int_{r_0}^{r} rK_0 \, (x) \, dr = \varphi$$

eqn. (14) becomes

$$-\frac{dV_{(r)}}{dr} = \frac{I_0 r_i}{2\pi r} - \frac{2nV_0\varphi}{\lambda^2 r} \tag{15}$$

The practical integration formula for φ is

$$\varphi = \sum_{r=r_0}^{r=r} \left[\frac{K_0 \, (x)}{2} \, (r_2^2 - r_1^2) \right] \tag{16}$$

(b) Curve fitting

The experimental results provide two of the terms contained in eqn. (11), namely $V_{(r)}$ and r. The remaining terms, *i.e.* nV_0 and λ, were determined by curve fitting as follows. The measured values of $V_{(r)}$ for a given culture were linearly normalized for $I_0 = 10^{-8}$ A, and plotted semilogarithmically against r. Justification for linear normalization will be found in Fig. 2. The regression line of the voltage–distance plot was drawn according to the least-square method. The plot was then compared with families of Bessel curves made out beforehand for various values of λ and nV_0, until a suitable degree of coincidence was obtained. The fit was considered satisfactory when the regression line of the experimental points coincided with that of the points of the theoretical Bessel curve comprised within the limits of r tested in the experiment. The values of

$$K_0(x) = \frac{\pi}{2} iH_0^{(1)}(ix)$$

were taken from tables of functions (Jahnke and Emde, 1938). Term R_i was calculated using eqn. (15), in which

$$-\frac{dV_{(r)}}{dr}$$

was measured graphically and φ was integrated in steps of $\Delta x = 0.04$, starting arbitrarily at $x_0 = 0.02$ in all cultures. The values of R_i and R_l were computed from eqns. (2) and (9) respectively.

SUMMARY

(*1*) A method for preparing practically pure cultures of cardiac myoblasts and fibroblasts is described. With this technique it has been possible to investigate the properties of three functionally distinct types of cell junction, and the effects of association of heterotypic cells.

(*2*) Under identical culturing conditions, the attenuation length of pure myoblast cultures was found to be 5 times greater than that of pure fibroblast cultures. This difference is due both to the lower overall specific resistance of the intracellular medium of myoblast cultures, and to the higher specific membrane resistance of these cells. The attenuation length of mixed cultures was intermediate between the two extremes.

(*3*) Electrotonic coupling was found between heterotypic cells (myoblasts and fibroblasts).

(*4*) The measured membrane potential of fibroblasts was 3 times higher when they were in intimate association with myoblasts in mixed cultures than in pure cultures. Conversely, the resting potential of stray myoblast contaminants in predominantly fibroblastic cultures was of the same magnitude as that of the surrounding fibroblasts.

(*5*) Neither myoblast–myoblast junctions, nor fibroblast–fibroblast junctions exhibited rectification.

(*6*) Typical nexuses were found at myoblast–myoblast junctions, but not at fibroblast–fibroblast and myoblast–fibroblast junctions. This suggests that electrotonic coupling may occur through junctional structures other than the nexus.

References p. 310–311

(7) At fibroblast–fibroblast and myoblast–fibroblast junctions the appearance of the points of closest proximity between the adjoining cells was suggestive of focal contact of the outer leaflets of the unit membranes. Even rotation of the section under the electron beam by means of a goniometer did not entirely clarify the precise nature of these focal contacts.

(8) The results at hand suggest that formation of nexuses at a cell junction requires that the partners in the junction be homotypic.

ACKNOWLEDGEMENTS

We wish to thank Prof. C. P. Enz (Department of Theoretical Physics, University of Geneva, Switzerland) for helping us in selecting the model and working out the equations thereof, and Prof. J. Posternak (Department of Physiology, University of Geneva, Switzerland) for enduring interest and helpful criticism throughout this work.

REFERENCES

AMBROSE, E. J., (1967); Possible mechanisms of the transfer of information between small groups of cells. In: A. V. S. DE REUCK AND J. KNIGHT (Eds.), *Cell Differentiation*, Ciba Foundation Symposium, Churchill, London, pp. 101–115.

BENNETT, M. V. L., (1968); Similarities between chemically and electrically mediated transmission. In: F. D. CARLSON (Ed.), *Physiological and Biochemical Aspects of Nerve Interaction*, Prentice-Hall, Englewood Cliffs, N.J.

BERNARD, C., AND GARGOUÏL, Y. M., (1963); Évolution de la dépolarisation du myocarde ventriculaire chez le foetus de rat. *C.R. Acad. Sci. (Paris)*, **256**, 4972–4974.

BERNARD, C., RAYMOND, G., GROS, D., AND GARGOUÏL, Y. M., (1968); Étude de la perméabilité membranaire du myocarde de l'embryon de rat, à l'aide de quelques inhibiteurs spécifiques. *J. Physiol. (Paris)*, **60**, 216.

BEUMER, J., DIRKX, J., AND BEUMER-JOCHMANS, M. P., (1957); Role of cations in phage adsorption to sensitive bacteria. *Nature (Lond.)*, **180**, 83–85.

BLONDEL, B., ROIJEN, I., AND CHENEVAL, J.-P., (1969); Heart cell cultures: a simple method for increasing the proportion of myoblasts. *Science*, in the press.

CHAMBERS, R., AND CHAMBERS, E. L., (1961); *Explorations into the Nature of the Living Cell*. Harvard University Press, Cambridge, Mass.

CLAUSEN, T., RODBELL, M., AND DUNAND, P., (1967); The metabolism of isolated fat cells. VII. Sodium-linked, energy-dependent and ouabain-sensitive potassium accumulation in ghosts. *J. biol. Chem.*, in the press.

CORABOEUF, E., AND WEIDMANN, S., (1954); Temperature effects on the electrical activity of Purkinje fibres. *Helv. physiol. pharmacol. Acta*, **12**, 32–41.

CRILL, W. E., RUMERY, R. E., AND WOODBURY, Y. W., (1959); Effects of membrane current on transmembrane potentials of cultured chick embryo heart cells. *Amer. J. Physiol.*, **197**, 733–735.

DEVIS, R., AND JAMES, D. W., (1964); Close association between adult guinea pig fibroblasts in tissue culture, studied with the electron microscope. *J. Anat. (Lond.)*, **98**, 63–68.

DULBECCO, R., (1963); Transformation of cells *in vitro* by viruses. Science, **142**, 932–936.

DULBECCO, R., AND VOGT, M., (1954); Plaque formation and isolation of pure lines with poliomyelitis viruses. *J. exp. Med.*, **99**, 167–182.

FÄNGE, R., PERSON, H., AND THESLEFF, S., (1957); Electrophysiologic and pharmacological observations on trypsin-disintegrated embryonic chick hearts cultured *in vitro*. *Acta physiol scand.*, **38**, 173–183.

GEORGE, E. P., (1961); Resistance values in a syncytium. *Aust. J. exp. Biol. med. Sci.*, **39**, 267–274.

GIRARDIER, L., HYDE, A., MATTER, A., AND BLONDEL, B., (1967); Étude de la propagation de l'excitation dans des cultures de cellules myocardiques de rat. *J. Physiol. (Paris)*, **59**, 410–411.

HARARY, I., AND FARLEY, B., (1963); *In vitro* studies on single beating rat heart cells. I. Growth and organization. *Exp. Cell. Res.*, **29**, 451–465.

HO, R. J., AND JEANRENAUD, B., (1967); Insulin-like action of ouabain. I. Effect on carbohydrate metabolism. *Biochim. biophys. Acta (Amst.)*, **144**, 61–73.

JAHNKE, E., AND EMDE, F., (1938); *Tables of Functions with Formulae and Curves.* 3rd (revised) ed., Teubner, Leipzig, Berlin.

KERNAN, R. P., (1965); In E. EDWARD BITTAR (Ed.), *Cell K.* Butterworth, London.

LEHMKUHL, D., AND SPERELAKIS, N., (1963); Transmembrane potentials of trypsin-dispersed chick heart cells cultured *in vitro. Amer. J. Physiol.*, **205**, 1213–1220.

LETARTE, J., AND RENOLD, A. E., (1968); Effects of cations upon glucose transport in isolated fat cells. In: H. PEETERS (Ed.), *Protides of the Biological Fluids*, Vol. 15, Elsevier, Amsterdam, pp. 241–250.

LOEWENSTEIN, W. R., (1966); Permeability of membrane junctions. *Ann. N.Y. Acad. Sci.*, **137**, 441–472.

MARK, G. E., AND STRASSER, F. F., (1966); Pacemaker activity and mitosis in cultures of new-born rat heart ventricle cells. *Exp. Cell. Res.*, **44**, 217–233.

MATTER, A., GIRARDIER, L., HYDE, A., AND BLONDEL, B., (1968); Untersuchungen zur Entwicklung des sarkoplasmatischen Retikulums in kultivierten Herzmuskelzellen. *Verh. anat. Ges. (Jena)*, in the press.

MOSCONA, A., (1962); Analysis of cell recombination in experimental synthesis of tissues *in vitro. J. cell. comp. Physiol.*, **60**, *Suppl. 1*, 65–80.

MOSINGER, B., AND KUJALOVA, V., (1966); Potassium-dependent lipomobilizing effect of adrenaline on incubated adipose tissue. *Biochim. biophys. Acta (Amst.)*, **116**, 174–177.

POTTER, D. D., FURSHPAN, E. J., AND LENNOX, E. S., (1966); Connections between cells of the developing squid as revealed by electrophysiological methods. *Proc. nat. Acad. Sci. (Wash.)*, **55**, 328–336.

REVEL, J. P., AND KARNOVSKY, M. J., (1967); Hexagonal array of subunits in intercellular junctions of the mouse heart and liver. *J. Cell Biol.*, **33**, C7–C12.

RINGER, S., (1890); Concerning experiments to test the influence of lime, sodium, and potassium salts on the development of ova and growth of tadpoles. *J. Physiol. (Lond.)*, **11**, 79–84.

STEINBERG, M. S., (1958); On the chemical bonds between animal cells. A mechanism for type-specific association. *Amer. Naturalist*, **92**, 65–81.

TANAKA, I., AND SASAKI, Y., (1966); The electrotonic spread in cardiac muscle of the mouse. *J. gen. Physiol.*, **49**, 1089–1110.

TYLER, A., (1947); An auto-antibody concept of cell structure, growth and differentiation. *Symp. Soc. Study Develop. Growth*, **6**, 7–19.

WEIDMANN, S., (1952); The electrical constants of Purkinje fibres. *J. Physiol. (Lond.)*, **118**, 348–360.

WEISS, P., (1947); The problem of specificity in growth and development. *Yale J. Biol. Med.*, **19**, 235–278.

WOODBURY, J. W., AND CRILL, W. E., (1961); On the problem of impulse conduction in the atrium. In: ERNST FLOREY (Ed.), *Nervous Inhibition*, Pergamon, Oxford, pp. 124–135.

The Functional Organization within the Ommatidium of the Lateral Eye of *Limulus*

T. G. SMITH* AND F. BAUMANN**

INTRODUCTION

For a variety of historical and technical reasons, the lateral eye of the horseshoe crab, *Limulus polyphemus*, has been a favorite organ for investigating the manner and the means by which light evokes visually related potential changes within single photoreceptor cells and by which these signals are transmitted along neuronal pathways to the brain. Many of these reasons and much of what is known about these processes have recently been reviewed (Wolbarsht and Yeandle, 1967).

In this paper we shall present some selected observations made with intracellular microelectrode recordings from cells lying in single ommatidia when they are stimulated by light or by extrinsic electrical current applied through a microelectrode. In addition, we will present evidence consistent with the following conclusions. Light affects primarily the retinular cells, hence, they are the photoreceptor cells of the ommatidium (Tomita, 1956; Waterman and Wiersma, 1954). Light evokes from these cells a depolarization of complex waveform which may properly be called a receptor potential (Davis, 1961). The mechanisms by which light generates this receptor potential lie mainly, if not exclusively, within the retinular cell membrane (Tomita, 1956).

In contrast to the retinular cells, the eccentric cell is a second-order neuron in the visual pathway (Hartline *et al.*, 1952b; Tomita, 1956; Waterman and Wiersma, 1954). It is not affected directly by light (Waterman and Wiersma, 1954). The light-evoked depolarization of the eccentric cell, a generator or synaptic potential (Davis, 1961), is a consequence of prior activity in the retinular cells. Specifically, the receptor potential of the retinular cells produces the generator potential of the eccentric cell mainly, if not exclusively, by means of a rectifying, electrotonic "tight" junction between the two cells (Tomita, 1956, 1957, 1958; Tomita *et al.*, 1960; Waterman and Wiersma, 1954).

Once the generator potential depolarizes the eccentric cell's spike generating locus situated in its axon to a threshold value, action potentials are produced which conduct without decrement to the optic lobe of the brain (Hartline *et al.*, 1952a, b, 1961;

* Laboratory of Neurophysiology, National Institute of Neurological Diseases and Stroke, National Institutes of Health, Bethesda, Maryland 20014 (U.S.A.).
** Institut de Physiologie, Université de Genève, Genève (Switzerland).

References p. 347–349

Hartline and Ratliff, 1957). The effect of the generator potential on the spike generator can be modulated *via* the lateral inhibition which the eccentric cell of one ommatidium exerts on eccentric cells of neighboring ommatidia (Hartline *et al.*, 1952b, 1961; Hartline and Ratliff, 1957; Tomita, 1958) and *via* the self-inhibition which an eccentric cell exerts on itself (Purple and Dodge, 1965, 1966); however, these latter integrative processes have not been investigated in the experiments reported here and will not be considered further.

Finally, a model of the organization of a single ommatidium in the form of an equivalent electrical circuit will be presented. This model can simulate both the manner in which the cells behave to applied currents and the interactions between ommatidial cells.

Some of the results of this paper have been published in previous reports (Borsellino *et al.*, 1965; Smith, 1966; Smith *et al.*, 1965).

METHODS

The experiments to be reported were performed on lateral eyes excised from adolescent or adult *Limulus polyphemus* obtained from the Marine Biological Laboratory at Woods Hole, Massachusetts. In any given experiment, a lateral eye was transected in a plane perpendicular to the corneal surface and the preparation was mounted in a chamber containing Woods Hole sea water (Cavanaugh, 1956), with the long axis of the ommatidia lying in a horizontal plane. The exposed ommatidia were then probed sequentially with micropipettes.

The micropipettes were drawn from Corning #7740 Pyrex glass on a Livingston micropipette puller and filled by diffusion with 3 M KCl. Both single- and double-barrel microelectrodes with external tip diameters of about one micron were used. The resistance of the single-barrel electrodes was between 10 and 20 $M\Omega$ and that of each of the double-barrel electrodes between 15 and 40 Ω. The latter had a coupling resistance of 0.5–2 $M\Omega$ and a coupling capacitance of about 10 pF. Only those single-barrel electrodes which could pass current in excess of 10^{-8} A and those double-barrel electrodes which could pass current in excess of 10^{-7} A without significant rectification or increased noise were used in the experiments.

Electrical connection to the micropipettes was made by Ag–AgCl electrodes. The reference electrode was also an Ag–AgCl wire which made contact with the extracellular fluid by a 3 M KCl–agar bridge. The preparation and electrodes were incorporated in the circuit diagrammed in Fig. 1. This circuit is a slight variant of the Wheatstone bridge used by previous investigators and whose operation has been described elsewhere (Frank and Becker, 1964). Here, OMMTD represents an ommatidium and R_1 and R_2 the resistances of two single-barrel microelectrodes. A_1 and A_2 were Bak wideband electrometers; A_3, A_4 and A_5 were Tektronix Type D DC-Differential amplifiers or their equivalent; and A_6 and A_7 were Tektronix Type CA amplifiers or their equivalent. Amplifier A_6 was operated in the chopped mode and its output delivered to one beam of a Tektronix 502 oscilloscope (C.R.O.). All amplifiers and the C.R.O. were DC-coupled. By means of a switch (Sw.) either the

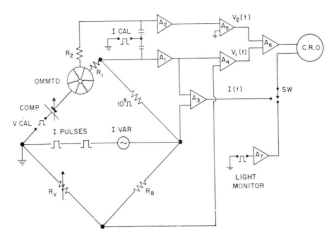

Fig. 1. Schematic diagram of circuit employed in single-barrel microelectrode experiments. See Methods for description.

extrinsic current (A_3) or the light stimulus (A_7) could be monitored on the other beam of the C.R.O. In those experiments where the current–voltage characteristics of the cell were traced directly on the oscilloscope, the current signal was applied to the horizontal amplifier of the C.R.O. and the voltage signal to the vertical amplifier (Furshpan and Potter, 1959). The current through the microelectrode was varied by applying a slowly changing (*ca.* 0.1 cps) signal by I VAR.

In those experiments using double-barrel microelectrodes, the circuitry was the same as that described elsewhere (Fig. 3 in Smith *et al.*, 1967). The potentials from the microelectrodes and photocell were continuously monitored on an ink recorder.

Either a tungsten or Xenon light source was used to stimulate the eye. Usually, the image of the source was focused by an optical train onto the side of a single ommatidium. Occasionally, the eye was stimulated through the lens of a single ommatidium. Thus far, no differences have been found in the responses evoked by the two methods. This finding is consistent with the absorption spectra of the screening pigmented cells (Wasserman, 1967). The light stimulus was controlled by means of a shutter with a rise-time of 1 msec. Pulses of light as short as 5 msec and steps of light could be delivered to the eye. The intensity of the light was controlled with neutral density filters. The time course of the light stimulus was monitored by a photocell located between the source and the neutral density filters.

All the records illustrated were taken on 35-mm film from the C.R.O. The temperature of the preparation chamber was maintained at near 15°.

RESULTS

(1) The distinguishing electrophysiological characteristics of cell types in the ommatidium

A knowledge of the histology of the ommatidium of the *Limulus* lateral eye is essential for understanding the potentials which can be recorded from its cells with microelectrodes. The details of this histology have been described and illustrated elsewhere (Behrens and Wulff, 1965; Demoll, 1914; Hartline *et al.*, 1952b; Kikuchi and Minagawa, 1961; Kikuchi *et al.*, 1965; Lasansky, 1967; MacNichol, 1956, 1958; Miller, 1957; Patten, 1912; Watase, 1887). For present purposes, it is sufficient to recall that the ommatidium is composed of four cell types: a layer of pigmented cells which form the outer shell of the ommatidium, a number of unpigmented glial cells, some 8–20 segmentally arranged retinular cells, and usually one eccentric cell.

In most electrophysiological investigations, few of the ommatidia's histological details can be observed, even when a high-power dissecting microscope and bright illumination are employed. Moreover, when the tip of a microelectrode blindly probes an ommatidium, a considerable variety of spontaneous and light-evoked potentials can be recorded. Many of these potentials are doubtlessly due to artifacts (*e.g.*, mechanical distortion of the microelectrode tips; recording from injured cells; partially intracellular, partially extracellular recordings, etc.). On the basis of the experience of this and other laboratories (Behrens and Wulff, 1965, 1967; Dowling, 1968; Fuortes, 1958, 1959a, b; Fuortes and Poggio, 1963; Fuortes and Yeandle, 1964; Kikuchi and Ueki, 1965; Smith, 1966; Stieve, 1965; Tomita, 1957, 1958; Tomita *et al.*, 1960; Yeandle, 1957, 1958), however, the cell types of the ommatidium can be identified with reasonable accuracy on the basis of their electrophysiological characteristics.

(a) Retinular cells

In keeping with their numerical majority, intracellular recordings are most commonly obtained from retinular cells. In agreement with most of the previously re-

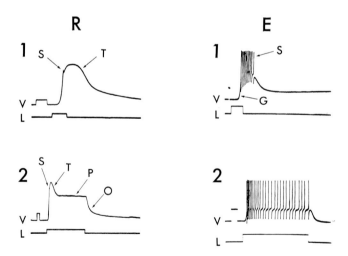

Fig. 2. Intracellular recordings from retinular (Column R) and from eccentric (Column E) cells. Responses (*V*) to pulses of light (*L*). In this and succeeding figures, the pulses at beginning of voltage (*V*) trace are voltage–time calibrations. Calibrations are 10 mV in all cases; 50 msec in R1 and 2, and in E2, 5 msec in E1. Letters with arrows indicate spike (S), transient (T), plateau (P), "off" response (O), generator potential (G) and spikes (S).

ported results, we find that the stable, resting potential of well-penetrated, dark-adapted retinular cells lies between —40 and —60 mV (Behrens and Wulff, 1965; Benolken, 1961; Kikuchi and Tazawa, 1960; Tomita, 1956). In addition, the response of retinular cells to light stimuli consists of a graded depolarization or receptor

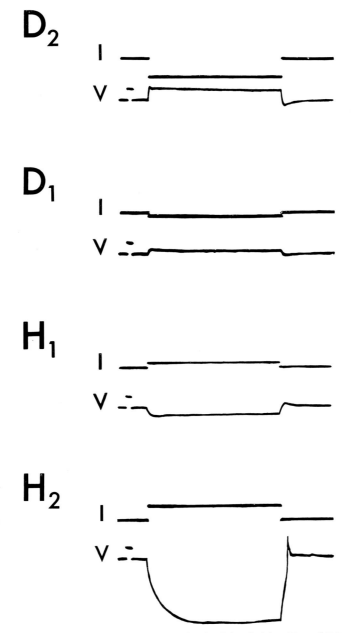

Fig. 3. Voltage (V) response of retinular cell to two levels of depolarizing (D_1 and D_2) and of hyperpolarizing (H_1 and H_2) extrinsic current (I). Identical gain throughout. V, cal. 10 mV, 100 msec. Current in D_2 is 2 nA.

References p. 347–349

potential. Examples of receptor potentials evoked by short and long pulses of bright light are illustrated in Fig. 2, Column R. The response has at least four components. Following the onset of the light, these components are an initial spike (S), a graded transient (T), a steady or plateau (P) depolarization and, after cessation of the light stimulus, an "off" (O) or repolarization phase (Behrens and Wulff, 1965, 1967; Benolken, 1961; Borsellino et al., 1965; Dowling, 1968; Fuortes, 1958; Fuortes and Poggio, 1963; Hartline et al., 1952b; Kikuchi and Tazawa, 1960; MacNichol, 1956, 1958; Smith, 1966; Stieve, 1965; Tomita, 1956). Occasionally, the receptor potential has superimposed spikes (Fig. 10A); however, these action potentials are always less than 10 mV in peak-to-peak amplitude (Behrens and Wulff, 1965, 1967; Fuortes, 1958; MacNichol, 1956, 1958; Tomita, 1957). Less often, the amplitude of the transient component of the receptor potential exceeds the resting membrane potential, i.e., the membrane potential becomes inside positive (Benolken, 1961; Fuortes, 1958; Kikuchi and Tazawa, 1960). In our experience such reversals of membrane potential usually occur in a dark-adapted eye in response to the first stimulus with a bright light or when very bright stimuli are applied infrequently (less than 0.1/sec).

Retinular cells also respond characteristically to extrinsic current applied through a microelectrode. With small current, the membrane charges and discharges with little or no evidence of active responses (Fig. 3, D_1 and H_1). Large depolarizing current, however, often evokes a single, small, regenerative, spike-like transient at the onset of the current (Fig. 3, D_2). In other retinular cells, depolarizing current evokes multiple action potentials which are less than 10 mV in amplitude (Fig. 15, D_1-R and D_2-R). In some retinular cells, large hyperpolarizing current charges the membrane very slowly and without inflections (Fig. 3, H_2). In other cells, however, large hyperpolarizing current evokes the so-called hyperpolarizing response (Grundfest, 1961; Reuben et al., 1961), whose onset is a function of both the magnitude and the duration of the applied current (Fig. 11, H_2-R_1, H_3-R_1; Fig. 15, H_2-R, H_3-R). The hyperpolarizing response apparently results from a large increase in the resistance of the membrane (Grundfest, 1961; Reuben et al., 1961). The sudden removal of a large hyperpolarizing current leads to a rapid discharge of the membrane potential, followed by a brief oscillating, depolarization with a spike-like transient similar to that evoked by depolarizing current (Fig. 3, H_2). The rapid discharge of the membrane potential underlies part of the hysteresis of the current–voltage curves (see below).

Another feature of retinular cells with large resting and receptor potentials is the non-linearity of their current–voltage (I–V) characteristics, when measured in the dark or in steady light (Borsellino et al., 1965; Smith, 1966). As shown in Figs. 4 and 5, hyperpolarization of the membrane increases the slope resistance and depolarization between resting potential and near-zero membrane potential decreases the resistance. In the dark, further depolarization reveals another region of apparently high resistance (Fig. 5, D). As can be seen, the I–V curves also have considerable hysteresis; however, this property of the retinular cell will not be discussed further in this paper.

Steady light stimuli have characteristic effects on the retinular cell I–V curves. For example, the tangential or slope resistance measured at the steady-state membrane

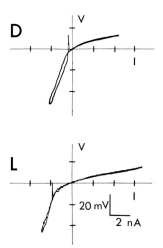

Fig. 4. Current (*I*)–voltage (*V*) curves from retinular cell in dark (D) and in steady light (L). Marks on axes set at increments of calibrations in the fourth quadrant of L. Origin taken as steady-state membrane potential and zero applied current.

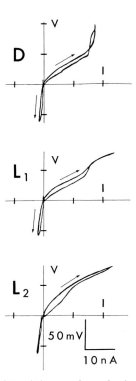

Fig. 5. Retinular cell current (*I*)–voltage (*V*) curve determined with double-barrel microelectrode in dark (D) and with steady light of moderate (L_1) and of bright (L_2) light intensity. Arrows indicate direction of charging of membrane. Origin is steady-state membrane potential. Marks on axes are increments of calibrations in the fourth quadrant of L_2.

potential in the light can be decreased to as little as 10% of the slope resistance at steady-state membrane potential in the dark. When examined with small current, however, the basic shape of the I–V curve is but little affected by light (Fig. 4, cf. D and L). Often, the curve traced in steady light can, after translation along the X–Y axes, be superimposed on the curve traced in the dark. The most striking change in the I–V characteristic brought about by light occurs in the region of the curve examined with large depolarizing current. Here, the apparently high resistance region of the curve found in the dark (Fig. 5, D) is reduced by moderate light intensities (Fig. 5, L_1) and abolished by very bright light (Fig. 5, L_2).

While these properties of the retinular cell membrane have been useful in studying the mechanisms by which light evokes the receptor potential (Smith et al., 1968a, b), for present purposes it is sufficient to note that the doubly rectifying I–V curve in the dark (Fig. 5, D) and the effect of steady light on the I–V curves in retinular cells (Fig. 5) are essentially the same as those found in the ventral eye of Limulus (Smith et al., 1968a), where the photoreceptor cells are not electrotonically coupled to one another. Furthermore, the passive I–V characteristics of the dark-adapted ventral eye photoreceptor membrane can be simulated reasonably well by two semiconductor diodes arranged back-to-back and in series (unpublished observations). For these reasons, we have chosen to represent schematically the membrane lying *directly* between the intracellular and extracellular spaces of the retinular cell (the "γ" membrane* of Fig. 21) with two diodes in series (Fig. 21, B and C).

As has been shown previously, changing the membrane potential with current can alter both the amplitude and the polarity of the receptor potential (Kikuchi et al., 1962; Smith, 1966). Fig. 6 illustrates the results of passing sufficiently long current to bring the membrane potential to a steady-state value and then stimulating the retinular cell with a short pulse of bright light. The records of Column A, on a slow-time base, show the full time-course of both current and light-induced potential changes. The dotted line in each row indicates zero-membrane potential. The records of Column B, on a time base five times faster than that of Column A, show only the receptor potentials corresponding to the records in Column A. Row R illustrates the receptor potential in the absence of extrinsic current. The vertical line extending through the records of Column B marks the identical time in all records that corresponds to the peak of the transient in Row R. Hyperpolarization of the retinular cell (Row H) increases the amplitude of the potential change of the response; however, the level to which the receptor potential depolarizes the cell is the same as that in Row R, *viz.*, to near-zero membrane potential. Depolarization of the cell with current initially reduces the amplitude (D_1 and D_2) and eventually reverses the polarity (D_3) of the receptor potential. However, the membrane potential level which is reached at the peak of the transient, even when reversed in sign, is approximately the same in all records. This is not true of the initial spike (D_1 and D_2), which reaches a membrane potential level on the positive side of zero. In D_3, it is not clear whether the

---

* In this paper we shall use the α, β, γ and σ designation of Borsellino et al., (1965) for the various ommatidial membranes and their respective conductances or resistances.

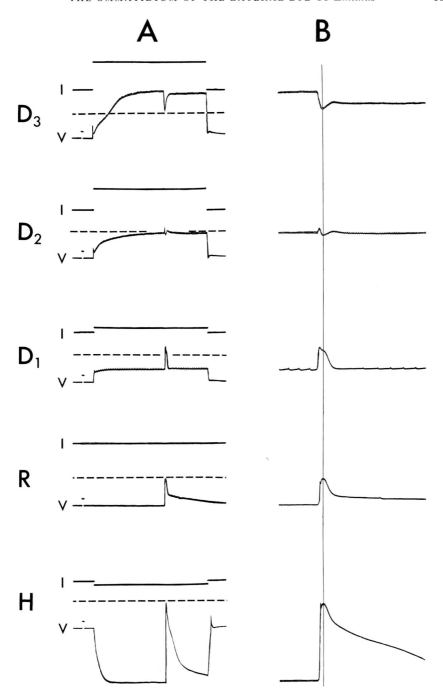

Fig. 6. Interaction of light pulse and long current pulse in one retinular cell with two single-barrel microelectrodes. Column A shows full response (*V*) at slow sweep speed with V, cal 10 mV, 100 msec. *I* in D₃ is 20 nA. Column B shows responses at same gain but sweep speed 5 times A. *R* is response without extrinsic current. *H* is with hyperpolarizing current and D_{1-3} with increasing depolarizing current. Dotted line in A is at zero-membrane potential. Vertical line in B marks all records at the same point in time as peak of transient in R. See text.

spike is present, and if so, if it is reversed in polarity. Despite this uncertainty with respect to the spike, these results indicate that the reversal potential for the receptor potential is near-zero membrane potential. We have examined also the effects of changing membrane potential on receptor potentials evoked by longer pulses of light. We find that the reversal potential of the plateau component of the receptor potential is also near-zero membrane potential (not illustrated).

We take these results, *viz.* that light leads to a large decrease in the slope resistance of the retinular cell membrane when examined at the steady-state membrane potential, that light produced significant changes in the overall *I–V* curves of these cells and that the polarity of the receptor potential reverses near-zero membrane potential, as strong evidence that the retinular cell is directly sensitive to light and is therefore a photoreceptor cell.

(b) Eccentric cells

Microelectrodes encounter eccentric cells much less frequently than retinular cells (Behrens and Wulff, 1965; Fuortes, 1958; MacNichol, 1958; MacNichol *et al.*, 1953; Tomita, 1956; Tomita *et al.*, 1960), and stable penetrations of eccentric cells are associated with resting potentials of more than —40 mV. The response of the eccentric cell to light stimuli has been well documented (Behrens and Wulff, 1965, 1967; Fuortes, 1958, 1959a, b; Hartline *et al.*, 1952b; MacNichol, 1956, 1958; MacNichol *et al.*, 1953; Purple and Dodge, 1965, 1966). It consists of a graded de-

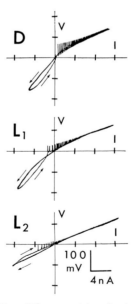

Fig. 7. Eccentric cell current (*I*)–voltage (*V*) curves determined with double-barrel microelectrode in the dark (D) and with continuous moderate (L$_1$) and bright (L$_2$) light. Origin taken as steady-state membrane potential and zero extrinsic current. Marks on axes at increments of calibrations in L$_2$. Arrows indicate direction of charging and discharging of membrane potential.

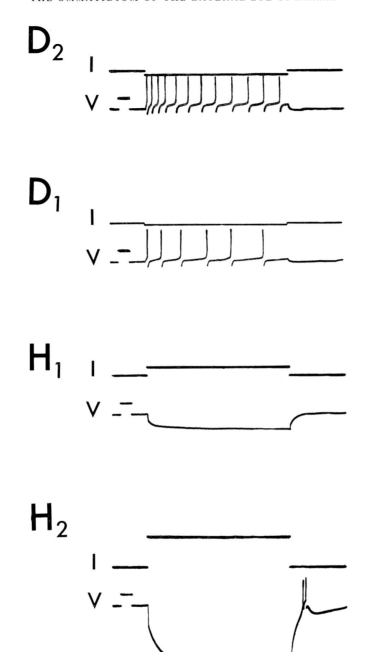

Fig. 8. Voltage (*V*) response of eccentric cell to two levels of depolarizing (*D₁* and *D₂*) and of hyperpolarizing (*H₁* and *H₂*) with extrinsic current (*I*). Identical gain throughout. *V*, cal is 20 mV and 100 msec. Current in *H₂* is 3nA.

polarization of the membrane (a generator potential, G; Fig. 2, Column E) and super-imposed action potentials (S) of large amplitude. The spikes apparently arise in the eccentric cell axon and do not actively invade the eccentric cell soma and dendrite (Fuortes, 1959a; MacNichol, 1956; Purple and Dodge, 1965, 1966; Tomita, 1956, 1957). The frequency of the spikes is determined by the amplitude of the generator potential (Fuortes, 1958, 1959a; MacNichol, 1956, 1958; MacNichol *et al.*, 1953), whose time course is similar to that of the graded receptor potential of the retinular cell (*cf.*, Fig. 2 R and E).

In contradistinction to the retinular cell, the current–voltage characteristic meas-ured from the eccentric cell is often linear or shows only slight rectification with small current (Fig. 7). The decreased resistance with large depolarization may be a consequence of the increase in spike activity, delayed rectification or both. Also the shape of the $I-V$ curve is changed by light (Fig. 7; see below). In addition, with large hyperpolarizing current pulses, the eccentric cell shows an initial, rapidly charging curve followed by a slower phase of charging (Fig. 8, H_2; Fig. 9, H_1 and H_2). The latter is similar in time-course to that seen in retinular cells; however, the eccentric cell does not generate a hyperpolarizing response. The sudden removal of large hyper-polarizing current leads, like the retinular cell, to a rapid recovery of membrane potential, an overshoot and spikes (Fig. 8, H_2). Depolarization of the eccentric cell evokes spikes, whose steady-state firing rate is a linear function of the current applied and the membrane-potential change produced (Fuortes, 1958, 1959a; Hartline *et al.*, 1952a; MacNichol, 1956, 1958; MacNichol *et al.*, 1953; Fig. 8, D_1 and D_2).

The effect of changing the membrane potential of eccentric cells on the generator potential, illustrated in Fig. 9, differs in several significant respects from the results of the same manipulation on the receptor potential in retinular cells (*cf.* Fig. 6). Fig. 9, Line R, illustrates the generator potential evoked by a bright light pulse in the absence of applied current. Hyperpolarization (H_1 and H_2) increases the amplitude of the generator potential; however, the membrane potential level reached at the peak of the generator potential is below that reached in the absence of current (*cf.*, lines H_1 and H_2 with R). Depolarization (D_1 and D_2) reduces the amplitude and raises the level reached by the peak amplitude of the response. The generator potential, however, does not reverse its polarity, even with membrane potential changes of 150 mV (Line D_3; membrane potential + 100 mV) (Fuortes, 1959a). At such mem-brane potential levels, the amplitude of the generator potential becomes vanishingly small, even though the cell's resistance still remains fairly large (*cf.* Fig. 7). This inability to reverse the polarity of the eccentric cell generator potential is consistent with the interpretation that the eccentric cell membrane conductance is not directly affected by light (Waterman and Wiersma, 1954). Taken at first glance, the decrease in slope resistance of the eccentric cell $I-V$ curve with light (Fig. 7) might suggest that the eccentric cell is *directly* sensitive to light; however, as we will discuss later, this change may be a secondary effect due to the changes in retinular cell membrane conductance evoked directly by light and to the electrotonic junctions between retinular and eccentric cells.

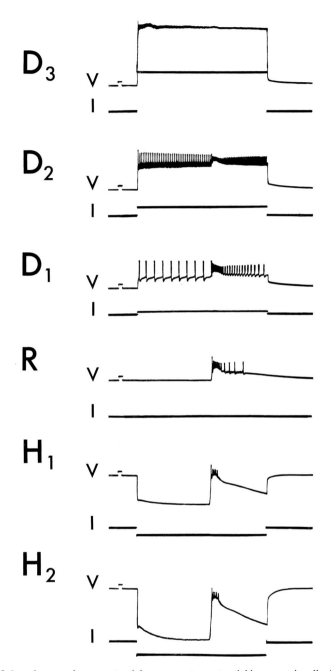

Fig. 9. Effect of changing membrane potential on generator potential in eccentric cell with two single-barrel microelectrodes. R shows response (V) to short pulse of light in the absence of extrinsic current (I). H_1 and H_2 display effect of two levels of hyperpolarization and D_{1-3} of three levels of depolarization. V, cal is 10 mV, 100 msec. I in D_3 is 13 nA.

(2) The interactions between cells within a single ommatidium

With some difficulty the tips of two separate microelectrodes can be placed within two different cells of a single ommatidium. From such microelectrodes, the potentials evoked either by light or by current injected through one or the other microelectrode can be recorded simultaneously. Thereby, information can be obtained on the nature of transmission of signals between different cells within an ommatidium (Behrens and Wulff, 1965; Borsellino *et al.*, 1965; Smith *et al.*, 1965; Stieve, 1965).

(a) Retinular–retinular interactions

The simultaneously evoked receptor potentials from two different retinular cells are shown in Fig. 10A. Often, there are only small differences in the details of the two waveforms. Invariably, however, if action potentials are present, they are synchronous in the two cells (Behrens and Wulff, 1965; Borsellino *et al.*, 1965; Smith *et al.*, 1965; Stieve, 1965).

When small current is passed through one electrode (R_1), a potential change occurs in both cells; however, the *IR*-drop is smaller in the neighboring, unstimulated cell (R_2) (Fig. 11, D and H_1; Fig. 12, H_1, D_1, D_2). With depolarization sufficiently large to evoke spikes, they are synchronous in both cells (Fig. 11, D; Fig. 12, D_1 and D_2). Small hyperpolarizing current evokes only passive charging of the membrane potential of both cells (Fig. 11, H_1; Fig. 12, H_1). By definition, the ability of current of either polarity to spread easily from one cell to another indicates the presence of electrotonic junctions between them (Bennett *et al.*, 1967; Furshpan, 1960; Furshpan and Potter, 1959).

Large hyperpolarizing current evokes a hyperpolarizing response in the stimulated cell (R_1) only. Concomitant with the development of the hyperpolarizing response

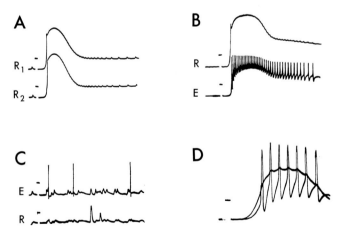

Fig. 10. (A) Response in two simultaneously recorded retinular cells (R_1 and R_2) in same ommatidium to short pulse of light. Onset of light (not shown) at end of *V*-cals. *V*, cal 10 mV, 10 msec. (B) Simultaneously recorded response to retinular (R) and eccentric (E) cell in same ommatidium. *V*, cal 10 mV, 10 msec. (C) Simultaneous recordings of quantum bumps in eccentric (E) and retinular cell (R). *V*, cal 10 mV, 10 msec. (D) Longest latency difference observed in simultaneous recordings from retinular and eccentric cells when stimulated by bright light pulse. *V*, cal 10 mV, 5 msec.

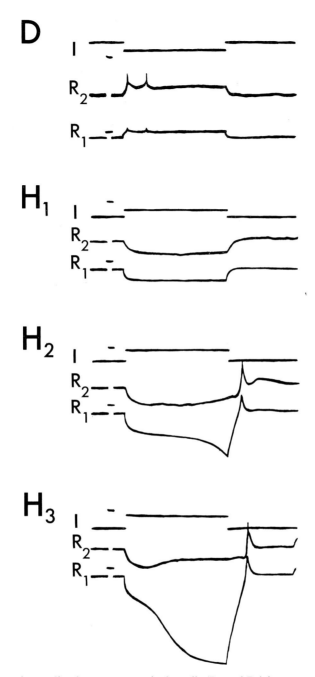

Fig. 11. Electrotonic coupling between two retinular cells (R_1 and R_2) in same ommatidium in the dark. Shown by effects of passing depolarizing (D) and three levels of hyperpolarizing (H_{1-3}) current (I) through microelectrode in R_1 and observing IR-drops in both R_1 and R_2. Note coupling throughout D and H_1, but uncoupling in H_2 and H_3 coincident with development of hyperpolarizing response in R_1. V, cal 10 mV and 100 msec in both R_1 and R_2; note higher gain in R_2. I in H_3 is 1.5 nA.

References p. 347–349

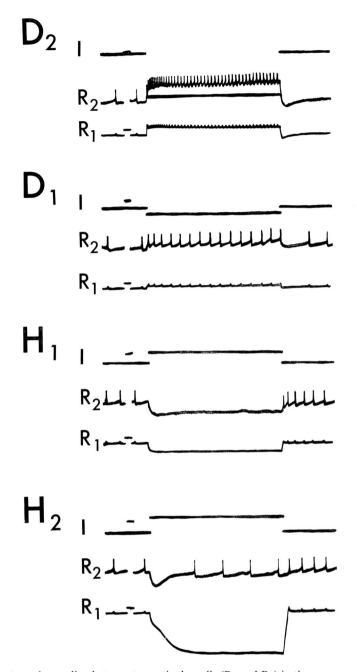

Fig. 12. Electrotonic coupling between two retinular cells (R_1 and R_2) in the same ommatidium in the presence of continuous illumination. Shown by passing depolarizing (D_1 and D_2) and hyper-polarizing (H_1 and H_2) current (I) through R_1 and observing IR-drops and synchronous spikes in both R_1 and R_2. Note uncoupling in H_2 with disappearance of spikes in R_1 during hyperpolarizing response. V, cal 10 mV, 100 msec in both R_1 and R_2; note higher gain in R_2. I in H_2 is 1.8 nA.

in the stimulated cell (R_1), the potential change in the unstimulated cell (R_2) declines (Fig. 11, H_2 and H_3; Fig. 12, H_2). Moreover, if spikes reappear in R_2, they cannot be seen in R_1 during its hyperpolarizing response (Fig. 12, H_2). With the sudden removal of the large hyperpolarizing current, R_1 repolarizes rapidly, with a characteristic transient depolarization, (Fig. 11, H_2 and H_3; Fig. 12, H_2) and with an increase in the frequency of spikes, which are again synchronous in the two cells. These observations indicate that the resistance of the electrotonic junction between the retinular cells also increases during the hyperpolarizing response, thereby uncoupling them.

Furthermore, this electrophysiological uncoupling of the connections between retinular cells on hyperpolarization is a useful indication that the microelectrode tips are indeed in different retinular cells. When, by chance, the two microelectrodes are within a single retinular cell, the hyperpolarizing response evoked *via* current through one microelectrode is recorded with both microelectrodes and the responses are, within experimental error, of the same magnitude (not illustrated). Moreover, in such cells, our results indicate that an individual retinular cell is essentially isopotential over the extent of intracellular region of its cell body.

The *I–V* curves of two retinular cells both in the dark and in the light, and for small current through R_1, are shown in Fig. 13. The uncoupling of the cells with hyperpolarization is apparent. In addition, it can be seen that a given potential change in R_1 produces a smaller change in R_2 in the light than in the dark. This is illustrated quantitatively, for depolarization, in Fig. 18, graph 1. This apparent decrease in the coupling between retinular cells with light will be discussed later.

The *I–V* curves of two retinular cells, over a larger range of current and voltage, are illustrated in Fig. 14. Evidently the electrotonic junction between retinular cells also undergoes an increased resistance with large depolarizing current and the cells become less well coupled since the increasing *IR*-drop in R_1 is accompanied by a decreasing *IR*-drop in R_2.

Essentially identical results to those illustrated in Figs. 11–14 are obtained when current is passed through the other retinular cell (R_2). Thus the retinular cells are electrically symmetrical with respect to their neighbors. Furthermore, as might be expected, one finds a wide range in the degree to which cells are coupled in the experimental population. For example, the ratio of the potential evoked in the cell into which the current is passed (R_1) to the potential recorded in another cell (R_2) may lie between two and ten to one. We interpret this variation as reflecting, in part, the anatomical proximity of and, hence, the number of retinular cells intercalated between the two retinular cells being studied.

These several observations indicate that the retinular cells of a single ommatidium form an electrotonic network arranged in a cylindrical array (Borsellino *et al.*, 1965; Tomita, 1956, 1957, 1958; Tomita *et al.*, 1960). Moreover, the results suggest the equivalent circuit of adjacent retinular cells illustrated in Fig. 21, B. The *R*'s indicate the intracellular spaces of retinular cells and the ground symbol the extracellular medium. The diode-pairs, labelled γ, representing the membrane lying directly between the inside and outside of the cell, have been discussed (see above). The diode-pair representation, labelled β, for the membrane of the electrotonic

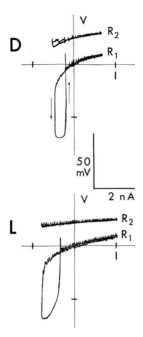

Fig. 13. Current (I)–voltage (V) curves recorded simultaneous in two retinular cells (R_1 and R_2) when current passed through R_1. In the dark (D) and in continuous light (L) the origin is taken as the steady-state potential in R_1. Gain of R_1 and R_2 the same. Arrows indicate direction of charging and discharging in R_1. Note R_2 uncouples from R_1 with hyperpolarization.

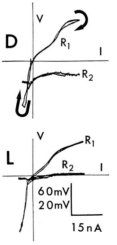

Fig. 14. Current (I)–voltage (V) curves recorded simultaneously with double-barrel microelectrode in R_1 and single-barrel electrode in R_2. Current gain the same for R_1 and R_2. Voltage gain low in R_1 (60 mV cal) and high in R_2 (20 mV). Current through R_1. In the dark (D) and in steady light (L) the origin is the steady-state potential of R_1. Note that R_1 and R_2 uncouple with hyperpolarization and with large depolarizations of R_1.

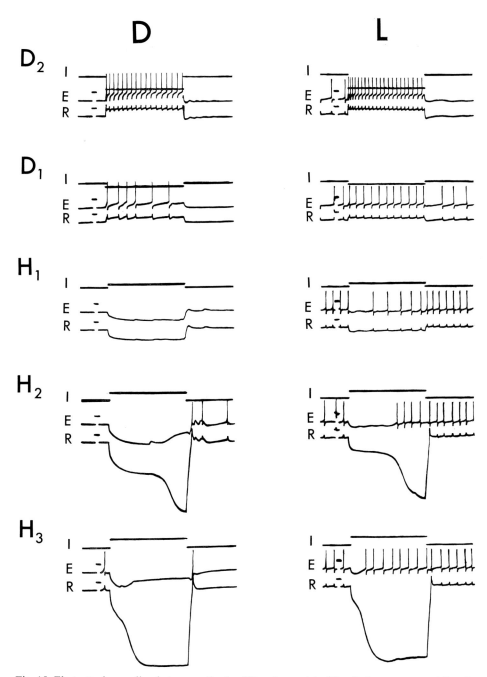

Fig. 15. Electrotonic coupling between retinular (R) and eccentric (E) cells in same ommatidium in the dark (Column D) and with continuous light (Column L). Shown by passing depolarizing (rows D_1 and D_2) and hyperpolarizing (rows H_{1-3}) current (I) through retinular cell. Note IR-drops and synchronous spikes in both R and E with small potential changes (H_1, D_1, D_2), but uncoupling and loss of spikes with hyperpolarizing response in R (H_2 and H_3). V,cal 10 mV, 100 msec. I in H_2 is 2 nA.

junction between adjacent retinular cells is consistent with our observations that the cells uncouple with both large hyperpolarization and large depolarization and that each retinular cell is electrically symmetrical with respect to its neighbors, since uncoupling with large current is apparently a property of all retinular cells.

Perhaps worth noting is that the β-electrotonic junction may actually be composed of two γ-like membranes in series with one another; in which case, β should be represented by four diodes, two facing in one direction and interspersed with two diodes facing in the opposite direction. Whether or not the electrotonic junction is directly affected by light would be indicative of whether β is a two- or four-diode system. The observation that the retinular cells are apparently less well connected in the light than in the dark suggests that the conductance of β is not significantly affected directly by light and that the two-diode representation is sufficient.

(b) Retinular–eccentric interactions

The simultaneously recorded receptor potential of a retinular cell and generator potential of an eccentric cell are illustrated in Fig. 10, B and D. In well penetrated cells, the amplitude of the retinular cell receptor potential is invariably larger than that of the eccentric cell generator potential, while the spikes, which are synchronous in the two cells, are larger in the eccentric cell.

As has been previously reported (Behrens and Wulff, 1965; Stieve, 1965), the relative latencies to onset of the receptor potential and generator potential are variable across preparations and occasionally in the same preparation. In our experiments with bright lights, however, the most common finding is that the latencies are identical within the error of measurement. The greatest difference in latency we have observed is illustrated in Fig. 10, D.

In well penetrated cells in the dark-adapted eye, the so-called quantum bumps (Adolph, 1964; Fuortes, 1959b; Fuortes and Yeandle, 1964; Stieve, 1965; Yeandle, 1957, 1958) are synchronous in the retinular and eccentric cells and the largest quantum bumps are seen in retinular cells (Fig. 10C).

The effects on the retinular and eccentric cells of passing current through the microelectrode in the retinular cell, both in the dark and in the light, are illustrated in Fig. 15. The results and conclusions are similar to those found with two retinular cells, viz., the cells are electrotonically coupled (rows D_1, D_2 and H_1), but become uncoupled during the hyperpolarizing response of the retinular cell (Fig. 15, rows H_2 and H_3); the spikes are synchronous in both cells (all rows), except during the hyperpolarizing response (Fig. 15, Column L, rows H_2 and H_3); and the two cells are apparently less well coupled in the light than in the dark (Fig. 15, cf. Columns D and L; Fig. 18, graph 2).

The consequences of passing current through the eccentric cell microelectrode, on the other hand, are different in several significant respects (Fig. 16). Hyperpolarizing pulses produce the customary two stages of charging in the eccentric cell; however, the eccentric cell does not generate a hyperpolarizing response and, at no level of hyperpolarization studied, do the cells uncouple (Fig. 16, H_2). These results suggest that the slow phase of charging in the eccentric cell may actually reflect the charging in the retinular cell through the electrotonic junctions (see below). In addition, when depolarizing potential changes are evoked in the eccentric cell, the potential changes produced in retinular cells are often smaller than those evoked with comparable hyperpolarizing potential changes.

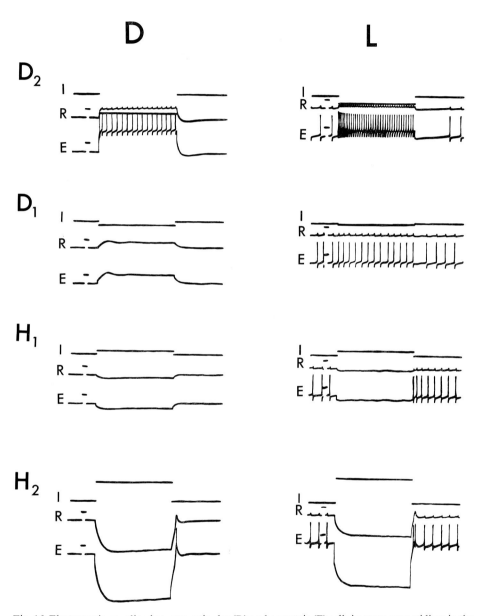

Fig. 16. Electrotonic coupling between retinular (R) and eccentric (E) cells in same ommatidium in the dark (Column D) and with continuous light (Column L). Shown by passing depolarizing (rows D_1 and D_2) and hyperpolarizing (rows H_1 and H_2) current (I) through eccentric cell. Note absence of hyperpolarizing response and uncoupling with hyperpolarization (H_2) and synchrony of spikes. V,cal 10 mV, 100 msec. Current in L, H_2 is 6 nA.

In Fig. 17 are illustrated the *I–V* curves examined with small current in the dark (Column D) and in the light (Column L) when the current is applied directly to the retinular cell (row R) or to the eccentric cell (row E). While there is some variability in the degree of coupling across the retinular cell–eccentric cell pair population, it is less than that seen between retinular cells. Moreover, the ratios of potentials evoked by small current in one cell to that of the coupled cell in the dark are quite high and range between 3 : 2 and 3 : 1.

These several observations indicate that positive charge flows more readily from retinular to eccentric cells than in the opposite direction and suggest that an adjacent retinular cell and eccentric cell, along with their electrotonic junction, may be represented by the equivalent circuit of Fig. 21, C.

In Fig. 21, C, the *R* and *E* represent the intracellular spaces of the retinular and eccentric cells, respectively; γ is the retinular cell membrane adjacent to the extracellular space, σ is the eccentric cell membrane and α the electrotonic junction. The diode-pair representation of γ has been discussed. The junction, α, is represented by a single diode in order to be consistent with the direction of the easy flow of conventional current and the lack of a hyperpolarizing response and intercellular uncoupling with large hyperpolarizing current applied to the eccentric cell. The eccentric cell membrane is represented as a conductance (σ) since the *I–V* curves measured from eccentric cells are nearly linear (Fig. 7; Fig. 17, row E) and the devi-

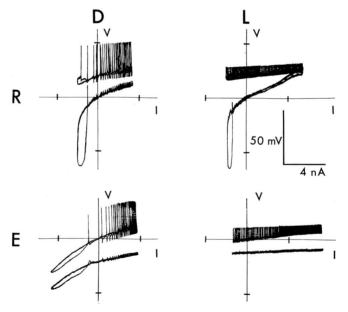

Fig. 17. Current (*I*)–voltage (*V*) curves recorded simultaneous in eccentric (upper trace of each record) and in retinular (lower trace) cells in the dark (Column D) and in continuous light (Column L). Origin is steady-state potential of cell through which current injected; therefore, in Row R current was through retinular cell and in Row E through eccentric cell. Gain the same throughout. Note uncoupling only with hyperpolarization in retinular cell and decreased coupling between cells in the presence of light.

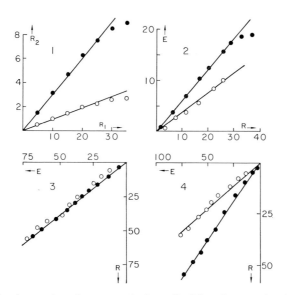

Fig. 18. Intercellular interactions between retinular cells (R) and eccentric cells (E) in the dark (filled circles) and in the light (open circles). All coordinates are in millivolts. Cell through which current passed on abscissa; other cell on ordinate. Graph 1: relationship between depolarizing potential changes in two retinular cells (R_1 and R_2). Graph 2: relationship between depolarization in retinular (R) and eccentric (E) cells. Graphs 3 and 4: relationships between hyperpolarization of eccentric (E) and retinular (R) cells. See text.

ations from linearity are probably explicable on the basis of the coupling to retinular cells (see below). A necessary condition of the circuit of Fig. 21, C is that the value of σ in ohms be very large, otherwise the rectification with large depolarization in retinular cells in the dark (Figs. 5 D and 14 R_1) could not be obtained (see below).

Whether or not the electrotonic junction, a, between retinular and eccentric cells is directly affected by light is not entirely certain because of contradictory evidence. For example, the degree to which light affects the flow of hyperpolarizing current from eccentric to retinular cells is illustrated in Fig. 18, graphs 3 and 4. In some experiments (graph 3), light apparently has little effect on the relationship between the potential evoked in eccentric cells to that in retinular cells, except perhaps for small potential changes (< 25 mV). This suggests that a- and γ-membrane conductances increase proportionately with light. In other cells (graph 4), a given potential change in the eccentric cell evokes a smaller change in retinular cells in the light than in the dark. This suggests that the main effect of light is on γ and that a changes only to the extent that the depolarization of the retinular cell forward-biases the a-diode.

We usually find that a depolarizing potential evoked in retinular cells produces a larger potential change in eccentric cells in the dark than in the light, which suggests that a is not directly affected by light (Fig. 18, graph 2). At first glance, this might be taken as evidence for a direct photic effect on the eccentric cell membrane, σ; however, this could be due to a leakage of current through the forward-biased a's and the increased γ conductances of the remainder of the retinular cells of the ommatidium.

However, the bulk of the evidence weighs against a direct photic effect on the σ membrane; the most convincing is the inability to reverse the generator potential (Fig. 9) in the face of the rectifying properties of the α membrane (Fig. 21, C). If, as we assume, the α junction between the retinular and eccentric cell may be represented by a single diode (Fig. 21, C), then very large depolarizing current applied to the eccentric cell would effectively back-bias the α-diode thereby increasing its resistance. This increased resistance would then block the flow of depolarizing current from the retinular cell to the eccentric cell during stimulation with light. In that situation, any direct effect of light on the eccentric cell should be apparent as a reversed generator potential; however, since there is no generator potential, we conclude that light does not affect the eccentric cell membrane directly.

We should point out, however, that, although it is clear that the α-membrane behaves as a single rectifier over the range of membrane potentials investigated (see above and Figs. 15, 16, 17, 18 and 21, C), our assumption that the α-membrane behaves as a single rectifier with very large depolarizations applied to the eccentric cell is an inferential extrapolation of our data. A crucial test of this assumption would be to pass large depolarizing current through one microelectrode in an eccentric cell while monitoring the potential changes in that same eccentric cell with another electrode and in an adjacent retinular cell with yet a third electrode. We would expect that increasing the depolarizing current in the eccentric cell would lead to a progressive increase in the depolarization of the retinular cell but, eventually, the retinular cell would cease to depolarize concomitantly. That, is we would expect a result similar to that shown in Fig. 14, D.

Despite repeated attempts, we have been unable to penetrate simultaneously an eccentric cell with two microelectrodes and a retinular cell with a third microelectrode. Since this crucial data is lacking, we must leave open the question of alternative explanations for the results of Fig. 9. We believe, however, our conclusion that light does not affect the eccentric cell directly to be the most consistent with the data in hand.

If this conclusion is valid, the relationship between the light-evoked potential changes in retinular and eccentric cells bear on the direct affect of light, if any, on the α-membrane. Here, where we assume that all retinular cells are approximately equipotential, the complications of the experiment shown in Fig. 18, graph 2, are diminished. As illustrated in Fig. 19, there is a linear relationship between the depolarizations evoked by light in retinular and eccentric cells, *i.e.*, equal incremental depolarizations in retinular cells lead to equal incremental depolarizations in the eccentric cell over most of the physiological range of steady-state membrane potential. If therefore, σ is unaffected by light, these results indicate that α is not directly affected by light either. As mentioned above, however, there may be a secondary increase in the conductance of α due to a forward biasing of the α-diode.

(c) The ommatidial network

With regard to the overall intercellular organization of the photoreceptor unit, the cumulative data indicate that the ommatidium is an electrotonic network and

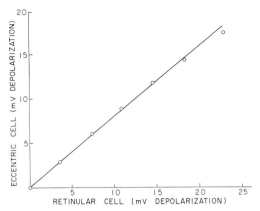

Fig. 19. Relationship between light induced depolarizations in retinular and eccentric cell. Origin is in presence of dim light and each successive point represents a 4-fold increase in light intensity. Each point is average steady-state potential.

that the equivalent circuit of that network may be represented by Fig. 21, A. There, each cell is represented as electrotonically connected to its nearest neighbors. In Fig. 21, A, the junctions are shown as conductances; however, the nature of each circuit element is indicated in Fig. 21, B and C.

For the ommatidial network, one can write the node and mesh equations and, using experimentally determined values, solve for the magnitudes of the individual slope conductances both in the light and in the dark. The methods used in these computations have been previously reported (Borsellino *et al.*, 1965). From the pooled average of experimental data, the results of these computations are shown in Table I. These data indicate that, with illumination, there are significant changes in γ, the retinular cell membrane conductance. The affects of light on the conductances of α, β, and σ are probably not statistically significant.

The results of Table I also suggest the mechanism by which a given potential change in one retinular cell or an eccentric cell evokes a smaller potential change in another retinular cell in the light than in the dark (Fig. 18). If one considers only the coupling conductance (α or β) and the conductance of the membrane of the cell immediately adjacent to the cell through which current is passed to constitute a simple voltage-divider network, then the voltage change in the stimulated cell is the input (V_{in}) and the voltage in the unstimulated cell is the output (V_{out}) of the network (*cf.* Borsellino *et al.*, 1965). Then the coupling ratio (ϱ) between V_{out} and V_{in} is

$$\varrho_\varepsilon = \frac{\beta}{\beta + \gamma}$$

when current is passed through the eccentric cell and the potentials are recorded from that cell and from a contiguous retinular cell. When current is passed through one retinular cell and potentials are recorded from that retinular cell and from an adjacent retinular cell, the ratio (ϱ_R) cannot be accurately expressed by a simple formula (Borsellino *et al.*, 1965); however, to a first approximation,

$$\varrho_R \sim \frac{a}{a + \gamma}$$

If, therefore, light increases the conductance of γ without significantly changing a or β, $\varrho_\mathcal{E}$ and ϱ_R will be less in the light than in the dark and, in one sense, the cells are less well coupled. The same result would obtain if the conductance of a and β were to decrease and that of γ unchanged with light; however, this is apparently not the case (Table I).

If coupling is defined in terms of the magnitude of the coupling conductances and if a and β are not significantly changed by light, in another sense, then, the coupling between adjacent cells is independent of light. On the other hand, for any given potential change in a cell stimulated with current there is actually *more* current flowing through its coupling conductances in the light than in the dark. Thus, in yet another sense, the cells are better coupled in the light than in the dark. Whether, therefore, one concludes that light affects the coupling between the cells in an ommatidium depends on the way "coupling" is defined.

The conclusion that the retinular cell membrane is the main or perhaps the exclusive light-sensitive element of the ommatidium in no way localizes that element to any specific portion of the retinular cell. A too literal reading of Fig. 21,A might interpret γ to represent only the non-rhabdomeric membrane resistance. This interpretation is decidedly incorrect: γ represents the resistance of any portion of the retinular cell membrane that communicates *directly* with the extracellular space. The recent finding that a significant portion of rhabdomeric membrane connects directly to the extracellular space (Lasansky, personal communication), suggests that that membrane may be involved in the generation of the receptor potential.

A particularly gratifying result in Table I is the relative magnitude of the σ and γ resistances in the dark, *viz.*, the resistance of σ is approximately 20 times that of γ. This result makes compatible our observation that the γ resistance increases markedly with large depolarizing current in the dark (Fig. 5, D), even in the face of a diode-like connection (a) between the retinular and eccentric cells which would be forward-biased by such current (Fig. 21, C). Therefore, even if γ increased 10-fold, it would still remain the dominant load to current passed through the retinular cell.

The results of Table I also suggest that the conductances of a and γ may constitute a significant load to current applied to the eccentric cell, *i.e.* a relative large fraction of such current exists through the retinular cell membrane (γ) to the extracellular space. If this is the case, then the a's and γ's should contribute significantly to the I–V curve measured from the eccentric cell. In this regard, a computation of interest can be made from a modified version of the node and mesh equations for the circuit shown in Fig. 21, A, which takes into account the non-linearities of the circuit elements shown in Fig. 21, B and C. For example, it can be shown that it is theoretically possible for the current–voltage curve measured from the eccentric cell to be approximately linear, even though it is connected through non-linear electrotonic junctions (a) to the retinular cells, whose membranes are also non-linear (γ).

This calculation may make the results of Fig. 7 consistent with the hypothesis

TABLE I

EFFECT OF LIGHT ON OMMATIDIAL NETWORK CONDUCTANCES

Calculated from node and mesh equations for Fig. 21A (Borsellino *et al.*, 1965).
Values in μmhos $\pm$ 1 S.D. See text.

	Dark	Light
α	0.03 $\pm$ 0.004	0.07 $\pm$ 0.02
β	0.09 $\pm$ 0.01	0.08 $\pm$ 0.02
γ	0.02 $\pm$ 0.0003	0.06 $\pm$ 0.02
σ	0.001 $\pm$ 0.02	0.001 $\pm$ 0.02

that the eccentric cell is not directly affected by light. As previously mentioned, the decrease in the slope of the eccentric cell *I–V* curve during illumination might suggest that this cell's membrane (σ) does undergo a direct increase in conductance. The above calculation, however, indicates that the observations of Fig. 7 may be explained on the basis of a conductance change only in the retinular cell membrane and of the electrotonic connections between retinular and eccentric cells. Specifically, the increased conductance with light measured from the eccentric cell (Fig. 7) may only reflect the conductance change occurring in the retinular cell membrane (γ).

(d) Origin and size of spikes

Finally, we would remark on the origin and size of the spikes recorded from ommatidial cells. Under conditions similar to those of our experiments, the data of other investigators indicated that regenerative and propagated action potentials arise only from eccentric cell axons (Hartline *et al.*, 1952b; MacNichol, 1956, 1958; MacNichol *et al.*, 1953; Tomita, 1956, 1957, 1958; Tomita *et al.*, 1960; Waterman and Wiersma, 1954). Moreover, the direction of the rectification of the α-membrane (Fig. 21, C) suggests one reason for the diminished amplitude or absence of spikes recorded in retinular cells (Figs. 10, 15, 16). Equally important in this regard may be the electrical characteristics of the α- and γ-membranes, *viz.*, that the effective con-

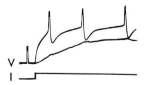

Fig. 20. Filtering action of retinular–eccentric electrotonic junction resistance and retinular cell membrane capacitance. Cells hyperpolarized with steady current in eccentric cell. A step of depolarizing current (*I*) applied to eccentric cell. In V, upper trace with large spikes from eccentric cell, lower trace from retinular cell. Note rapid response from eccentric cell and slow response with attenuated spikes in retinular cell. *V*, cal 10 mV, 5 msec.

ductance of the α-membrane and the effective capacitance of the γ-membrane behave as a low-pass filter to current injected in the eccentric cell and the potential recorded in the retinular cell. The consequence of such a high-frequency filtering action is illustrated in Fig. 20, where the cells are coupled by passing a steady hyperpolarizing current to the eccentric cell. A depolarizing step of current, sufficient to evoke spikes but not to uncouple the cells, rapidly depolarizes the eccentric cell; however, the retinular cell charges very slowly. Moreover, the eccentric cell spikes appear only as small ripples on the retinular cell trace.

DISCUSSION

In this paper we have presented a selected body of the data gathered from micro-electrode recordings in the lateral eye of *Limulus polyphemus*. The data have been selected by a number of criteria which depend upon measurable electrophysiological variables (*e.g.*, the magnitudes of membrane potential, response to light, membrane rectification, etc.). Based on these criteria and on previously reported experiments where the cells were marked with dyes (Behrens and Wulff, 1965, 1967; Kikuchi and Ueki, 1965), we have classified the visual cells studied as retinular cells or eccentric cells (Behrens and Wulff, 1965, 1967; Fuortes, 1958; Kikuchi and Ueki, 1965; Stieve, 1965; Tomita, 1957, 1958; Tomita *et al.*, 1960; Yeandle, 1957, 1958). In addition, for both cell types, we have chosen for detailed analysis only those in the best physiological condition obtainable in our hands. From the cells that satisfy the above criteria, we have chosen examples which best illustrate a hypothesis which is the most internally consistent with our best data.

This hypothesis of ommatidial photophysiology is not novel with us. Its separate components, as well as the overall thesis, have developed as a consequence of the anatomical and physiological investigations of the *Limulus* lateral eye over the past two decades. The hypothesis is this:

(*1*) The retinular cells are the primary photoreceptor or sensory cells of the lateral eye (Tomita, 1956; Waterman and Wiersma, 1954). The action of light on these cells is the production of a depolarizing potential change of complex waveform across their membranes (Tomita, 1956). In Davis' terminology this depolarization should be called a receptor potential (Davis, 1961).

(*2*) The eccentric cell is the second-order neuron in the visual pathway (Hartline *et al.*, 1952b; Tomita, 1956; Waterman and Wiersma, 1954) and is not intrinsically sensitive to light (Waterman and Wiersma, 1954).

(*3*) The receptor potential sets up a potential gradient between the retinular and eccentric cells, which results in a flow of current between these two cells through an electrotonic junction formed by a fusion of their contiguous membranes (Tomita, 1956, 1957, 1958; Tomita *et al.*, 1960; Waterman and Wiersma, 1954).

(*4*) The current entering the eccentric cell soma and dendrite evokes a graded depolarization across its membranes which spreads electrotonically to the axon of the cell

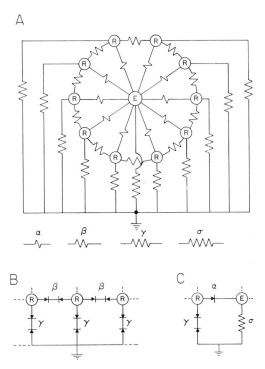

Fig. 21. (A) Equivalent circuit for intercellular network of a single ommatidium. Ⓡ and Ⓔ represent intracellular compartments of retinular and eccentric cells, respectively; and ground symbol represents extracellular compartment. The various electrical connections are indicated as conductances, which correspond to key below diagram. The nature of these connections is indicated in B and C. (B) Equivalent circuit for retinular–retinular connections. γ is retinular cell membrane to extracellular space; β is electrotonic junction between adjacent retinular cells. (C) Equivalent circuit for retinular–eccentric connections; γ is as before; σ is eccentric cell membrane to extracellular space; and α is electrotonic junction between retinular and eccentric cell. See text.

(Hartline *et al.*, 1952b; MacNichol, 1956, 1958; MacNichol *et al.*, 1953; Tomita, 1956, 1957, 1958; Tomita *et al.*, 1960; Waterman and Wiersma, 1954). When the axon is depolarized to a threshold value, action potentials or spikes are generated which travel without decrement to the brain (Fuortes, 1959a; Hartline *et al.*, 1952b; Mac-Nichol, 1956, 1958; MacNichol *et al.* 1953). These spikes, however, do not actively invade the eccentric cell soma and dendrite (Fuortes, 1959a; MacNichol, 1956, 1958; MacNichol *et al.*, 1953). In Davis' terminology, the graded depolarization may be called either a post-synaptic potential or a generator potential (Davis, 1961). Bowing to historical precedent, we will use the latter term.

In the remainder of this Discussion we shall review the evidence presented in this paper and elsewhere in support of this hypothesis and indicate some of the details of the mechanisms involved.

Ommatidial organization. The ommatidium has long been considered the visual or photoreceptor unit of the compound eye (Demoll, 1914; Hartline *et al.*, 1952b; Patten, 1912; *cf.* also Wolbarsht and Yeandle, 1967). The cumulative evidence of recent electrophysiological and anatomical experiments, however, suggest an intimate organization between the cellular constituents of a single ommatidium. Specifically, this evidence indicates that the cells of an ommatidium form a tightly coupled electrotonic network and that physiological activity in any one ommatidial cell can influence the responsiveness of its neighbors.

The essential electrophysiological evidence is straightforward and unequivocal, *viz.*, when small current of either polarity is passed between the inside of any given cell of the ommatidium and the extracellular fluid, a similar but smaller potential change is produced in the other cells of the same ommatidium (Behrens and Wulff, 1965; Borsellino *et al.*, 1965; Smith *et al.*, 1965; Figs. 11–18). The essential anatomical evidence is likewise straightforward; *viz.*, "tight" junctions exist between contiguous cells within the same ommatidium (Lasansky, 1967). The conclusion appears inescapable that adjacent retinular cells in an ommatidium are joined by electrotonic junctions and, in addition, that all the retinular cells are separately joined to the (usually) single eccentric cell of the ommatidium *via* electrotonic junctions.

Beyond these essentials, however, there are a number of characteristics in which these electrotonic junctions are distinctive and, perhaps, unique. For example, as we have noted, large depolarizations and hyperpolarizations of a retinular cell produce a large increase in the resistance of that cell's membrane (Figs. 5, 14) and that coincidentally the retinular cell becomes uncoupled from its neighbors (Figs. 11–14). In addition, the junctions between adjacent retinular cells are electrically symmetrical. These results indicate that the equivalent circuit elements of the electrotonic junction between adjacent retinular cells and of the retinular cell membrane connecting the inside of the cell directly to the extracellular fluid may both be represented by two back-to-back diodes. These are shown in Fig. 21,B as the β connections and the γ components.

In the Results we indicated that our data are not sufficient to decide between a two- and a four-diode representation for β; however, should the two-diode model be correct, this would indicate that the fusion of the outer components of the bimolecular leaflets at the tight junctions is associated with a loss of part of the membrane's rectifying properties.

This possible loss of part of the rectifying properties of a membrane at a tight junction is also suggested by the nature of the coupling between retinular and eccentric cells. Here, as illustrated by the α in Fig. 21,C, the junction is singly rectifying such that conventional current passes more easily from the retinular to the eccentric cell than *vice versa*. This junction is basically similar to that found at the crayfish giant motor synapse (Furshpan and Potter, 1959).

Therefore, the electrical organization of an ommatidium is similar to that represented schematically in Fig. 21,A, where each cell is electrotonically connected to its nearest neighbors. We have illustrated these connections as conductances; however, the nature of each circuit element is indicated in Fig. 21,B and C.

Over the course of the past 10 years an impressive number of electrotonic synapses have been found in a wide variety of species and organs (*cf.* Bennett *et al.*, 1967, for bibliography). To our knowledge, however, the lateral eye of the horseshoe crab, the retina of the locust (Shaw, 1967a) and the retina of the dione honeybee (Shaw, 1967b) are the only sensory organs that have such synapses. In addition, most of the electrotonic junctions examined previously have linear current–voltage characteristics. The lateral eye of *Limulus* is apparently only the third junction found to have rectification (Bennett *et al.*, 1967; Furshpan, 1960; Furshpan and Potter, 1959) and the first to have double rectification.

Recently there has been a good deal of interest in those factors which may regulate or influence the presence or degree of electrotonic coupling between cells. For example, electrotonic coupling may correlate with the stage of differentiation or growth of embryonic tissue (Potter *et al.*, 1965) or may be altered by manipulation of the ionic or osmotic environment of the tissue, by treatment with enzymes and by damage of cells in an electrotonically coupled tissue (Lowenstein *et al.*, 1967). In most of the cases studied, the basic membrane mechanisms which underlie electrotonic coupling are unknown and once cells have been uncoupled by experimental manipulation, the process is usually irreversible. While the basic membrane mechanisms underlying electrotonic coupling in the *Limulus* ommatidium are also obscure, the coupling is a function of the potential difference across the junction and uncoupling by appropriate adjustment of the junctional potential difference is quite reversible (Figs. 11–17). These characteristics suggest that the *Limulus* ommatidium might be a tractable preparation in which to study the regulation of electrotonic coupling.

We should point out, however, that other procedures can apparently uncouple ommatidial cells irreversibly. When, for example, an ommatidial cell is damaged either by inadvertant injury with a micropipette (unpublished observation) or by extreme electrical stimulation (Behrens and Wolff, 1967), the remaining cells in the ommatidium continue to function normally. If the cells of an ommatidium are ordinarily as closely coupled as our results indicate, then damage and depolarization of one cell of the group must uncouple it from its neighbors. Otherwise, the damaged cell would constitute a severe electrical load on its neighbors and seriously alter their function, but this is apparently not the case (Behrens and Wolff, 1967; this paper).

The light-sensitive element. There have been a number of different opinions expressed in the literature as to the locus of the light-sensitive element in the ommatidium (*cf.* Wolbarsht and Yeandle, 1967). To our minds, the preponderance of the anatomical, physiological and comparative biological data is in favor of the retinular cell membrane as the *primary* site of generation of visually related potential changes.

The rhabdomere, which is commonly thought to be the locus of the visual pigment (Langer and Thorell, 1966), rhodopsin, is mainly a constituent of the retinular cell (Lasansky, 1967; Miller, 1957) and, indeed, is probably formed by specialized portions of the retinular cell membrane. The eccentric cell makes a small, but not insignificant, contribution to the rhabdomere (Lasansky, 1967); however, these portions of the eccentric cell membrane may play a more mechanical and electrical than photoreceptive function.

There are at least five lines of electrophysiological evidence that argue in favor of identifying the retinular cell as the primary photosensitive cell:

(1) Given the electrotonic junctions and the direction of rectification between the retinular and eccentric cells, the fact that the retinular cell receptor potential is of larger amplitude than the eccentric cell generator potential indicates that the potential gradient for depolarizing current is *from* the retinular cell *to* the eccentric cell. The finding that the largest quantum bumps occur in the retinular cells is also consistent with this interpretation. Often some of the quantum bumps recorded in the eccentric cell are larger than those simultaneously recorded from the impaled retinular cell; however, we would suggest these bumps arise from retinular cells which are connected directly to the eccentric cell but which lie at a locus in the ommatidium that is remote to the impaled retinular cell.

(2) The polarity of the receptor potential reverses between the inside and the outside of the retinular cell, which indicates that the receptor potential generator lies in the retinular cell membrane (Tomita, 1956, 1957, 1958; Tomita *et al.*, 1960).

(3) The polarity of the receptor potential in the retinular cell reverses at near-zero membrane potential (Kikuchi *et al.*, 1960; Fig. 6) which also locates the generator in the retinular cell membrane. This is in contradistinction to the generator potential of the eccentric cell, which does not reverse polarity even when the membrane potential is 100 mV, inside positive (Fig. 9). At such membrane potential levels, where the eccentric cell is presumably uncoupled from the retinular cells, no generator potential is evoked. This observation is not only against the eccentric cell being a primary photoreceptor (Waterman and Wiersma, 1954) but also is inconsistent with a chemical synapse between the retinular and eccentric cell (Tomita *et al.*, 1960). In either of these latter two cases, the generator potential should have reversed polarity when the membrane potential is 100 mV, inside positive. Thus the eccentric cell is not a primary photoreceptor but the second-order neuron in the visual pathway and is apparently connected to the retinular cells only by electrotonic junctions.

(4) In contrast to the eccentric cell, which does not give a response to light when uncoupled from retinular cells, the retinular cells do respond to light when uncoupled from eccentric cells. This uncoupling may be achieved in one of two ways. In the first, the retinular cell, when hyperpolarized with a steady current, uncouples from the eccentric cell (Fig. 15, H_2 and H_3), but still responds vigorously to light (Fig. 6, H). In the second case, the eccentric cell can be killed by a sufficiently large current passed through a microelectrode, yet retinular cells in the same ommatidium still respond to light (Behrens and Wulff, 1967).

(5) The solution of the node and mesh equations for the ommatidial network indicate that the conductance of the membrane which connects the inside of the retinular cell directly to the extracellular space changes on illumination; however, the conductance of the eccentric cell membrane apparently does not change with light. The status of the junctional resistances is uncertain (Borsellino *et al.*, 1965; this paper) but probably they are not directly affected by light.

Finally, the comparative biology of invertebrate eyes would indicate that the retinular cell is the photoreceptor. Specifically, most if not all compound eyes in other species have only retinular cells and yet give receptor potentials similar to those of *Limulus* (*cf.* Goldsmith, 1964; Naka and Kishida, 1966). Indeed, the ventral eye of *Limulus* itself has no eccentric cells and its photoreceptor cells behave remarkably like retinular cells of the lateral eye (Millechia *et al.*, 1966; Smith *et al.*, 1968a).

While we interpret the above evidence as indicating the retinular cell to be the photoreceptor, we know of no compelling evidence which delimits any particular macroscopic portion of that cell's membrane as the sole site of the receptor potential generator. Within the sensitivity of presently available techniques, any portion of retinular cell membrane that communicates directly with the extracellular space could be involved. Moreover, with the recent evidence that a significant fraction of rhabdomeric membrane may be in direct contact with the extracellular space (Lasansky, personal communication) this membrane may well be actively involved in the receptor potential. Furthermore, we know of no evidence which indicates any intrinsic physiological difference between rhabdomeric and non-rhabdomeric membrane. If, therefore, there is specialization of the retinular cell membrane, it may be on a scale smaller than that suggested by the rhabdomeric–nonrhabdomeric dichotomy, namely, a mosaic of different types of membrane at a submicroscopic or molecular level. Such a specialized organization would be consistent with the suggestions that the rhodopsin may actually be a membrane constituent (Hagins and McGaughy, 1968; Smith and Brown, 1966) and that the receptor potential is generated across the retinular cell membrane (Tomita, 1956, 1957, 1958; Tomita *et al.*, 1960; this paper). Moreover, such an organization places constraints on mechanisms of transduction of light-to-electrical energy, in that the question of energy transduction becomes a question of how one patch of receptor membrane, containing rhodopsin, after absorbing photons, can affect a nearby patch of receptor membrane concerned with the generation of the receptor potential (Smith and Brown, 1966; Smith *et al.*, 1968b).

To us, a submicroscopic specialization of the receptor membrane avoids some of the problems inherent in a specialization at the rhabdomere–nonrhabdomere level. For example, if light were absorbed exclusively by the rhabdomere and the receptor potential produced solely by nonrhabdomeric membrane, it might be difficult to explain how the rhabdomeric membrane can communicate a signal to the non-rhabdomeric membrane over a distance of several microns with a latency of only a few milliseconds.

Our suggestion that there may be no intrinsic difference between rhabdomeric and nonrhabdomeric membrane does not indicate that the rhabdomere does not play a dominant role in the photoreceptor. The fact that the majority of the retinular cell membrane lies in the rhabdomere implies its dominance (Lasansky, 1967; Miller, 1957). Indeed, postulating that the rhabdomeric membrane actively participates in the production of the receptor potential as well as in the absorption of light increases the importance of the rhabdomere.

Physiological implications. If the results and conclusions of this paper are substantially correct, they have a number of implications for the photophysiology of the lateral eye ommatidium. The most obvious are those stated in the hypothesis, *viz.*, the retinular cells are the photoreceptors, the eccentric cell is a second-order neuron in the visual pathway and visually related signals are transmitted from the retinular to the eccentric cell *via* an electrotonic junction. Of a number of other consequences, we shall discuss two.

The first concerns the effect of the electrotonic junction between a retinular cell and the eccentric cell on the fidelity and efficiency of transmitting information through an ommatidium. Apparently the burden of generating the primary photosignal rests solely with the retinular cell and, so long as it can maintain its activity, the eccentric cell activity is bound to follow *pari passu*. Thus, the communication between the cells is not subject to the hazards of chemical transmitter depletion or of post-synaptic membrane desensitization found at chemical synapses (Katz, 1962; Katz and Thesleff, 1957; *cf.* also Eccles, 1964). Moreover, the complex machinery and expenditure of energy required for the production, release and breakdown of a chemical transmitter are avoided. It may be, therefore, that, in addition to synchronizing the activity of a group of cells (*cf.* Bennett *et al.*, 1967), electrotonic junctions also optimally insure the transmission of signals, particularly continuous ones, from one cell to another. In addition, the rectifying property of the retinular–eccentric junction also increases the efficiency of transmitting depolarizing signals from one retinular cell to the axon of the eccentric cell by reducing the back-leakage of positive charge from the eccentric cell to other retinular cells.

Another consequence of the results of this paper concerns the regulation of the sensitivity of the eye to photic stimulation. In the first place, the I–V characteristic of the retinular cell membrane suggests a means by which that membrane regulates its own sensitivity (*cf.* Naka and Kishida, 1966). Thus, if a given increment in light intensity evokes a fixed increment of receptor current, the more depolarized the membrane, the smaller will be the incremental change in membrane potential. In addition, because of the electrotonic junction between adjacent retinular cells, depolarization of one retinular cell by light will also depolarize its neighbors, thereby reducing the resistance of their γ-membranes and hence their sensitivity to light. The electrotonic network of cells would therefore tend to average the activity and prevent large disparities of behavior among the several ommatidial cells.

In summary, we have presented a number of selected observations made with intracellular recordings in single ommatidia of the lateral eye of *Limulus*. We have attempted to characterize some of the distinctive features of recording from retinular cells and from eccentric cells when they are stimulated by light and by extrinsic current. In addition, we have presented and discussed the evidence indicating that the retinular cell is the primary photoreceptor cell. We have also presented and discussed the evidence which indicates that the eccentric cell is not inherently photosensitive and is, therefore, the second-order neuron in the visual pathway. Finally, we have presented the evidence for and discussed the physiological consequences of the electrotonic organization of the ommatidium, where each cell is joined to its immediate neighbors by rectifying tight junctions.

SUMMARY

In this paper the following items are presented and discussed:

(*1*) The distinguishing characteristics of the electrical activity recorded with intracellular microelectrodes from retinular and from eccentric cells in the lateral eye of *Limulus polyphemus*.

(*2*) The evidence indicating that the retinular cell is the primary photoreceptor.

(*3*) The evidence which indicates the eccentric cell is not inherently photosensitive and is, therefore, the second-order neuron in the visual pathway.

(*4*) The evidence which indicates that adjacent retinular cells are connected by a doubly-rectifying, electrotonic "tight" junction.

(*5*) The evidence which indicates that individual retinular cells are joined to eccentric cells *via* a singly rectifying, electrotonic "tight" junction.

(*6*) An equivalent circuit of the electrotonic network of the ommatidium.

ACKNOWLEDGEMENTS

We wish to express our thanks for the hospitality of the Marine Biological Laboratory, Woods Hole, Mass. (U.S.A.) and of the Department of Biology and Research Laboratory of Electronics, Massachusetts Institute of Technology, Cambridge, Mass. (U.S.A.), where many of the experiments reported here were performed. Our thanks also to those many colleagues who provided helpful discussion, criticism and suggestions. Our especial thanks to Prof. A. Borsellino and Dr. M. G. F. Fuortes for their generous permission to use in Table I the results of their calculations on their and our pooled data.

REFERENCES

ADOLPH, A., (1964); Spontaneous slow potential fluctuations in the *Limulus* photoreceptors. *J. gen. Physiol.*, **48**, 297–322.

BEHRENS, M. E., AND WULFF, V. J., (1965); Light-initiated responses of retinular and eccentric cells in the *Limulus* lateral eye. *J. gen. Physiol.*, **48**, 1081–1093.

BEHRENS, M. E., AND WULFF, V. J., (1967); Functional autonomy in the lateral eye of the horseshoe crab, *Limulus polyphemus*. *Vision Res.*, **7**, 191–196.

BENNETT, M. V. L., PAPPAS, G. D., GIMENEZ, M., AND NAKAJIMA, Y., (1967); Physiology and ultrastructure of electrotonic junctions IV. Medullary electromotor nuclei in Gymnotid fish. *J. Neurophysiol.*, **30**, 236–300.

BENOLKEN, R. M., (1961); Reversal of photoreceptor polarity recorded during graded receptor potential response to light in the eye of *Limulus*. *Biophys. J.*, **1**, 551–564.

BORSELLINO, A., FUORTES, M. G. F., AND SMITH, T. G., (1965); Visual responses in *Limulus*. *Cold Spr. Harb. Symp. quant. Biol.*, **30**, 429–443.

CAVANAUGH, G. F., (Ed.), (1956); *Formulae and Methods, Vol. V*, Marine Biological Laboratory, Woods Hole, Mass.

DAVIS, H., (1961); Some principles of sensory receptor action. *Physiol. Rev.*, **41**, 391–416.

DEMOLL, R., (1914); Die Augen von *Limulus*. *Zool. Jahrb. Abt. Anat.*, **38**, 443–464.

DOWLING, J. E., (1968); Discrete potentials in the dark-adapted eye of the crab *Limulus*. *Nature (Lond.)*, **217**, 28–31.

ECCLES, J. C., (1964); *The Physiology of Synapses*, Springer, Heidelberg.

FRANK, K., AND BECKER, M. C., (1964); Microelectrodes for recording and stimulating, In: W. L. NASTUCK (Ed.), *Physical Techniques in Biological Research*, Vol. 5, Academic Press, New York, pp. 22–87.

FUORTES, M. G. F., (1958); Electrical activity of cells in the eye of *Limulus. Amer. J. Ophthal.*, **46**, 210–223.

FUORTES, M. G. F., (1959a); Initiation of impulses in visual cells of *Limulus. J. Physiol. (Lond.)*, **148**, 14–28.

FUORTES, M. G. F., (1959b); Discontinuous potential evoked by sustained illumination in the eye of *Limulus. Arch. ital. Biol.*, **97**, 243–250.

FUORTES, M. G. F., AND POGGIO, G. F., (1963); Transient responses to sudden illumination in cells in the eye of *Limulus. J. gen. Physiol.*, **46**, 435–452.

FUORTES, M. G. F., AND YEANDLE, S., (1964); Probability of occurrence of discrete potential waves in the eye in *Limulus. J. gen. Physiol.*, **47**, 443–463.

FURSHPAN, E. J., (1960); Electrical transmission at an excitatory synapse in the vertebrate brain. *Science*, **144**, 878–880.

FURSHPAN, E. J., AND POTTER, D., (1959); Transmission at the giant motor synapse of the crayfish. *J. Physiol. (Lond.)*, **145**, 289–325.

GOLDSMITH, T. H., (1964); The visual system of insects. In: M. ROCKSTEIN (Ed.), *Physiology of Insecta*, Academic Press, New York, pp. 397–462.

GRUNDFEST, H., (1961); Ionic mechanisms in electrogenesis, *Ann. N.Y. Acad. Sci.*, **94**, 405–457.

HAGINS, W. A., AND McGAUGHY, R. E., (1968); Membrane origin of the fast photovoltage of squid retina. *Science*, **159**, 213–215.

HARTLINE, H. K., COULTNER JR., N. A., AND WAGNER, H. G., (1952a); Effects of electric current on responses of single photoreceptor units in the eye in *Limulus. Fed. Proc.*, **11**, 65–66.

HARTLINE, H. K., WAGNER, H. G., AND MacNICHOL JR., E. F., (1952b); The peripheral origin of nervous activity in the visual system. *Cold Spr. Harb. Symp. quant. Biol.*, **17**, 125–141.

HARTLINE, H. K., AND RATLIFF, F., (1957); Inhibitory interaction of receptor units in the eye of *Limulus. J. gen. Physiol.*, **40**, 357–376.

HARTLINE, H. K., RATLIFF, F., AND MILLER, W. H., (1961); Inhibitory interaction in the retina [and its significance in vision. In: E. FLOREY (Ed.), *Nervous Inhibition*, Pergamon, Oxford, pp. 241–284.

KATZ, B., (1962); The transmission of impulses from nerve to muscle and the subcellular unit of synaptic activity. *Proc. Roy. Soc. B*, **155**, 455–479.

KATZ, B., AND THESLEFF, S., (1957); A study of the "desensitization" produced by acetylcholine at the motor end-plate. *J. Physiol. (Lond.)*, **138**, 63–80.

KIKUCHI, R., AND TAZAWA, M., (1960); Effect of intensity, duration and interval of stimulus on retinal slow potential. In Y. KATSUKI (Ed.), *Electrical Activity of Single Cells*, Igakushoin, Tokyo.

KIKUCHI, R., AND MINAGAWA, S., (1961); Effect of barium ions upon the action potentials of the photoreceptor. *J. Physiol. Soc., Jap.*, **23**, 498–499.

KIKUCHI, R., NAITO, K., AND TANAKA, I., (1962); Effect of sodium and potassium ions on the electrical activity of single cells in the lateral eye of the horseshoe crab. *J. Physiol. (Lond.)*, **161**, 319–343.

KIKUCHI, R., IHNUMA, M., AND TACHI, S., (1965); Different cellular components in ommatidia of horseshoe crab, *Tachypleus tridentatus. Naturwissenschaften*, **52**, 265.

KIKUCHI R., AND UEKI, K., (1965); Double discharge recorded from single ommatidia of horseshoe crab, *Tachypleus tridentatus. Naturwissenschaften*, **52**, 458–459.

LANGER, H., AND THORELL, B., (1966); Microspectrophotometric assay of visual pigments in single rhabdomes of the insect eye, in C. G. BERNHARD (Ed.), *The Functional Organization of the Compound Eye*, Pergamon, Oxford, pp. 145–149.

LASANSKY, A., (1967); Cell junctions in ommatidia of *Limulus. J. Cell Biol.*, **33**, 365–383.

LOWENSTEIN, W. R., NAKAS, M., AND SOCOLAR, S. J., (1967); Junctional membrane uncoupling: Permeability transformations at cell membrane junction. *J. gen. Physiol.*, **50**, 1865–1891.

MacNICHOL JR., E. F., (1956); Visual receptors as biological transducers, In: R. G. GREWELL AND L.J. MULLINS (Eds.), *Molecular Structure and Functional Activity of Nerve Cells*, American Institute of Biological Sciences, **Publ. No. 1**, 34, Washington, D.C., pp. 34–52.

MacNICHOL, E. F., (1958); Subthreshold excitatory processes in the eye of *Limulus. Exptl. Cell Res.*, **Suppl. 5**, 411–425.

MacNICHOL, E. F., WAGNER, H. G., AND HARTLINE, H. K., (1953); Electrical activity recorded within single ommatidia of the eye of *Limulus. XIX Int. Physiol. Congr., Abstr. of Comm.*, pp. 582–583.

MILLECCHIA, R., BRADBURY, J., AND MAURO, A., (1966); Single photoreceptor cells in *Limulus poly-phemus*. *Science*, **154**, 1199–1201.

MILLER, W. H., (1957); Morphology of the ommatidia of the compound eye of *Limulus. J. Biophys. Biochem. Cytol.*, **3**, 421–428.

NAKA, K. I., AND KISHIDA, K., (1966); Retinal action potentials during dark and light adaptation, In C. G. BERNHARD (Ed.), *The Functional Organization of the Compound Eye*, Pergamon, Oxford, pp. 251–266.

PATTEN, W., (1912); *The Evolution of Vertebrates and their Kin*. Blackiston, Philadelphia.

POTTER, D. D., FURSHPAN, E. I., AND LENNOX, E. J., (1966); Connections between cells of the develop-ing squid as revealed by electrophysiological methods. *Proc. natl. Acad. Sci. (Wash.)*, **55**, 328–333.

PURPLE, R. L., AND DODGE, F. A., (1965); Interaction of excitation and inhibition in the eccentric cell in the eye of *Limulus. Cold Spr. Harb. Symp. quant. Biol.*, **30**, 529–537.

PURPLE, R. L., AND DODGE, F. A., (1966); Self-inhibition in the eye of *Limulus*, In C. G. BERN-HARD (Ed.), *The Functional Organization of the Compound Eye*, Pergamon, Oxford, pp. 451–454.

REUBEN, H. P., WERMAN, R., AND GRUNDFEST, H., (1961); The ionic mechanism of hyperpolarizing responses in lobster muscle fibers. *J. gen. Physiol.*, **45**, 243–265.

SHAW, S. R., (1967a); Simultaneous recording from two cells in the locust retina. *Z. vergl. Physiol.*, **55**, 183–194.

SHAW, S. R., (1967b); Coupling between receptors in the eye of the drone honeybee. *J. gen. Physiol.*, **50**, 2480–2481.

SMITH, T. G., (1966); Receptor potentials in retinular cells in *Limulus. Res. Lab. Elec. Quant. Prog. Rept., Mass. Inst. Techn.*, **81** (XIX, Neurophysiology), 242–248.

SMITH, T. G., BAUMANN, F., AND FUORTES, M. G. F., (1965); Electrical connections between visual cells in the ommatidium of *Limulus. Science*, **147**, 1446–1448.

SMITH, T. G., AND BROWN, J. E., (1966); A photoelectric potential in invertebrate cells. *Nature (Lond.)*, **212**, 1217–1219.

SMITH, T. G., WUERKER, R. W., AND FRANK, K., (1967); Membrane impedance changes during synaptic transmission in cat spinal motoneurons. *J. Neurophysiol.*, **30**, 1072–1096.

SMITH, T. G., STELL, W. K., AND BROWN, J. E., (1968a); Conductance changes associated with receptor potentials in *Limulus* photoreceptors, *Science*, **162**, 454–456.

SMITH, T. G., STELL, W. L., BROWN, J. E., FREEMAN, J. C., AND MURRAY, G. C., (1969b); A role for the sodium pump in photoreception. *Science*, **162**, 456–458.

STIEVE, H., (1965); Interpretation of generator potential in terms of ionic processes. *Cold Spr. Harb. Symp. quant. Biol.*, **30**, 451–456.

TOMITA, T., (1956); The nature of action potentials in the lateral eye of the horseshoe crab as revealed by simultaneous intra- and extracellular recordings. *Jap. J. Physiol.*, **6**, 327–340.

TOMITA, T., (1957); Peripheral mechanism of nervous activity in eye of *Limulus. J. Neurophysiol.*, **21**, 245–254.

TOMITA, T., (1958); Mechanism of lateral inhibition in the eye of *Limulus. J. Neurophysiol.*, **21**, 419–429.

TOMITA, T., KIKUCHI, R., AND TANAKA, I., (1960); Excitation and inhibition in lateral eye of horseshoe crab, In Y. KATSUKI (Ed.), *Electrical Activity of Single Cells*, Igakushoin, Tokyo.

WASSERMAN, G. S., (1967); Density spectrum of *Limulus* screening pigment. *J. gen. Physiol.*, **50**, 1075–1077.

WATASE, S., (1887); On the morphology of the compound eye of anthropods. *Studies Biol. Lab. Johns Hopk. Univ.*, **4**, 287–334.

WATERMAN, T. H., AND WIERSMA, C. A. G., (1954); The functional relation between retinular cell and optic nerve in *Limulus. J. Exp. Zool.*, **126**, 59–85.

WOLBARSHT, M. L., AND YEANDLE, S. S., (1967); Visual processes in the *Limulus* eye. *Ann. Rev. Physiol.*, **29**, 513–542.

YEANDLE, S., (1957); *Ph. D. Thesis*, The Johns Hopkins University.

YEANDLE, S., (1958); Evidence of quantized slow potentials in the eye of *Limulus. Amer. J. Ophthal.*, **46**, 82–87.

Author Index

Subject index

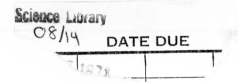